PROGRESS IN CLINICAL AND BIOLOGICAL RESEARCH

Series Editors

Nathan Back   Vincent P. Eijsvoogel   Kurt Hirschhorn   Sidney Udenfriend
George J. Brewer   Robert Grover   Seymour S. Kety   Jonathan W. Uhr

RECENT TITLES

Please contact the publisher for information about previous titles in this series.

PRIMARY CHEMOTHERAPY IN CANCER MEDICINE

PRIMARY CHEMOTHERAPY IN CANCER MEDICINE

Proceedings of an International Symposium on Chemotherapy Preceding Surgery or Irradiation in Cancer Medicine held in Valkenburg a/d Geul, The Netherlands, January 31–Feburary 2, 1985

Editors

D.J. Theo Wagener
Department of Internal Medicine
Division of Medical Oncology
St. Radboud University Hospital
Nijmegen, The Netherlands

Geert H. Blijham
Department of Internal Medicine
University Hospital Annadal
Maastricht, The Netherlands

Jan B.E. Smeets
Medical Department
Farmitalia Carlo Erba
Benelux, Brussels, Belgium

Jacques A. Wils
Department of Internal Medicine
Laurentius Hospital
Roermond, The Netherlands

ALAN R. LISS, INC. • NEW YORK

Address all Inquiries to the Publisher
Alan R. Liss, Inc., 41 East 11th Street, New York, NY 10003

Library of Congress Cataloging-in-Publication Data

International Symposium on Chemotherapy Preceding
    Surgery or Irradiation in Cancer Medicine (1985:
    Valkenburg, Limburg, Netherlands)
    Primary chemotherapy in cancer medicine.

    Includes bibliographies and index.
        1. Cancer—Chemotherapy—Congresses.   2. Cancer—
Adjuvant treatment—Congresses.   I. Wagener, Damianus
Johannes Theodorus. II. Title. [DNLM: 1. Antineoplastic
Agents—therapeutic use—congresses. 2. Neoplasms—
drug therapy—congresses.
W1 PR668E v. 201 / QZ 267 I614p 1985]
RC 271.C5I553   1985   616.99'4061   85-23061
ISBN 0-8451-5051-0

Contents

Contributors

E.J. Aartsen, Department of Internal Medicine, Netherlands Joint Study Group for Ovarian Cancer, University Hospital, 3500 CG Utrecht, The Netherlands [217]

Reto Abele, Division of Oncology, University Hospital, CH-1211 Geneva 4, Switzerland [169]

Mukyi Al-Sarraf, Department of Medicine, Wayne State University, Detroit, MI 48201 [177]

Frederick C. Ames, Department of Surgery, University of Texas M.D. Anderson Hospital, Houston, TX 77030 [105]

R. Baird, Division of Medical Oncology, Cancer Control Agency of British Columbia, Vancouver, British Columbia, Canada V5Z 4E6 [77]

E. Bajetta, Istituto Nazionale Tumori, 20133 Milan, Italy [369]

F. Bammatter, Division of Medical Oncology, University Hospital, Zurich, Switzerland [351]

Geert H. Blijham, Department of Internal Medicine, University Hospital Annadal, 6201 BX Maastricht, The Netherlands [3,89,213]

Ronald H. Blum, Rita and Stanley H. Kaplan Cancer Center, New York University Medical Center, New York, NY 10016 [119]

George R. Blumenschein, Department of Medical Oncology, University of Texas M.D. Anderson Hospital, Houston, TX 77030; present address: Cancer Treatment Center, Arlington, TX 76012 [105]

Gianni Bonadonna, Istituto Nazionale Tumori, 20133 Milan, Italy [369]

J. Bouma, Department of Internal Medicine, Netherlands Joint Study Group for Ovarian Cancer, University Hospital, 3500 CG Utrecht, The Netherlands [217]

H. Bron, Gynecologic Oncology Group, Comprehensive Cancer Center Limburg, The Netherlands [213]

H. Buhr, Division of Surgical Oncology, Ruprecht-Karls-Universität, Heidelberg, Federal Republic of Germany [253]

Aman U. Buzdar, Department of Medical Oncology, University of Texas M.D. Anderson Hospital, Houston, TX 77030 [105]

R. Buzzoni, Istituto Nazionale Tumori, 20133 Milan, Italy [369]

Hubert Calderoli, Department of Radiotherapy, Centre Hospitalier et Universitaire, Strasbourg, 67091 Cedex, France [95]

F. Cavalli, Division of Oncology, University Hospital, CH-1211 Geneva 4, Switzerland; present address: Division of Oncology, Ospedale San Giovanni, CH-6500 Bellinzona, Switzerland [169]

A. Coldman, Division of Medical Oncology, Cancer Control Agency of British Columbia, Vancouver, British Columbia, Canada V5Z 4E6 [77]

The number in brackets is the opening page number of the contributor's article.

Jay S. Cooper, Rita and Stanley H. Kaplan Cancer Center, New York University Medical Center, New York, NY 10016 **[119]**

John Crissman, Department of Pathology, Wayne State University, Detroit, MI 48201 **[177]**

H. de Koning Gans, Gynecologic Oncology Group, Comprehensive Cancer Center Limburg, The Netherlands **[213]**

C.F. De Oliveira, Free University Hospital, Amsterdam, The Netherlands **[225]**

E.B. Dorman, Departments of Otolaryngology, Radiation Therapy, and Medical Oncology, Boston Veterans Administrative Medical Center, Boston University School of Medicine, Boston, MA 02215 **[191]**

Harold O. Douglass, Jr., Rita and Stanley H. Kaplan Cancer Center of New York University Medical Center and the Gastrointestinal Tumor Study Group, New York, NY 10016 **[295]**

Jeffrey Eckhardt, Division of Surgical Oncology, John Wayne Clinic, Jonsson Comprehensive Cancer Center, UCLA School of Medicine, Los Angeles, CA 90024 **[25]**

A. Eekhout, Gynecologic Oncology Group, Comprehensive Cancer Center Limburg, The Netherlands **[213]**

Frederick R. Eilber, Division of Surgical Oncology, John Wayne Clinic, Jonsson Comprehensive Cancer Center, UCLA School of Medicine, Los Angeles, CA 90024 **[25,59]**

Nina Einhorn, Department of Gynaecological Oncology, Epidemiological Unit, Department of Obstetrics and Gynaecology, Karolinska Hospital, S-104 01 Stockholm, Sweden **[207]**

John Elliott, Department of Oncology II, Finsen Institute, DK-2100 Copenhagen, Denmark **[141]**

John F. Ensley, Department of Medicine, Wayne State University, Detroit, MI 48201 **[177]**

S. Fofonoff, Departments of Otolaryngology, Radiation Therapy, and Medical Oncology, Boston Veterans Administrative Medical Center, Boston University School of Medicine, Boston, MA 02215 **[191]**

E. Frei III, Dana-Farber Cancer Institute, Joint Center for Radiotherapy, Harvard Medical School, Boston, MA 02115 **[127]**

D. Fritze, Division of Surgical Oncology, Ruprecht-Karls-Universität, Heidelberg, Federal Republic of Germany **[253]**

James H. Goldie, Division of Medical Oncology, Cancer Control Agency of British Columbia, Vancouver, British Columbia, Canada V5Z 4E6 **[5,77]**

R. Grossenbacher, Division of Oncology, University Hospital, CH 1211 Geneva 4, Switzerland; present address: ORL Klinik, Kontonsspital, CH 9000 St. Gallen, Switzerland **[169]**

Armando E. Guiliano, Division of Surgical Oncology, John Wayne Clinic, Jonsson Comprehensive Cancer Center, UCLA School of Medicine, Los Angeles, CA 90024 **[25,59]**

Nicole Guiochet, Department of Radiotherapy, Centre Hospitalier et Universitaire, Strasbourg, 67091 Cedex, France **[95]**

J. Haest, Gynecologic Oncology Group, Comprehensive Cancer Center Limburg, The Netherlands **[213]**

Heine H. Hansen, Department of Oncology II, Finsen Institute, DK-2100 Copenhagen, Denmark **[141]**

D. Hauri, Department of Urology, University Hospital, Zurich, Switzerland **[351]**

A.P.M. Heintz, Department of Internal Medicine, Netherlands Joint Study Group for Ovarian Cancer, University Hospital, 3500 CG Utrecht, The Netherlands **[217]**

Ch. Herfarth, Division of Surgical Oncology, Ruprecht-Karls-Universität, Heidelberg, Federal Republic of Germany **[253]**

R. Herrmann, Division of Surgical Oncology, Ruprecht-Karls-Universität, Heidelberg, Federal Republic of Germany **[253]**

Bridget T. Hill, Department of Cellular Chemotherapy, Imperial Cancer Research Fund Laboratories and Department of Medical Statistics, Charing Cross Hospital, London, England **[159]**

V. Hofmann, Division of Medical Oncology, University Hospital, Zurich, Switzerland **[351]**

H.P. Honegger, Division of Oncology, University Hospital, CH-1211 Geneva 4, Switzerland; present address: Department of Medical Oncology, Stadspital Triemli, CH-8063 Zurich, Switzerland **[169]**

Waun Ki Hong, Section of Medical Head and Neck Oncology, The University of Texas System Cancer Center, M.D. Anderson Hospital and Tumor Institute, Houston, TX 77030 **[191]**

W.J. Hoogenraad, Department of Internal Medicine, Division of Medical Oncology, St. Radboud University Hospital, 6500 HB Nijmegen, The Netherlands **[301]**

H.J. Hoogland, Gynecologic Oncology Group, Comprehensive Cancer Center Limburg, The Netherlands **[213]**

Gabriel N. Hortobagyi, Department of Medical Oncology, University of Texas M.D. Anderson Hospital, Houston, TX 77030 **[105]**

H. Huiskes, Gynecologic Oncology Group, Comprehensive Cancer Center Limburg, The Netherlands **[213]**

Patrick Hurteloup, Centre Hospitalier et Universitaire, Strasbourg, France; present address: Farmitalia Carlo Erba, Paris, 92800 CX 11, France **[95]**

James F. Huth, Division of Surgical Oncology, John Wayne Clinic, Jonsson Comprehensive Cancer Center, UCLA School of Medicine, Los Angeles, CA 90024 **[25,59]**

P. Iten, Department of Surgery, University Hospital, Zurich, Switzerland **[351]**

John Jacobs, Department of Otolaryngology, Wayne State University, Detroit, MI 48201 **[177]**

D.D. Karp, Departments of Otolaryngology, Radiation Therapy, and Medical Oncology, Boston Veterans Administrative Medical Center, Boston University School of Medicine, Boston, MA 02215 **[191]**

A.H. Keijser, Breast Cancer Group of the Comprehensive Cancer Centre Limburg (IKL), Maastricht, The Netherlands; present address: Department of Radiotherapy, R.T.I.L., 6419 PC Heerlen, The Netherlands **[89]**

Roger Keiling, Department of Radiotherapy, Centre Hospitalier et Universitaire, Strasbourg, 67091 Cedex, France [95]

David Kelsen, Solid Tumor Service, Memorial Sloan-Kettering Cancer Center, Department of Clinical Medicine, Cornell University Medical College, New York, NY 10021 [241]

Jeannie Kinzie, Department of Radiation Oncology, Wayne State University, Detroit, MI 48201 [177]

J.A. Kish, Department of Medicine, Wayne State University, Detroit, MI 48201 [177]

H.O. Klein, Medical Clinic, University of Cologne, 5000 Köln 41, Federal Republic of Germany [283]

Krsto Kolarić, Central Institute for Tumors and Allied Diseases, Zagreb, Yugoslavia [259]

J. Kornman, Gynecologic Oncology Group, Comprehensive Cancer Center Limburg, The Netherlands [213]

J. Kozonis, Mount Vernon Hospital, Mt. Vernon, NY; and Evangelismos Hospital, Athens, Greece [317]

H. Kruisselbrink, Department of Internal Medicine, Division of Medical Oncology, St. Radboud University Hospital, 6500 HB Nijmegen, The Netherlands [301]

Claude Krzisch, Department of Radiotherapy, Centre Hospitalier et Universitaire, Strasbourg, 67091 Cedex, France [95]

F. Lalisang, Gynecologic Oncology Group, Comprehensive Cancer Center Limburg, The Netherlands [213]

F. Largiadèr, Department of Surgery, University Hospital, Zurich, Switzerland [351]

Nancy Leslie, Department of Radiation Oncology, Dana-Farber Cancer Institute, Joint Center for Radiotherapy, Harvard Medical School, Boston, MA 02115 [127]

Christopher J. Logothetis, Department of Medicine, M.D. Anderson Hospital and Tumor Institute, Houston, TX 77030 [341,359]

B. Luboinski, Institut Gustave Roussy, Villejuif, France [199]

Dorothy McCauley, Rita and Stanley H. Kaplan Cancer Center, New York University Medical Center, New York, NY 10016 [119]

K. Macrae, Imperial Cancer Research Fund Laboratories and Department of Medical Statistics, Charing Cross Hospital, London, England [159]

Arnold Malcolm, Dana-Farber Cancer Institute, Joint Center for Radiotherapy, Harvard Medical School, Boston, MA 02115; present address: Department of Radiation Oncology, Vanderbilt University Hospital, Nashville, TN 37232 [127]

C. Mangioni, Free University Hospital, Amsterdam, The Netherlands [225]

Alec Megibow, Rita and Stanley H. Kaplan Cancer Center of New York University Medical Center and the Gastrointestinal Tumor Study Group, New York, NY 10016 [295]

B. Mermillod, Division of Oncology, University Hospital, CH-1211 Geneva 4, Switzerland; present address: SAKK Central Office, CH-3012 Bern, Switzerland [169]

U. Metzger, Department of Surgery, University Hospital, Zurich, Switzerland [351]

Joseph Mirra, Division of Pathology, John Wayne Clinic, Jonsson Comprehensive Cancer Center, and Department of Pathology,UCLA School of Medicine, Los Angeles, CA 90024 [59]

Eleanor D. Montague, Department of Radiotherapy, University of Texas M.D. Anderson Hospital, Houston, TX 77030 [105]

P. Moorman, Gynecologic Oncology Group, Comprehensive Cancer Center Limburg, The Netherlands [213]

Donald L. Morton, Division of Surgery/Orthopedics, John Wayne Clinic, Jonsson Comprehensive Cancer Center, and Department of Pathology, UCLA School of Medicine, Los Angeles, CA 90024 [59]

Franco M. Muggia, Rita and Stanley H. Kaplan Cancer Center, New York University Medical Center, and the Gastrointestinal Tumor Study Group, New York, NY 10016 [119, 295, 377]

J.D.K. Munting, Breast Cancer Group of the Comprehensive Cancer Centre Limburg (IKL), Maastricht, The Netherlands; present address: Department of Surgery, De Wever Hospital, 6419 PC Heerlen, The Netherlands [89]

Andre Naus, Department of Biochemistry, St. Laurentius Hospital, 6043 CV Roermond, The Netherlands [133]

J.P. Neijt, Department of Internal Medicine, Netherlands Joint Study Group for Ovarian Cancer, University Hospital, 3500 CG Utrecht, The Netherlands [217]

Bo Nilsson, Department of Gynaecological Oncology, Epidemiological Unit, Department of Obstetrics and Gynaecology, Karolinska Hospital, S-104 01 Stockholm, Sweden [207]

Anita Nirenberg, Comprehensive Cancer Centers, Inc., Beverly Hills, CA 90210 [39]

J. Nomicos, Mount Vernon Hospital, Mt. Vernon, NY; and Evangelismos Hospital, Athens, Greece [317]

G.M. O'Donoghue, Departments of Otolaryngology, Radiation Therapy, and Medical Oncology, Boston Veterans Administrative Medical Center, Boston University School of Medicine, Boston, MA 02115 [191]

P. Oliynyk, Dana-Farber Cancer Institute, Joint Center for Radiotherapy, Harvard Medical School, Boston, MA 02115 [127]

Kell Østerlind, Department of Oncology II, Finsen Institute, DK-2100 Copenhagen, Denmark [141]

R. Overholt, Dana-Farber Cancer Institute, Joint Center for Radiotherapy, Harvard Medical School, Boston, MA 02115 [127]

A. Papaioannou, Mount Vernon Hospital, Mt. Vernon, NY; and Evangelismos Hospital, Athens, Greece [317]

S. Pecorelli, Free University Hospital, Amsterdam, The Netherlands [225]

Anders Gersel Pedersen, Department of Oncology II, Finsen Institute, DK-2100 Copenhagen, Denmark [141]

G. Plataniotis, Mount Vernon Hospital, Mt. Vernon, NY; and Evangelismos Hospital, Athens, Greece [317]

A. Polychronis, Mount Vernon Hospital, Mt. Vernon, NY; and Evangelismos Hospital, Athens, Greece [317]

L.A. Price, Imperial Cancer Research Fund Laboratories and Department of Medical Statistics, Charing Cross Hospital, London, England; present address: Head and Neck Unit, Royal Massden Hospital, SW3 London, England [159]

J. Ragaz, Division of Medical Oncology, Cancer Control Agency of British Columbia, Vancouver, British Columbia, Canada V5Z 4E6 [77]

P. Rebbeck, Division of Medical Oncology, Cancer Control Agency of British Columbia, Vancouver, British Columbia, Canada V5Z 4E6 [77]

Gerald Rosen, Comprehensive Cancer Centers, Inc., Beverly Hills, CA 90210 [39]

G. Schettler, Division of Surgical Oncology, Ruprecht-Karls-Universität, Heidelberg, Federal Republic of Germany [253]

P. Schillings, Department of Internal Medicine, Division of Medical Oncology, St. Radboud University Hospital, 6500 HB Nijmegen, The Netherlands [301]

P. Schlag, Division of Surgical Oncology, Ruprecht-Karls-Universität, Heidelberg, Federal Republic of Germany [253]

L. Schouten, Breast Cancer Group of the Comprehensive Cancer Centre Limburg (IKL), 6211 LN Maastricht, The Netherlands [89]

S. Sheetz, Departments of Otolaryngology, Radiation Therapy, and Medical Oncology, Boston Veterans Administrative Medical Center, Boston University School of Medicine, Boston, MA 02215 [191]

Kerstin Sjövall, Department of Gynaecological Oncology, Epidemiological Unit, Department of Obstetrics and Gynaecology, Karolinska Hospital, S-104 01 Stockholm, Sweden [207]

Arthur T. Skarin, Division of Medical Oncology, Dana-Farber Cancer Institute, Joint Center for Radiotherapy, Harvard Medical School, Boston, MA 02115 [127]

Jan B.E. Smeets, Medical Department, Farmitalia Carlo Erba, Benelux, Brussels, Belgium

J. Stoot, Gynecologic Oncology Group, Comprehensive Cancer Center Limburg, The Netherlands [213]

S. P. Strijk, Department of Internal Medicine, Division of Medical Oncology, St. Radboud University Hospital, 6500 HB Nijmegen, The Netherlands [301]

H. Stroeken, Breast Cancer Group of the Comprehensive Cancer Centre Limburg (IKL), Maastricht, The Netherlands; present address: Department of Surgery, Hospital Sittard, 6131 BN Sittard,The Netherlands [89]

S. Strong, Departments of Otolaryngology, Radiation Therapy, and Medical Oncology, Boston Veterans Administrative Medical Center, Boston University School of Medicine, Boston, MA 02215 [191]

A.J. Subandono, Free University Hospital, Amsterdam, The Netherlands [225]

A.H.M. Taminiau, Department of Orthopaedic Surgery, University Hospital, 2300 RC Leiden, The Netherlands [53]

M. Tsamouri, Mount Vernon Hospital, Mt. Vernon, NY; and Evangelismos Hospital, Athens, Greece [317]

P. Tushuizen, Gynecologic Oncology Group, Comprehensive Cancer Center Limburg, The Netherlands [213]

Irwan Utama, Department of Pulmonary Diseases, St. Laurentius Hospital, 6043 CV Roermond, The Netherlands [133]

P. Valagussa, Instituto Nazionale Tumori, 20133 Milan, Italy [369]

Paul van den Broek, Department of Otorhinolaryngology, University Hospital, Nijmegen, The Netherlands [155]

J.W. van der Eijken, Onze Lieve Vrouwe Gasthuis, Amsterdam, The Netherlands [53]

H. van Geuns, Gynecologic Oncology Group, Comprehensive Cancer Center Limburg, The Netherlands [213]

M. van Lent, Department of Internal Medicine, Netherlands Joint Study Group for Ovarian Cancer, University Hospital, 3500 CG Utrecht, The Netherlands [217]

A.C.M. van Lindert, Department of Internal Medicine, Netherlands Joint Study Group for Ovarian Cancer, University Hospital, 3500 CG Utrecht, The Netherlands [217, 225]

A.T. van Oosterom, Department of Clinical Oncology, University Hospital, 2300 RC Leiden, The Netherlands [53, 225]

Luke M. van Putten, Radiobiological Institute TNO, P.O. Box 5815, 2280 HV Rijswijk, The Netherlands [15]

C.W. Vaughan, Departments of Otolaryngology, Radiation Therapy, and Medical Oncology, Boston Veterans Administrative Medical Center, Boston University School of Medicine, Boston, MA 02215 [191]

M.E.L. v.d. Burg, Free University Hospital, Amsterdam, The Netherlands [225]

J. v.d. Meulen, Gynecologic Oncology Group, Comprehensive Cancer Center Limburg, The Netherlands [213]

J.B. Vermorken, Free University Hospital, Amsterdam, The Netherlands [225]

Tom A. Verschueren, Radiotherapeutisch Instituut Limburg, 6419 PC Heerlen, The Netherlands [133]

A.R. von Hochstetter, Department of Pathology, University Hospital, Zurich, Switzerland [351]

P.A. Voûte, Department of Oncology, Emma Kinderziekenhuis, 1018 HJ Amsterdam, The Netherlands [53]

J. Vreeswijk, Gynecologic Oncology Group, Comprehensive Cancer Center Limburg, The Netherlands [213]

D.J. Theo Wagener, Department of Internal Medicine, Division of Medical Oncology, St. Radboud University Hospital, 6500 HB Nijmegen, The Netherlands [301]

Arthur Weaver, Department of Surgery, Wayne State University, Detroit, MI 48201 [177]

J. Welch, Departments of Otolaryngology, Radiation Therapy, and Medical Oncology, Boston Veterans Administrative Medical Center, Boston University School of Medicine, Boston, MA 02215 [191]

Th. Wiggers, Breast Cancer Group of the Comprehensive Cancer Centre Limburg (IKL), Maastricht, The Netherlands; present address: Department of Surgery, University Hospital Annadal, 6201 BX Maastricht, The Netherlands [89]

B. Willett, Departments of Otolaryngology, Radiation Therapy, and Medical Oncology, Boston Veterans Administrative Medical Center, Boston University School of Medicine, Boston, MA 02215 [191]

Jacques A. Wils, Department of Internal Medicine, Laurentius Hospital, 6043 CV Roermond, The Netherlands [89,133,213,385]

Th. Wobbes, Department of Internal Medicine, Division of Medical Oncology, St. Radboud University Hospital, 6500 HB Nijmegen, The Netherlands [301]

M. Wolfensberger, Division of Oncology, University Hospital, CH-1211 Geneva 4, Switzerland; present address: ORL Klinik, University Hospital, CH-8091 Zurich, Switzerland [169]

S.H. Yap, Department of Internal Medicine, Division of Medical Oncology, St. Radboud University Hospital, 6500 HB Nijmegen, The Netherlands [301]

P. Zola, Free University Hospital, Amsterdam, The Netherlands [225]

SECTION I
THEORETICAL AND EXPERIMENTAL ASPECTS

Primary Chemotherapy in Cancer Medicine, pages 3–4
© 1985 Alan R. Liss, Inc.

INTRODUCTORY REMARKS

G.H. Blijham
Department of Internal Medicine
University Hospital Annadal
Annalaan 1
6201 BX Maastricht

When we, in the fall of 1983, conceived the idea of organizing a symposium specifically dedicated to neoadjuvant chemotherapy, we discussed the possibility of adding the prefix "First" to the title, making this symposium the forever-famous First International Symposium on Chemotherapy Preceding Surgery or Irradiation in Cancer Medicine. However, we rejected this idea since we felt confident that no other scientists or institutions would have the courage or the creativity to organize a conference on this subject, anywhere near 1985. We were wrong. It is a tribute to the topic of this symposium that at the same time and completely independently a quite similar conference was in the process of being organized. It was only during the ASCO 1984 Meeting in Toronto that we became aware of the "First International Symposium on Neoadjuvant Chemotherapy", to be held in Vancouver in March, 1985. Since Vancouver is the hometown of some of the godfathers of neoadjuvant chemotherapy, we were anxious to see the program of that meeting: to our relief and satisfaction it appeared to coincide with ours at several points. So we now have the unique situation that both Europe and North America are being served with a symposium on the same subject and with, in part, the same invited speakers. I wish to consider this as an indication that European Oncology has now grown up to the standards set on the North American continent.

Neoadjuvant chemotherapy can be defined as chemotherapy given to patients with locoregionally confined disease, a percentage of whom can be cured by applying surgery and/or radiotherapy only. The potential advantages of such "up-front" chemotherapy are threefold. Firstly, according to

the computer model of Goldie and Coldman, dividing and
therefore mutating tumors may progress from chemotherapy-
sensitive to chemotherapy-resistant in only a few doublings;
early chemotherapy may therefore be curative for micrometastases whereas delayed chemotherapy is not. Secondly, by applying chemotherapy before removal of visible tumor, the
response can be evaluated; further postoperative adjuvant
chemotherapy may then be individualized according to the
outcome of such an in-vivo chemosensitivity assay. Finally,
preoperative shrinkage of the tumor may help the surgeon
and/or radiotherapist to reduce the extent of locoregional
therapy, thereby decreasing the degree of local morbidity
and mutilation.

Despite these obvious advantages, neoadjuvant chemotherapy has only been recently introduced in clinical research. This is in part due to scepticism related to the
efficacy of current chemotherapy protocols. Another area of
concern is related to the interference of early, aggressive
chemotherapy with the subsequent ability to deliver adequate
radiotherapy or surgery. One of the main purposes of this
symposium is to bring surgeons, radiotherapists and medical
oncologists together to careful consider the evidence both
for and against initial chemotherapy, in a variety of human
neoplasms.

I would like to finish this brief introduction with a
quotation from Ovidius, the famous Roman poet. He was, of
course, an expert on love, and considered love to be a disease often grave and sometimes incurable. He gave us good
advice, and this advice may be the leading theme of this
symposium: "stop it at the start, it's late for medicine to
be prepared when disease has grown strong through long delays".

Primary Chemotherapy in Cancer Medicine, pages 5-14
© 1985 Alan R. Liss, Inc.

THE RATIONALE FOR THE USE OF PREOPERATIVE CHEMOTHERAPY

James H. Goldie

Division of Medical Oncology Cancer Control
Agency of British Columbia, 600 West 10th
Avenue, Vancouver, British Columbia, Canada
V5Z 4E6

The basis for utilizing adjuvant chemotherapy is related to the supposition that clinically inapparent burdens of metastatic tumor are much more susceptible to being completely eradicated by chemotherapy than clinically advanced disease. A considerable amount of experimental evidence supports this belief, as well as studies on drug-sensitive classes of clinical tumors. A more specific question relating to the use of adjuvant chemotherapy, is the issue of the optimal timing of commencement of such treatment. If the likelihood of cure drops off very slowly with time then there is little indication for the initiation of chemotherapy as an urgent measure. If, however, there are biological processes operating within tumors that could rapidly change the probability of cure for a large proportion of patients, then a case can be made for the institution of chemotherapy as an almost emergency procedure. In this paper we will review some of the phenomena that could occur within a neoplastic cell population which would argue for the use of chemotherapy early, even before locoregional therapy is undertaken. We will give emphasis to the phenomenon of spontaneous mutations to drug resistance as a factor in determining tumor curability but will also briefly mention other processes that might have an effect on drug sensitivity.

Kinetic Processes Relating to Adjuvant Chemotherapy

Various kinetic models of tumor growth have suggested that small (i.e. microscopic) populations of tumor cells will have more favourable growth kinetics from the point of

view of chemotherapy than large tumor masses (1,2). With
many experimental solid tumors it can be shown that growth
fraction diminishes and doubling time increases as the tumor
population expands. These changes tend to correlate with a
declining sensitivity to chemotherapy. All other things
being equal, therefore, one might anticipate that the micrometastases present at the time adjuvant chemotherapy is
commenced should be more sensitive to drug treatment.

In addition to the effect related to size alone, experimental studies have suggested that removal of the primary
tumor may result in a temporary increase in growth fraction
and shortened doubling time of the residual metastatic
tumor (3,4). The mechanism of this change in kinetics is unknown but it could be postulated as being due to the removal
of some type of growth inhibitory factor being produced by
the primary tumor. As these kinetic changes would be compatible with an increase in drug sensitivity it has been proposed that chemotherapy administered during the perioperative period might be expected to be more beneficial on the
basis of this effect. While this is an attractive hypothesis
some caution should be exercised before assuming that enhanced growth potential on its own will necessarily result
in increased drug sensitivity. There are no reasons to believe that if a tumor cell is genetically resistant to a
specific type of chemotherapy that increasing its growth
rate is going to change this property. In fact, in the absence of chemotherapy capable of overcoming the drug resistant tumor cells simply increasing their growth rate might
be expected to be deleterious. However, if there exists
within the tumor significant numbers of quiescent tumor stem
cells that are relatively invulnerable to chemotherapy by
virtue of their position in the cell cycle (but are genetically drug sensitive), then recruitment of such quiescent
cells into the generation cycle at the time that chemotherapy is being administered would be beneficial.

Drug Resistance as a Basis of Treatment Failure

There is substantial evidence from laboratory studies
indicating that it is the emergence of drug resistant tumor
cells that constitutes a major barrier to chemotherapeutic
cure (5). These drug resistant phenotypes have a genetic
origin and arise as a consequence of random and spontaneous
mutations (6). Populations of cancer cells are characterized
by what might be called genetic instability and give rise at
a relatively high frequency to a broad range of drug-resis-

tant variants (7).

Although there are considerable data available from studies of experimental neoplasms, less is known regarding the causes of treatment failure in clinical treatment. The information that does exist is consistent with similar processes generating treatment failure in clinical chemotherapy (8). The phenomenon of spontaneous mutation to resistance can be studied using appropriate mathematical techniques (9). The usefulness of such an approach is that it permits one to examine in more detail the consequences of such phenomena and from there develop treatment strategies which can be subjected to experimental testing.

In any population of cancer cells there will be a continuous generation of phenotypic variant forms which will display a great range of sensitivity to the whole spectrum of antineoplastic agents. It is likely, under these conditions, that no two cells in the tumor population will have identical ranges of drug sensitivity and resistance. However, we would utilize an operational definiton of drug resistance and define it as phenotypic state of a particular cell which will allow it to escape killing by a specific pharmacologically achievable drug concentration. The resistance therefore is not absolute but is defined in terms of the drug concentration and drug type that is being tested against the cell. Higher or lower concentrations of the therapeutic agent would be expected to influence the probability of the cell undergoing lethal damage. In modelling this process we will simply assume that the drug concentration being applied represents some optimal value as defined by pharmacological and toxicological data.

Once a single drug resistant clone appears within the malignant cell population then that neoplasm is by definition incurable by the drug treatment regimen being used. Substantial destruction of the sensitive forms in the tumor may be achieved but ultimately the drug resistant mutant will grow out in the face of continually applied therapy and cause eventual treatment failure.

The time taken for any mutant cell type to develop and to become "fixed" within the neoplasm will be a very short interval. It is probable that this is no longer than a single generation time of the dividing cells within the tumor. Thus in any one individual case the transition from potential curability to incurability will occur as a sudden discontinuous event. The random nature of mutational processes makes it impossible to predict specifically when this will occur, but the longer the period of elapsed time then the greater probability that the event will have happened.

The question being addressed here is the predicted be- haviour of a whole set of neoplastic populations and what the impact of elapsed time will be in terms of the probabi- lity of cure (or percent cures achievable) of the complete set.

Our mathematical analysis of this process has indicated that for such a population of individual tumors the proba- bility of there being at least one drug resistant cell pre- sent goes from a low to a very high probability over an approximate two log increase in tumor cell burden (9). If we define the absence of any drug resistant cells as the minimal conditions required for chemotherapeutic cure, then this indicates that the probability of cure in a popu- lation of tumors will decline relatively quickly as the malignant cell population increases.

The plot of the function relating tumor burden to prob- ability of cure is depicted in Figure 1.

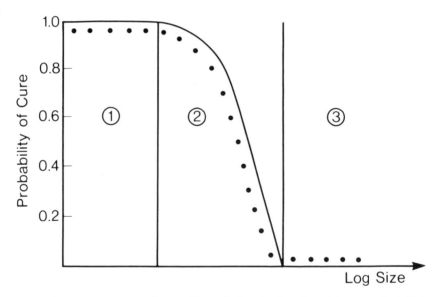

Fig. 1. The figure shows the plot of the function probabili- ty of cure versus tumor size. The data represent individual patients with a particular tumor burden. Group 1 is located in the early flat portion of the curve. Moderate increases in tumor size will not significantly change their likeli- hood of cure. The same is true for the group 3 patients who

are already in the near incurable portion of the curve.
Group 2 includes those patients whose burdens are distributed over the steep portion of the curve. Short delays in
the institution of treatment in this group will result in
significant movement "down" the cure curve. In the context
of this model chemotherapy with enhanced effectiveness can
be visualized as shifting the probability of cure curve to
the right and a less effective treatment a shift to the
left. That is, a totally ineffective treatment regimen would
not be displaced away from the Y axis and all tumor burdens
would be to the right of the curve and hence all patients
would be incurable.

The curve has a characteristic sigmoid shape with an
interval when there is a steep decline in the probability
of cure. The point at which downward inflection of the curve
begins will be dictated by the average mutation rate for the
tumor population being considered. A high mutation rate to
drug resistance will result in an earlier downward deflec-
tion of the curve and conversely a low mutation rate will
result in a later one.

At the time adjuvant chemotherapy is commenced we might
imagine that the distribution of subclinical tumor burdens
can be divided into three separate categories. As is illustrated in the figure the first category would constitute
those patients with minimal tumor burdens and who are on a
flat portion of the probability of cure curve. These patients have a very high probability of potential cure and
moreover, because of their position on the probability of
cure relatively short delays in the institution of treatment will not impact significantly on this probability for
the great majority of cases.

The second category of patients are those whose tumor
burdens are distributed over the steep portion of the probability of cure curve. On this steep part a single doubling
in tumor burden can result in a theoretical 25% decline in
the probability of cure. It is this group of patients that
we would anticipate would be the ones in whom short delays
in the institution of therapy might have an unexpectedly
large unfavourable effect on outcome.

Finally there would be a third category of patients,
who while still having subclinical burdens of disease, are
already incurable with our hypothetical drug treatment.
Treatment directed at this group would not be expected to
alter eventual outcome but might be expected to increase

disease-free survival. Again, the timing of initiation of chemotherapy would not be expected to be a crucial factor in this set of patients.

The argument in favour of preoperative or perioperative chemotherapy essentially comes down to the issue as to what proportion of the total number of patients with sub-clinical disease have burdens that are distributed along the steep portion of the probability of cure curve. If this is a negligible proportion of the total number of patients being considered then advancing forward in time the initiation of treatment would probably not produce discernible benefit.

If we assume an approximate uniform distribution of tumor burdens over the range of subclinical disease (i.e. from 1 cell to 10^9) then approximately 25% of the patients could be considered as falling somewhere on the curve before probability of cure declines to less than 1%. If the distributions of tumor burdens are weighted in one direction or the other then of course this percentage will be correspondingly greater or less.

At the present time we have no reliable techniques that would permit us to accurately estimate what this actual range distribution of tumor burden is. However, some sense of what the potential distributions may be can be developed from examining patterns of relapse time following loco-regional treatment and changes in long term disease free survival associated with earlier institution of chemotherapy.

Estimates of Tumor Burden Distributions in Premenopausal Breast Carcinoma

By utilizing the technique of "break point analysis" Skipper (10) has estimated the distribution of tumor burdens in patients with premenopausal breast carcinoma and with differing nodal status at the time of surgery. The principle of the break point analysis is that in the actu-arial survival curves of cancer patients one can often i-dentify a biphasic form to the curve. There is an initial relatively steep decline in disease free survival followed by a flattening of the curve. The patients represented by the flatter part of the curve have either been cured or have times to relapse significantly longer than the median for the group as a whole. The point in the survival curve where the flattening begins can be considered to represent patients who had very few to zero viable residual tumor cells following initial treatment. By correcting for the average doubling time of the neoplasms when they become clinically apparent one can extrapolate back from the survival curve to the hypothetical tumor size that was present at the time of initial therapy.

This method has been shown by Skipper to be accurate within a first approximation for estimating residual tumor burden in experimental neoplasms. In the absence of better techniques for estimating subclinical disease this represents an interesting approach in attempting to define a range of subclinical tumor mass in patients with breast cancer and other malignancies.

Skipper's analysis suggested in patients with Stage II breast carcinoma, 1 to 3 positive nodes, that the hypothetical distribution of tumor mass was slightly weighted towards the low end of the scale and towards the upper end, nonetheless there was a significant number of cases distributed over the entire range of subclinical volume. An unknown factor at present is: What is the upper limit of subclinical tumor burden that is curable with existing chemotherapy programs? If we accept Skipper's figure of 10^5 as representing this upper limit then one can estimate that approximately a third of the total number of patients will have burdens on some portion of the probability of cure curve, before it reaches negligible levels. If this estimate is accurate then it does imply that advancing the average time of initiation of chemotherapy by a period equivalent to one tumor volume doubling time should improve overall survival by an amount sufficient to be detectable in an appropriately sized clinical trial.

Clinical Trials Comparing Early versus Delayed Administration of Adjuvant Chemotherapy

Two studies in breast cancer have suggested that relatively short delays in the institution of chemotherapy appear to have a significant negative effect on long term treatment results. The well known study of Nissen-Meyer et al (11) found in one of their subgroups of patients in which the immediate postoperative chemotherapy was delayed for three to four weeks, that any benefit of the treatment in terms of long term disease free survival was abolished. Another study by Jones et al (12) suggested that patients who commenced their chemotherapy at four weeks or greater following surgery had a poorer outcome than patients who started on treatment within two weeks of operation.

In both these studies the apparent negative impact of slight delay was seen only on retrospective analysis. The studies had not been prospectively planned to evaluate delay. Likewise, even if the effect was real the data do not permit distinguishing the mechanism responsible for the treatment failure. Other processes than drug resistance could be involved, though the drug resistance model does predict for an effect on survival by small treatment delays.

This is a question that will certainly require answering by appropriate prospective studies, though a confounding variable in such studies is going to be the actual time difference between the early versus later adjuvant treatment. If this time period is relatively small then no differences may be discernible. We have noted this difficulty in our own institution where the existence of a preoperative chemotherapy arm in one adjuvant trial has generally increased awareness in the clinical community about the importance of early referral to the centre for consideration of adjuvant chemotherapy. Thus, the average interval between surgery and commencement of postoperative chemotherapy appears to be progressively declining which could make it more difficult to demonstrate statistically significant differences between the two approaches. Likewise, it would be ethically dubious to deliberately delay postoperative chemotherapy to a point (six to eight weeks) where the clinician might strongly suspect that elapsed time would begin to seriously compromise the effect of the drug treatment.

Summary

A considerable amount of experimental and clinical data support the idea that there is a strong relationship between tumor mass and potential curability by chemotherapy. Malignancies for which there could be no realistic expectation of cure when treated at the advanced stage, may be quite sensitive to cure if the treatment can be initiated at a time when the tumor burden is very small. The somatic mutation model of drug resistance and cancer chemotherapeutic effect predicts a steep relationship between tumor burden and curability. One clinical implication of such a relationship is that the time period over which a significant proportion of individual cases would move from a position of curability to incurability may be substantially shorter than what one would intuitively expect. This argues

for the earliest feasible utilization of appropriate chemotherapy as part of adjuvant treatment programs. This intro-
duces a component of urgency into establishing a correct
diagnosis and commencing appropriate anticancer drug treatment.

Such measures may have the potential for increasing
cure rates in a variety of human solid tumors for which adjuvant chemotherapy is deemed an appropriate technique.
With the demonstration of the relative safety of such approaches then many of the ethical concerns about the early
use of chemotherapy can be assuaged. One of the attractions
of the method of preoperative chemotherapy is that it offers
the possibility of improving cure rates in a variety of
common human malignancies without developing new classes of
antineoplastic drug or entirely novel treatment approaches.
The prompt institution of chemotherapy during the perioperative period may have greater impact on the natural history
of the disease than much more aggressive and complex treatment utilized in the later stages.

References

1. Steel, G.G,, and Lamerton, L.F. (1968). Cell population
   kinetics and chemotherapy. Natl. Cancer Inst. Monogr.,
   30: 29-50.
2. Swan, G.W. (1977). In: Some Current Mathematical Topics
   in Cancer Research, pp. 71-83. Ann Arbor, MI: University Microfilms Int.
3. Simpson-Herren, L., Sanford, A.H., and Holmquist, J.P.
   (1976). Effects of surgery in the cell kinetics of
   residual tumor. Cancer Treat. Rep., 60: 1744-1760.
4. Fisher, B., Gunduz, N., and Saffer, E.A. (1983). Influence of the interval between primary tumor removal and
   chemotherapy on kinetics and growth of metastases.
   Cancer Res., 43: 1482-1488.
5. Ling, V. (1982). Genetic basis of drug resistance in
   mammalian cells. In: N. Bruchovsky and J.H. Goldie
   (eds.), Drug and Hormone Resistance in Neoplasia, Vol.
   1. Boca Raton, FL: CRC Press.
6. Siminovitch, L. (1976). On the nature of hereditable
   variation in cultured somatic cells. Cell, 7: 1-11.
7. Nowell, P.C. (1982). Genetic instability in cancer
   cells: relationship to tumors cell heterogeneity. In:
   A.H. Owens, D.S. Coffey, and S.B. Baylin (eds.), Tumor
   Cell Heterogeneity Origins and Implications, pp. 351-
   369. New York: Academic Press, Inc.

8. Goldie, J.H. and Coldman, A.J. (1984). Genetic origin of drug resistance in neoplasms. Cancer Res., 44, 3643-53.

9. Goldie, J.H., and Coldman, A.J. (1979). A mathematic model for relating the drug sensitivity of tumors to their spontaneous mutation rate. Cancer Treat. Rep., 63: 1727-1733.

10. Skipper, H.E. (1979). Repopulation rates of breast cancer cells after mastectomy (Judged from break-points in remission duration curves). Booklet 12, Southern Research Institute, Birmingham, Ala.

11. Nissen-Meyer, R., Kjellgren, K., Malmio, K., Mansson, B., and Norin, T. (1978). Surgical adjuvant chemotherapy. Cancer (Phila), 41: 2088-2098.

12. Jones, S.E., Brooks, R.J., Takasugi, B.J., et al (1984). Current results of the University of Arizona adjuvant breast cancer trials (1974-84) In: Adjuvant Therapy of Cancer IV, Salmon, S.E. and Jones, S.E. (eds.), Grune and Stratton.

Primary Chemotherapy in Cancer Medicine, pages 15–21
© 1985 Alan R. Liss, Inc.

OPTIMAL TIMING OF ADJUVANT CHEMOTHERAPY IN MOUSE MODELS*

L.M. van Putten

Radiobiological Institute TNO, P.O. Box 5815
2280 HV Rijswijk, The Netherlands.

The study of adjuvant chemotherapy in experimental systems
differs widely from the clinical approach. Experimental
studies of transplantable tumors in rodents avails the
possibility of reproducing human disease types in the model
systems, thus opening the road to comparison of different
types of treatment, e.g., preoperative versus postoperative
adjuvant therapy. This is a major advantage, as it allows
us to obtain valid conclusions on mechanisms, resulting
from observations of a small homogeneous animal population
carrying a somewhat uniform disease. The problem is in the
"somewhat". In models, as in man, metastasis is not a uni-
formly reproducible process. After inoculation of a tumor
in mice, there is a marked heterogeneity in the time of
appearance of metastases. For that reason, we make use of
tumor inoculation in the foot pad of the mouse, since
growth at this location leads to early - and therefore to
relatively uniform - metastasis. However, appearance of
metastases after foot pad inoculation is only uniform in
comparison to inoculation at other sites. Unfortunately,
it remains far more heterogeneous than the pattern seen in
patients invalued in a clinical trial. If the time of removal of the primary tumor is then selected such that about
30% of the animals are without metastasis, of the remaining
animals approximately 20 to 40% will have metastases of a
size comparable to clearly manifest disease in man. It is
therefore obvious that we must be very critical when attempting to draw conclusions that may be valid for human
disease.

But that is not the only limitation. We usually study

metastatic disease in laboratory animals using either a
single tumor or several different tumors. I am happy to be
able to present to you some data on three animal tumors. If
the data on these three tumors were in agreement, we would
be confident of having found several generally valid rules
which might stand transference from one species to the
other. When you have reached the end of this paper, you
will agree that this is not the case; there may be some
generally valid rules, but it is obvious that there are also exceptions. The basis data on the three tumors are presented in Table 1.

TABLE 1

BASIC DATA ON THREE TUMORS STUDIED

Name	Lewis lung tumor	Mammary ca. 2661	Osteosarcoma C22LR
Host	C57Bl/Ka	CBA/Rij	(C57BLxCBA)F1
Origin	1951 Philadelphia	1961 Rijswijk	1957 Rijswijk
Passage	100	80	78-84
Flank inoculum	10^6	10^6	10^6
Foot pad inoculum	10^5	10^5	10^5
Metastasis to lung	100%	73%	100%
to lymph nodes	12%	93%	43%
Cyclophospha- mide dose mg.kg	100	200	50 or 100

LEWIS LUNG TUMOR

The Lewis lung tumor is sensitive to chemotherapy with
cyclophosphamide only when tumor volume is small. Subcuta-
neously inoculated tumors can be cured in 92% of the mice
if treatment is given three days after inoculation with 10^6

cells. Thirty-three percent of mice can be cured if treatment is given three days after an injection of 10^5 cells into the foot pad. In contrast, in the majority of mice neither cure nor growth delay is observed after chemotherapy if the tumor is first allowed to grow in either site until it is palpable. The effect of adjuvant treatment has been tested both before and after surgical removal of the primary tumor in the foot pad. Surgery without chemotherapy results in 90% mortality from pulmonary metastasis. As shown in Table 2, treatment before surgery is less effective than after surgery. There are not only fewer cures, but the growth delay of the relapsing tumors is also shorter. The most likely explanation for this paradoxical result probably relates to the well documented observation that measurable metastases of this tumor grow slowly while the primary tumors are present; the possibility of a competition for nutrients has been suggested. If this were also true at the time just prior to operation on the foot pad tumor, the poorer response to early chemotherapy could be caused by the lower sensitivity of resting cells to drug treatment. However, this mechanism has not been reported for other tumor models and since a more rapid growth of metastases after removal of the primary tumor is an infrequent phenomenon in clinical oncology, this model is probably not representative of the majority of human tumors.

TABLE 2

THE EFFECT OF TREATMENT WITH CYCLOPHOSPHAMIDE IN COMBINA-
TION WITH SURGERY

| Chemotherapy | Lewis lung | | | 2661 | | |
	ILS	ICR	p	ILS	ICR	p
Before surgery	15 days	25%	0.001	10 days	20%	0.01
After surgery	30 days	40%	0.001	20 days	0%	n.s.

ILS = % increase in life span of non-survivors.
ICR = % increase in cure rate.

Foot pad tumors were amputated at 3-4 weeks after implantation. Approximately 90% of surgical control mice died (all from pulmonary metastases). Chemotherapy was administered 2-3 days before surgery or 2-3 days after surgery.

MAMMARY CARCINOMA 2661

   This tumor is less sensitive to cyclophosphamide.
Treatment of mice three days after subcutaneous inoculation
of tumor in the flank or in the foot pad does increase the
cure rate; rather it only prolongs survival by 18 days for
the flank tumors and 36 days for the foot pad tumors. If
treatment is delayed till the tumors are palpable the growth
delay is reduced to 12 and 10 days, respectively. Adjuvant
therapy can increase the cure rate but only if treatment is
given before surgery, as indicated in Table 2.

   If the experimental mice are subdivided according to
size of the foot pad tumor, it appears that the benefit of
adjuvant therapy is seen mainly among the mice with large
foot pad tumors. In this group which had no survivors without adjuvant therapy, a major effect of adjuvant treatment
is noted in contrast to the group with small primary tumors
where mortality was unaffected by adjuvant treatment. Postoperative chemotherapy led to an increase in survival time
but not in cure rate (Mulder et al., 1983). The possibility
of a clinical counterpart to this model is a strong argument in favor of exploring the effects of chemotherapy before surgery.

TABLE 3

OSTEOSARCOMA
EFFECT OF ADJUVANT THERAPY

Dose 50 mg/kg cyclophosphamide

	Survivors/treated	
Control	4/24	
Treated day 3	4/24	

Dose 100 mg/kg cyclophosphamide

	Survivors/treated	
Control	15/45	33%
Treated day −3	29/38	76%
day +3	28/38	74%
day +10	19/24	79%

OSTEOSARCOMA C22LR

This tumor is very sensitive to cyclophosphamide chemotherapy; large flank tumors can be cured with two doses of cyclophosphamide. Adjuvant therapy at a dose of 50 mg/kg was without effect, but a dose of 100 mg/kg caused an increase in cure rate quite independent of the time of administration (see Table 3).

This response is clearly quite different from that seen in the two other tumors, but at present we have no explanation for this phenomenon and can not even speculate about a possible clinical counterpart.

In 1975, we reported on the paradoxical effect of treating tumors with chemotherapy after inoculation into the testicle (Van Putten et al., 1975). The reason for the experimental approach was a report that tumor inoculation at this site in hamsters would rapidly lead to lymph node metastasis (Rivenzon and Comisel, 1967). This was confirmed by our findings in mice ; in some cases we observed lymph node metastasis even if we amputated the injected testicle two hours after tumor cell inoculation, a finding that suggests a very rapid transport of some of the inoculated cells into the lymphatics. If high dose chemotherapy was given two hours after tumor cell inoculation into the testicle, a paradoxical effect of increased lung metastasis was noted (Table 4).

TABLE 4

LYMPH NODE AND LUNG METASTASIS OF OSTEOSARCOMA 18 DAYS AFTER INOCULATION INTO THE TESTICLE

Treatment	Number of mice	% mice with metastasis in lymph nodes	in lung
None	200	77	7
Cyclophospha- mide 250 mg/kg	44	16*	30+
CCNU 75 mg/kg	35	0*	26+

*: $p < 0.001$; +: $p < 0.01$ for difference with controls.

This occurred notwithstanding the high effectiveness of the cytostatic agents used. The chemotherapy often resulted in the complete cure of the testicular tumor, but the administration shortly after inoculation of the tumor cells was apparently ineffective against the migrating cells in the lymph nodes and actually enhanced the spread of the tumor to the lung. It is likely that tumors that are not sensitive to cyclophosphamide or nitrosoureas would, under similar conditions, show an even more marked spread than did this sensitive tumor.

This is an example of promotion of tumor cell spread, despite exposure to an agent of proven effectiveness against that tumor. In addition, there has been wide experience with promotion of tumor growth in mice by treatment of the animals with radiation before inoculation of the tumor cells (Hill and Bush, 1969; Brown, 1973,; Steel and Adams, 1977). Similar effects have been seen after treatment with cytostatic drugs (Van Putten et al., 1975). Recently, Poupon et al. (1984) reported on concomitant chemotherapy with nitrosoureas as a cause of enhanced tumor growth. Cyclophosphamide failed to show this effect.

CONCLUSIONS

The three tumor models studied have shown different types of dependence on timing of adjuvant chemotherapy. As mentioned they represent only three patients. However, it is possible to study these patients in great detail and to obtain insight into the wide variability of possible responses. It is hoped that this insight may contribute to the selection of optimal treatment models for clinical adjuvant therapy.

SUMMARY

In three mouse tumor models the effect of timing of adjuvant chemotherapy with a single dose of cyclophosphamide was studied. In one tumor, preoperative adjuvant therapy was better than postoperative therapy. In a second tumor, the reverse was the case, and in the third model there was no difference resulting from variation in the timing of cytostatic drug therapy. Obviously, the concept that a standard drug dose always gives a constant relative cell kill is not always a valid simplification of dose-effect relationships in chemotherapy.

* This study is based on the collection of experimental data in our institute by J.H. Mulder, J. de Ruiter, P. Lelieveld and M.B. Edelstein, T.F.C. Gerritsen, R.J.F. Middeldorp, T. Smink and L.K.J. Idsenga.

REFERENCES

Brown JM (1973) The effect of lung irradiation on the incidence of pulmonary metastases in mice. Br J Radiol 46: 613-618

Hill RP, Bush RS (1969) A lung colony assay to determine the radiosensitivity of the cells of a solid tumour. Int J Radiat Biol 15: 435-444

Mulder JH, De Ruiter J, Edelstein MB, Gerritsen TFC, Van Putten LM (1983) Model studies in adjuvant chemotherapy. Cancer Treat Rep 67: 45-50

Poupon MF, Pauwels C, Jasmin C, Antoine E, Lascaux V, Rosa B (1984) A inplicit pulmonary metastasis of rat rhabdomyosarcoma in response to nitrosourea treatment. Cancer Treat Rep 68: 749-758.

Rivenzon A, Comisel V (1967) Experimental model for the induction of tumoral lymph node metastasis in hamsters. Experientia 23: 756

Steel GG, Adams K (1977) Enhancement by cytotoxic agents of artificial pulmonary metastases. Br J Cancer 36: 653-658

Van Putten LM, Kram LKJ, Van Dierendonck HHC, Smink T, Füzy M (1975) Enhancement by drugs of metastatic lung nodule formation after intravenous tumour cell injection. Int J Cancer 15: 588-595

SECTION II
SARCOMAS

Primary Chemotherapy in Cancer Medicine, pages 25–37
© 1985 Alan R. Liss, Inc.

LIMB SALVAGE FOR MALIGNANT TUMORS OF BONE

Frederick R. Eilber, M.D., Armando E. Guiliano, M.D.
James F. Huth, M.D., and Jeffrey Eckhardt, M.D.
Division of Surgical Oncology, John Wayne Clinic,
Jonsson Comprehensive Cancer Center, UCLA School
of Medicine, Los Angeles, California 90024.

Malignant tumors of bone comprise less than 1% of all malignancies diagnosed annually. Historically, osteosarcoma has been considered to be the most common as well as the most lethal (Dahlin, Coventry 1967). Until the early 1970's, amputation was the preferred method, although attempts to salvage the affected limb were made occasionally. However, limb salvage was abandoned because of high local recurrence rates and the inherent instability of the bony replacements. During the late 1960's and early 1970's, two major developments made limb salvage more practical. The first was the discovery of chemotherapy regimens that increased the overall patient survival rate for osteosarcoma and Ewing's sarcoma. These results were most dramatic in osteosarcoma, improving overall survival from prechemotherapy rates of 10% to over 50% when the drugs were given as adjuvants following surgical resection (Carter, Friedman 1978). Advances in bioengineering soon followed. Metallic endoprosthesis of high strength and low weight were developed. Methylmethacrylate cement provided immediate firm fixation of these new prostheses.

With these two discoveries, multidisciplinary adjuvant pre- and postoperative programs could be developed for management of malignant primary bone tumors at UCLA beginning in 1972. The basic concept involved pretreatment with a combination of chemotherapy of proved effectiveness as an adjuvant and radiation therapy given sequentially before surgical excision of the involved bone. By pretreatment of these highly malignant bone tumors, we hoped to induce sufficient tumor-cell necrosis that would allow a surgical excision that was closer to the periphery of the tumor in order to preserve neurovascular structures and adjacent muscles.

By preservation of these vital structures, an endoprosthesis could be inserted into a functional extremity.

In this report, we describe our experience from the treatment of 172 primary malignant bone tumors from 1972 to 1984.

MATERIALS AND METHODS

The Divisions of Surgical Oncology and Orthopedics of the UCLA School of Medicine evaluated and treated 172 patients with malignant tumors of bone from 1972 to 1984. Treatment programs evolved into into three separate groups. The first, the control group, treated from 1972 to 1976, consisted of 57 patients who did not receive the preoperative therapy.

The second group, treated from 1975 to 1981, consisted of an additional consecutive series of 57 patients who were treated with preoperative intraarterial Adriamycin and 3500 rads of rapid-fraction radiation. Intraarterial Adriamycin was administered by a catheter inserted into the femoral artery by the Seldinger technique. Catheters in high-flow vessels such as the iliac, common femoral or axillary artery allowed infusion of Adriamycin to the lower extremity at a dose of 30 mg/24 hours X 3 days or 20 mg to an upper extremity for 3 days. Following the infusion, the catheters were removed and radiation of 3500 rads was begun at 250-rad fractions X 10 days. Treatment portals were AP/PA to the entire region, e.g. thigh or arm, excepting only a strip of skin opposite the biopsy site. Surgical excision of the involved bone and adjacent muscle took place approximately 1-2 weeks following completion of the radiation therapy.

All operations were performed through uninvolved tissue planes and included excision of the biopsy scar in continuity with the tumor. Confirmation of tumor-free margins was obtained by a surgical pathologist at the time of surgery. Long bones were transected 8 cm proximal to any scan or radiographic evidence of intramedullary tumor extension. Bony segments in this group were replaced by endoprostheses in 18 patients, by cadaver allografts in 22, and by rod and fusion in two. Eleven patients had excision alone with no bony replacment. Four of these 57 patients had primary amputation.

The third group, consisting of 58 patients, was treated from 1981 to 1984. These patients received treatment identical to that of the previous 57 except that the preoperative Adriamycin was followed by a the radiation dose of 1750 rads at 350-rad fractions X 5. Surgical procedures were identical, and in this group two patients had amputations, 47 received metallic endoprosthesis, and nine had excision without bony replacement.

A complete history and physical examination was obtained prior to therapy from all patients. Staging work-up included bone scans. CAT scans of the extremity were obtained for the past 6 years, as were chest x-rays, tomography, and CAT scans of the chest.

Table 1 lists the demographic characteristics of the patient population in the three treatment groups. The groups are comparable for male/female ratio (approximately 2:3 male to 1:3 female) and histologic subtypes (approximately 70-75% osteosarcomas). Other tumor types included four Ewing's sarcomas, eight malignant fibrohistiocytomas, and one metastatic epithelioid sarcoma. The primary tumor locations were comparable among the three groups, except that there was a higher percentage of tibia lesions in the control group that did not receive preoperative therapy. Limb salvage was possible in only two patients with tibial lesions.

Table 2 lists the additional staging information obtained before treatment of the three groups of patients. Again, the groups are relatively comparable in terms of patients who had primary disease only (Stage I), those treated for locally recurrent tumors (Stage II), and patients who presented with pulmonary metastases (Stage III). These groups were also staged by the Enneking Musculoskeletal Tumor Society Staging Procedure. Again, they were equal. By the Enneking procedure, Stage I patients have Grade I or Grade II bone tumors followed by an A or B, which represents the intramedullary or extramedullary extent of the disease (Enneking et al. 1980). Grade II tumors of either A or B, are considered to be high-grade lesions. In our three groups, approximately 80% of the lesions were high-grade.

Postoperative adjuvant chemotherapy was administered to some patients with high-grade lesions, which included the 140 patients with osteosarcoma. Adjuvant chemotherapy was given to an equal proportion of patients in all three treatment groups. Chemotherapy consisted of Adriamycin alternated with high-dose methotrexate every 2 weeks from 1973 to 1980. Adriamycin was given at a dose of 45 mg/m^2 on each of 2 consecutive days, followed in 2 weeks by high-dose methotrexate, 200 mg/kg of body weight, followed by citrovorum rescue. From 1980 to 1984,

Table 1 — LIMB SALVAGE: BONE TUMORS

	1972-76 Control (57)	1975-81 3500 (57)	1981-84 1750 (58)	TOTAL
Sex				
Male	34	36	35	105
Female	23	21	23	67
Histology				
Osteosarcoma	39 (68%)	45 (78%)	44 (75%)	128
Chondrosarcoma	14	4	6	24
Other	4	8	8	20
Location				
Femur	23	32	35	90
Tibia	17	1	1	19
Humerus	3	12	6	21
Ilium	10	10	7	27
Scapula	1	–	7	8
Other	3	2	1	6

our therapy program has consisted of the T-10 regimen of Rosen: alternating high-dose methotrexate (200 mg/kg of body weight) on each of two consecutive weeks with BCD — bleomycin (12 units/m^2), cyclophosphamide (600 mg/m^2), and Actinomycin D (450 μ g/m^2) — given on each of 2 consecutive days. Approximately 2 weeks later, the patients then received Adriamycin, 45 mg/m^2, given on each of 2 consecutive days. This cycle requires 6 weeks to administer, and 5-6 cycles are delivered (Rosen et al. 1982). Table 2 also lists the proportion of patients in each treatment group who received adjuvant chemotherapy.

Table 3 lists the various surgical procedures and bony replacements used for the three treatment groups. The control group received no preoperative therapy, and 30/57 (67%) required primary amputation. Ten patients received endoprostheses, 11 had excisions only, one had a cadaver allograft, and one had a rod and fusion. In the group that received 3500 rads of radiation,

Table 2 — LIMB SALVAGE: BONE TUMORS

	1972-76 Control (57)	1975-81 3500 (57)	1981-84 1750 (58)	TOTAL
Stage I	45	49	54	148
Stage II	7	1	2	10
Stage III	5	7	2	14
Enneking Stage:				
I (A,B)	15	4	11	30
II (A,B)	42 (74%)	53 (93%)	47 (81%)	128
Osteosarcoma	39	45	44	128
Adjuvant Chemotherapy:				
No	16	5	23	44
Yes	23	40	21	84
A-MTX	19	39	-	
T-10	4	1	21	

four patients (7%) required amputation. In the remaining patients, limb salvage was possible — 18 with endoprosthesis, 11 with excision only, 22 with cadaver allografts, and two with rod and fusion. In the third group, of the 58 patients treated with 1750 rads of radiation, limb salvage was possible in 96%, and only two patients required primary amputation. Diseased bone was replaced by endoprostheses in 47, and nine had excision without any bony replacement.

Assessment of the pretreatment effect on all tumors was made by Dr. Joseph Mirra of the Department of Pathology. Assessments were based on the evaluation of at least 10 slides per tumor, taken at various anatomic locations, and necrosis was defined as a lack of identifiable nuclei.

Table 3 — LIMB SALVAGE: BONE TUMORS

	1972-76 Control (57)	1975-81 3500 (57)	1981-84 1750 (58)	TOTAL
Amputation	34 (60%)	4 (7%)	2 (4%)	
Endoprosthesis	10	18	47	75
Excision	11	11	9	31
Cadaver Graft	1	22	–	23
Rod and Fusion	1	2	–	3

Table 4 — LIMB SALVAGE: BONE TUMORS

	1972-76 Control (57)	1975-81 3500 (57)	1981-84 1750 (58)
Amputation:			
Primary	35 (61%)	4 (9%)	2 (3%)
Secondary		7 (20%)	1 (5%)
Local Recurrence	6 (10%)	3 (5%)	5 (9%)
Osteo NED	12 (30%)	21 (46%)	30 (68%)
Chondro NED	12 (85%)	1 (25%)	5 (83%)

RESULTS

Although results of treatment in these three groups of patients does not represent a randomized trial, results were obtained from a consecutive series of patients treated by three treatment regimens. The first group of patients represents a control group that did not receive preoperative therapy but was treated by a surgical procedure. Thirty-four of the 57 patients (60%) required primary amputation to control the tumor. Of the patients in whom limb salvage was possible (23), none had osteosarcoma. In this group of 57 patients, 6 (10%) had local disease recurrence (Table 4).

In the second group, 57 patients treated from 1974 to 1981 with Adriamycin and 3500 rads of radiation, four required primary amputation despite pretreatment. In the remaining 53 limb salvage was possible, 18 by endoprosthesis, 11 by excision without bony replacement, 22 by cadaver allografts, and two by rod and fusion. Of these patients, three (5%) had a local disease recurrence. All cadaver allografts had to be revised or replaced in patients who lived more than 1 year.

In the third group, 58 patients treated from 1981 to 1984 with Adriamycin and 1750 rads of radiation, two (4%) had primary amputation. Limbs were salvaged in the remaining 56 (96%), 47 by endoprostheses and nine by excision alone. No cadaver allografts or rod and fusions were performed because of our poor experience in the previous group; five of these patients (9%) have had local disease recurrence. One patient had a secondary amputation because of complications; thus, the limb salvage rate for this group is 95%.

The pathology evaluation showed that tumor-cell necrosis was related to tumor grade. Of the patients with high-grade osteosarcoma, there was a median of 10% necrosis in the control group of patients. The 3500- and 1750-rad radiation-treated groups had an equal percentage of necrosis, with a median of approximately 85% and a range of 20-100%. There did not appear to be any reduction of tumor-cell necrosis with the reduced dose of radiation. In the other tumor types, tumor-cell necrosis was much more variable from the Ewing's sarcoma, with a high 95% median necrosis, to the chondrosarcomas, with an average of only 40% necrosis (Fig. 1).

The functional stability of the various bony replacements is shown in Figure 2, which shows that the cadaver allografts required reoperation at a higher rate with patient survival. Although some patients did not require revision of their cadaver allografts, in all instances this was because they expired before requiring revision. Of the endoprostheses used for distal femur replacement, the spherocentric-type knee required revision in approximately 30% of the patients, whereas the kinomatic rotating-hinge knee required it in less than 10%. Of the patients treated with 3500 rads preoperatively who had bony replacement, 70% have had an excellent functional result, but of those treated with 1750 rads, 90% have had a good to excellent functional result.

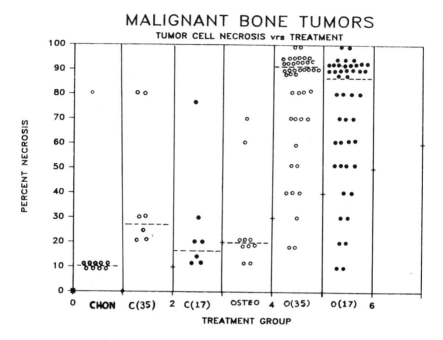

Figure 1

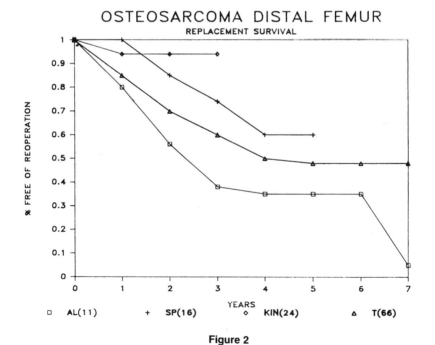

Figure 2

The overall survival rate of the three groups of patients is given in Table 4. Of those who had osteosarcoma, approximately 30% of the control, 46% of the 3500-rad group, and 68% of the 1750-rad group remain alive free of disease. An analysis of survival based on whether or not the patients received chemotherapy is given in Figure 3. The overall survival of patients with osteosarcoma who did not receive chemotherapy was less than 20%. From 1972 to 1981, all patients were advised to have chemotherapy — this was not a randomzied trial. The adjuvant chemotherapy consisted of Adriamycin and high-dose methotrexate. During this time, of 66 patients with Stage I disease (Stage II B osteosarcoma), the 50 who received Adriamycin and high-dose methotrexate had an overall survival rate of 50% at a median follow-up of 6 years. Of the 16 patients who did not receive adjuvant chemotherapy, the overall survival rate was less than 10%. Since 1981, a randomized prospective trial was undertaken to compare no adjuvant chemotherapy with the T-10 protocol of Rosen. This trial includes 50 patients with Stage II B osteosarcoma. The survival rate of the control group is 25% at 36 months, the same as that of the earlier historical control group. Of those patients receiving the T10 adjuvant chemotherapy, 70% remain alive free of disease at 36 months. This is a highly statistical difference, showing benefit for patients receiving adjuvant chemotherapy.

Overall survival for patients with osteosarcoma was also analyzed according to the type of primary tumor treatment (amputation versus limb salvage), as well as by results from adjuvant chemotherapy (Fig. 4). Again, there was improved 5-year survival (50%) for the 73 patients who received adjuvant chemotherapy, regardless of whether they had amputation (21) or limb salvage (53). Of the 33 patients who did not receive adjuvant chemotherapy, only 20% survived. Again, no difference was noted between those who had amputation (18) and those who had limb salvage (25).

DISCUSSION

There are three basic goals that must be achieved by any limb salvage program. First, the local recurrence rate must be no higher than that achieved with the alternative method of local control, amputation. Secondly, patients entered into a limb-salvage protocol should be at no greater risk for progression of disease or eventual disease recurrence, either because of a higher risk of local recurrence or because the program entails either

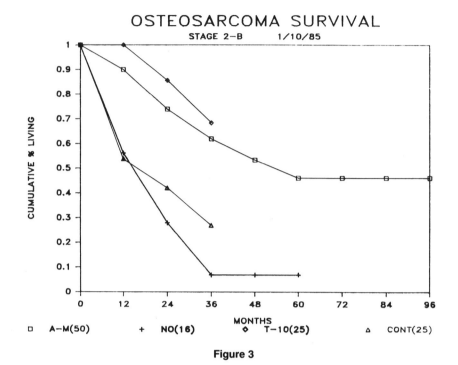

Figure 3

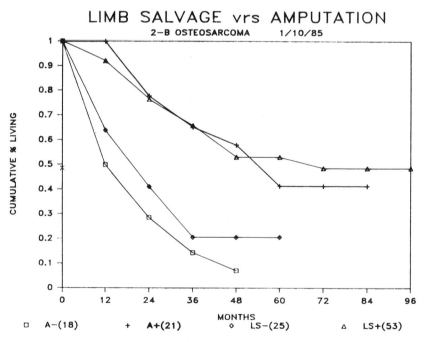

Figure 4

delay in treatment or employs ineffective treatment of the primary tumor. Thirdly, the means for reconstruction for limb salvage should be an enduring one and should not commit the patient to repetitive hospitalizations for management of local complications or complex revisional procedures.

The local recurrence rate in our series of patients who underwent limb salvage was 6%. This result is comparable to our historical control, i.e. patients with surgery alone (Harvei, Solheim 1981; Campanacci, Laus 1980). This rate was the same for both treatment groups, those who received 3500 rads or 1750 rads. The low rate of local recurrence in this series could be directly attributed to the preoperative Adriamycin and radiation therapy. We cannot be certain of this result, because this was not a randomized trial. However, Sim et al. reported a local recurrence rate of 23% for a limb salvage procedure without preoperative chemotherapy in the Mayo Clinic's experience (Trapeznikov et al. 1983). Simon and Heck reviewed 45 specimens and determined that if tumor invades the articular cartilege, a common occurrence in at least 30% of patients, it will extend into the capsule of the joint 50% of the time (Suman, Hecht 1982). Because of these findings, they recommend extraarticular resection for limb salvage patients. This tumor extension may be the reason for the high local recurrence rate seen in both the Russian and Mayo Clinic series of patients who did not receive presurgical treatment. Rosen reported that between 1973 and 1983, in good responders (greater than 50% necrosis to the T-10 chemotherapy) treatment success without radiation was only 43% (Rosen et al. 1982; Marcove, Rosen 1980). This finding suggests that with chemotherapy alone, there was no significant effect on the primary tumor for 50% of their patients.

Local complications are rare following primary amputative surgery. The complication rate among the limb-salvage patients was 30% in the 3500-rad group and 15% in the 1750-rad group. Most of the local complications in our series appeared to be associated with the higher dose of radiation and with the large medial and lateral incisions previously used routinely to resect the tumors (Eilber et al. 1984). Since 1981, with the reduction in radiation and the ability to use a single incision, most of the local problems have been eliminated. Furthermore, the improved fixation techniques and the metallic endoprosthesis with the kinematic rotating hinge have greatly reduced the complication and revision rates for distal femoral replacements since 1981.

Functional results following limb salvage procedures are dependent upon many factors, including the nature of any preoperative therapy, the tumor size and grade and the resection techniques, i.e. intraarticular or extraarticular, the design and fixation techniques of the prosthesis and the postoperative rehabilitation program, whether or not the patient is immobilized, and, possibly equally important, patient variables including weight, activity level, motion, and cooperation. The psychological and cosmetic advantages of having an extremity with enduring internal prostheses cannot be understated or underestimated. This is especially true for the upper extremity, where amputation about the shoulder girdle results in the loss of noninvolved normal functioning of the elbow and hand. None of our patients with upper extremity amputation became prosthetic wearers; none of the patients who required hip disarticulation or hemipelvectomy wore a prosthesis. Our results with cadaver allografts were disappointing. Of the 23 allografts that were placed, 50% had to be revised. Furthermore, there was no evidence by bone scan or repeated biopsy in any of the patients that the body incorporated of the allograft. Although other authors have reported successful incorporation of cadaver allografts in patients with malignant bone tumors, in most instances, the segment was relatively small, approximately 7–8 cm, and the patients did not receive adjuvant chemotherapy.

SUMMARY

With the use of preoperative therapy of chemotherapy and radiation, limb salvage has been possible in more than 95% of patients with highly malignant bone tumors. Without preoperative treatment, limb salvage is possible in only 40% of the patients. In our experience, improved limb salvage is a direct result of the preoperative therapy. We are not sure this preoperative therapy is the ideal one, or whether the intraarterial Adriamycin is superior to intravenous administration, or whether the dose of radiation is the proper one, or even whether radiation is necessary at all. These questions remain unanswered at this time. However, the pathologist's evaluation of the excised specimens shows that the preoperative treatment has definite beneficial effect for more than 80% of the patients on this program.

Local control is equal with either amputation or limb salvage. Additionally, the overall survival rate is identical for either limb salvage or primary amputation. The major factor for patient survival appears to be the systemic adjuvant chemotherapy.

Limb salvage as practiced at UCLA is as effective as amputation for control of malignant bone tumors. The selection of patients for our limb salvage program has not adversely affected the rate of disease progression or ultimate survival. The cosmetic and functional results of limb-salvage surgery is at least comparable to if not better than external prostheses. Finally, the only factor that appears to influence long-term survival in a positive manner is participation in a polydrug postoperative adjuvant chemotherapy program.

This work was supported by Grant CA29605, awarded by the National Cancer Institute, DHEW.

REFERENCES

Campanacci M, Laus M (1980). Local recurrence after amputation for osteosarcoma. J Bone Joint Surg (Br) 2:201.

Carter SK, Friedman M (1978). Osteogenic sarcoma — Treatment overview and some comments on interpretations of clinical trial data. Cancer Treat Rep 62:199.

Dahlin DC, Coventry MB (1967). Osteosarcoma: A study of six hundred cases. J Bone Joint Surg 49A:101.

Eilber FR, Morton DL, Eckhardt J, Grant T, Weisenburger T (1984). Limb salvage for skeletal and soft-tissue sarcomas: Multidisciplinary preoperative therapy. Cancer 53:2579.

Enneking WF, Spaniers SS, Goodman M (1980). Current concepts review: The surgical staging of musculoskeletal sarcoma. J Bone Joint Surg 62A: 1027.

Harvei S, Solheim O (1981). The prognosis in osteosarcoma: Norwegian national data. Cancer 48:1719.

Marcove RC, Rosen G (1980). En bloc resections for osteogenic sarcoma. Cancer 45:3040.

Rosen G, Capparros B, Huvos A, Kosloff C, Nirenberg A, Cacavio A, Marcove R, Lane J, Metha B (1982). Preoperative chemofor osteosarcoma: Selection of postoperative adjuvant chemotherapy based on the response of the primary tumor to chemotherapy. Cancer 49:1221.

Sim FC, Bowman WE, Chao EY (1982). Limb salvage for primary malignant bone tumors. In: "The 2nd International Workshop on the Design and Application of Tumor Prostheses for Bone and Joint Reconstruction," Vienna: Egerman and Co., p 153.

Suman MA, Hecht JD (1982). Invasion of joints by primary bone sarcomas in adults. Cancer 50:1649.

Trapeznikov NN, Yeremina LA, Amiraslanov AT, Sunakov PA (1983). Complex treatment of osteosarcoma patients. In: "The 2nd International Workshop on the Design and Application of Tumor Prostheses for Bone and Joint Reconstruction," Vienna, Egerman and Co., p 55.

Primary Chemotherapy in Cancer Medicine, pages 39–51
© 1985 Alan R. Liss, Inc.

NEOADJUVANT CHEMOTHERAPY FOR OSTEOGENIC SARCOMA: A FIVE
YEAR FOLLOW-UP (T-10) AND PRELIMINARY REPORT OF NEW STUDIES
(T-12)

Gerald Rosen, M.D. and Anita Nirenberg, R.N.,C.

Comprehensive Cancer Centers, Inc.
407 N. Maple Drive
Beverly Hills, California   90210

ABSTRACT

During the past 10 years, (November, 1973 through November, 1983) 208 patients with fully malignant primary osteogenic sarcoma of an extremity were treated with preoperative
chemotherapy on 4 successive treatment protocols. Continuous
improvements in the disease-free survival of patients were
attributed to refinements in the chemotherapy regimens.
These refinements were made after direct observation of the
response of the primary tumor to chemotherapy. At a minimum
follow-up time of over 38 months for 87 patients treated on
the T-10 chemotherapy protocol, 67 (77%) have remained alive
and continuously free of disease, and 71/87 (81.6%) are
currently free of disease at a median follow-up time of 5
years. Overall complete response rate of the primary tumor
to preoperative chemotherapy was 48%. Fifty-one patients
were treated on a pilot protocol (T-12) from November, 1981,
to November, 1983. The main difference was that after preoperative high dose methotrexate and combination bleomycin,
cytoxan and dactinomycin therapy, patients having a good
histologic response of the primary tumor (21/51 or 41%) had
their chemotherapy stopped at 15 weeks and did not receive
platinum or Adriamycin chemotherapy. 38/51 (75%) on T-12
remained continuously free of disease and 39/51 (76%) are
currently alive and free of disease. There were 2 local
recurrences on the T-10 protocol and 6 on the T-12 protocol.
Excluding local recurrences 71/85 (84%), patients treated on
T-10 are currently alive and free of disease and 38/45 (84%)
patients treated on T-12 are alive and free of disease (at a
median follow-up of 24 months for T-12). This preliminary

study indicates that preoperative chemotherapy may be used to select a subset of patients (who respond well to preoperative high dose methotrexate) who can have therapy terminated early, sparing those patients the undesirable side effects and cost of additional therapy with platinum and Adriamycin.

INTRODUCTION

During the past several years, there has been considerable controversy over the role of chemotherapy in the management of patients with osteogenic sarcoma.[1,2] While one group has maintained that the natural history of the disease has changed to that of a better prognosis with surgery alone, the majority of large series of patients with osteogenic sarcoma did not demonstrate such a favorable change.[3,4] Some groups reported that the early use of chemotherapy for the treatment of osteogenic sarcoma in the adjuvant or postoperative setting, did not appear to raise the overall 5 year survival to above 50%.[4,5,6] Others had consistently reported results in the adjuvant treatment of osteogenic sarcoma which were considerably higher.[7,8] Objections to the former studies[5,6] included the fact that high dose methotrexate with leucovorin rescue was not used at its optimal dosage.[9] The dose of 12 gm/m^2 of methotrexate, particularly for younger children who excrete the drug more efficiently than adults, and the introduction of the combination of bleomycin, cyclophosphamide, and dactinomycin (BCD) resulted in an increase in the reported disease-free survival from approximately 50% to over 75% on our second generation (T-7) protocol.[7,10] The use of high dose methotrexate at this schedule as well as the BCD combination and the subsequent introduction of another active drug in the treatment of osteogenic sarcoma, cisplatinum, has resulted in effective treatment protocols that were prototypes of the originally described T-7 chemotherapy protocol, namely the T-10 chemotherapy protocol.[8] Confirmation of the effectiveness of these treatment protocols used for adjuvant chemotherapy for osteogenic sarcoma have recently been reported by two large cooperative groups, both in this country and abroad.[11,12] In particular, a study utilizing adjuvant chemotherapy modeled after the T-10 chemotherapy protocol vs. no adjuvant chemotherapy has recently been performed by the Pediatric Oncology Group (POG). That study was prematurely terminated when it was determined that patients receiving no adjuvant chemotherapy had an overwhelmingly significantly poorer disease-free survival than those patients receiving adjuvant chemotherapy with high dose methotrexate at the dose of 12 gm/m^2 with leucovorin rescue, Adriamycin, BCD, and cisplatinum. Of 19 patients followed with no adjuvant chemotherapy, 15 patients relapsed, whereas only 8 patients relapsed of the 49 evaluable patients given immediate postoperative adjuvant chemotherapy. This study was significant (P=0.00006) and settles once and for all the question of whether or not adjuvant chemotherapy is of value in the treatment of osteogenic sarcoma and confirms that the natural history of the untreated disease still leads to a survival of less than 20% with surgery alone.[11] In a similar nonrandomized study, the German-Austrian Cooperative Osteogenic Sarcoma Study Group (COSS-80) demonstrated that there is an increase in the disease-free survival for patients with osteogenic sarcoma when treated with adjuvant or preoperative chemotherapy. They reported a disease-free survival in the range of 75% for such patients. They concluded that the increased percentage of patients surviving free of disease compared to their prior study (COSS-77) was attributed to the addition of methotrexate at the dose of 12 gm/m^2 as we had concluded in our T-7 chemotherapy study. There was no difference in the two arms of the study comparing the combination BCD vs. cisplatinum.[12]

Preoperative chemotherapy, or neoadjuvant chemotherapy as it has been termed, for osteogenic sarcoma is now receiving wide-spread acceptance. The initial concept introduced by Rosen and Marcove in 1974 had various therapeutic advantages associated with it.[13] Primarily, it allowed direct observation of the effect of drugs on the primary tumor which helped establish safe and effective dose schedules. Before custom prostheses were readily available, it allowed time to make a custom made endoprosthesis for some of those patients who underwent the first limb salvage surgical procedures for osteogenic sarcoma. With experience, it became evident that the use of preoperative chemotherapy to shrink the primary tumor had an advantage for the surgeon performing en bloc resection of the tumor. Very large or pathologically fractured and bleeding tumors could be made to regress, and lose their neovascularity helping to better define tissue planes and decrease bleeding at the time of surgery.

Perhaps the most important advantage of preoperative chemotherapy evolved in the T-10 chemotherapy protocol.[8] In 1978, it had become apparent that those patients who had a complete response of their primary tumor to preoperative

chemotherapy with high dose methotrexate and BCD or Adriamycin, had a 100% disease-free survival if they did not
develop a local recurrence. All of the relapses took place
in patients who did not have a complete response to preoperative chemotherapy. A complete response was defined as
a complete clinical response as well as the finding of only
a few microscopic foci of viable tumor, or no viable tumor at
all on complete histologic examination of the resected primary tumor. The T-10 chemotherapy protocol called for the
addition of cisplatinum and Adriamycin chemotherapy postoperatively for patients that had only a partial response to
preoperative chemotherapy. Those having a complete response
were expected to remain disease-free survivors if treated
with only the same chemotherapy (high dose methotrexate, BCD,
and Adriamycin) postoperatively. These latter patients did
not require the addition of the potentially renal toxic, and
ototoxic drug cisplatinum.

A pilot study, (T-12), was a refinement of the T-10
chemotherapy protocol in which patients having a complete
response to preoperative chemotherapy with high dose methotrexate and BCD, had their chemotherapy terminated after a
total of only 15 weeks of pre and postoperative chemotherapy.
Those patients who were good responders to preoperative chemotherapy with high dose methotrexate were thus spared any
exposure at all to both Adriamycin and cisplatinum, the drugs
that have the most serious long term toxicity associated with
them. On the other hand, patients responding incompletely to
preoperative high dose methotrexate and BCD did go on to
receive the full course of cisplatinum and Adriamycin
therapy similar to that in the T-10 chemotherapy protocol
(Fig 1).

METHODS

Chemotherapy

In November, 1981, a pilot fourth generation protocol
(T-12) was started in which patients were treated with preoperative high dose methotrexate, and the BCD combination.
Those that had a complete response to preoperative chemotherapy had only one BCD treatment and two high dose methotrexate treatments postoperatively and had their treatment
terminated at only 15 weeks (Fig 1). The T-12 protocol tried
to pose the question 'Is a complete response to preoperative

CHEMOTHERAPY FOR OSTEOGENIC SARCOMA — TREATMENT PROTOCOL (T-12)

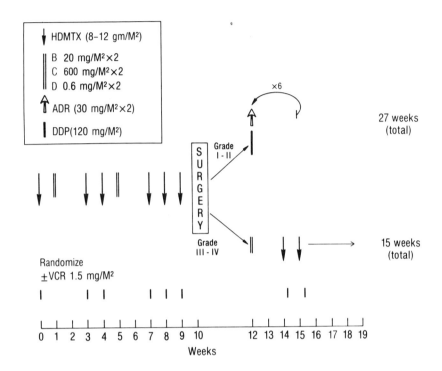

Figure 1

The T-12 pilot chemotherapy protocol. Patients having a
complete histologic response of the primary tumor to preoperative chemotherapy had their chemotherapy stopped after a
total of only 15 weeks of chemotherapy. Those patients never
received Adriamycin or cisplatinum. Allowing for differences
arising from the more liberal use of limb salvage surgery,
there was no difference in the survival of patients treated
on T-12 when compared to the earlier T-10 protocol which
required up to 40 weeks of chemotherapy for all patients
(Table 2).

chemotherapy an indication that the patient has had enough
chemotherapy to be curative?'

The exact details of the T-10 protocol as well as the
intricate details of the administration of high dose methotrexate with leucovorin rescue have been previously reported
in great detail.[8,9,14]

Patients

Included were patients who were referred to the author
or the author's clinic and were treated there with preoperative chemotherapy for osteogenic sarcoma during the
reported time period. During the T-10 and T-12 protocols, 7
patients referred with primary tumors had immediate surgery
for either uncontrollable (bed ridden) pain, or prior
surgical procedures for suspected benign tumors. Thirteen
additional patients were referred only for chemotherapy after
definitive surgery for the primary tumor was performed. The
treatment results in this group of concomitant "non-preop-
erative chemotherapy" patients is also presented.

All patients had fully malignant (III-IV/IV) osteogenic
sarcoma of an extremity. They had no evidence of pulmonary
metastasis or bone metastasis at the time of referral.
Seven patients had prior treatment with either chemotherapy
or radiation therapy. Most of those patients had what was
considered low doses of methotrexate, or one or two doses of
Adriamycin. Some patients had inadequate doses of radiation
therapy as well. These 7 patients were included, however,
because at the time of referral, they had large, advanced,
evaluable tumors, and the effect of preoperative chemotherapy
on them could be adequately judged. These latter patients
were considered very poor risk patients and would be excluded
from most protocols, but were included because of their
evaluable tumor, and the fact that we did not want to pre-
judice our data by stating that preoperative chemotherapy
should be confined only to patients with small or early
lesions.

Five patients were excluded from this study because of
refusal of postoperative chemotherapy with cisplatinum and
Adriamycin. Of those 5 patients, 2 are reported to be
continuously free of disease at this time. Of the 138
patients treated on the T-10 and T-12, 17 were above the age
of 21. Of the latter group of adults, the age ranged from

22 to 57. Patients above the age of 60 with osteogenic sarcoma arising in Paget's disease were excluded. Also excluded was one 50 year old patient who was lost to follow-up after surgery for his primary tumor (last noted to be free of disease). The youngest patient treated was 3 years of age.

Patients dying of complications of treatment (both surgical and drug) are counted as not surviving free of disease (or treatment failures).

RESULTS

Of 87 patients given preoperative chemotherapy on the T-10 chemotherapy protocol, 67 (77%) remained alive and continuously free of disease, and 71/87 (81.6%) are currently free of disease at a follow-up period of over 3 to 6 years. In the T-10 chemotherapy protocol group, 2 of the treatment failures included one postoperative surgical death and one death secondary to disseminated varicella. A further complication of therapy included a secondary leukemia in one of the T-10 patients. That patient is currently in complete remission from his leukemia for over 2½ years with no evidence of recurrent osteogenic sarcoma. It should be noted that since 1977 when guidelines for the safe and effective use of high dose methotrexate were firmly established and practiced in our clinic, there have been no incidents of severe drug toxicity or drug deaths.[9]

In the pilot T-12 chemotherapy protocol, 51 patients were treated with preoperative chemotherapy and 38 (75%) are surviving continuously disease free. At this brief median follow-up period of 2 years, 39/51 (76%) are alive and free of disease. There is no statistically significant difference between the survival of T-12 and T-10 treated patients (Table 1). Allowing for the fact that there were 6 local recurrences on T-12 and only 2 on T-10, the efficacy of the T-12 protocol is identical to T-10 (Table 2).

TABLE 1

Preoperative Chemotherapy for Osteogenic Sarcoma

Protocol	≠Patients	≠CDFS*	(%)	≠ANED**	(%)
T-10	87	67	(77)	71	(82)
T-12	51	38	(75)	39	(76)
Total	138	105	(76)	110	(80)

*CDFS Continuous disease free survival

**ANED Alive with no evidence of disease

TABLE 2

Preoperative Chemotherapy for Osteogenic Sarcoma
Excluding 8 Patients with Documented Local Recurrences

Protocol	≠Patients	≠CDFS*	(%)	≠ANED**	(%)
T-10	85	67	(79)	71	(84)
T-12	45	38	(84)	38	(84)
Total	130	105	(81)	109	(84)

*CDFS Continuous disease free survival

**ANED Alive with no evidence of disease

Of the concomitant small group of 20 patients presenting after surgery and receiving postoperative adjuvant
chemotherapy, 15 (75%) are continuously free of disease,
and 16 (80%) currently alive and free of disease. All 20 of
these patients were obliged to continue their adjuvant
chemotherapv with cisplatinum and Adriamycin following high
dose methotrexate and BCD treatment (Table 3).

TABLE 3

Preoperative Chemotherapy for Osteogenic Sarcoma
Concomitant Patients not Receiving Preoperative Chemotherapy

Protocol	≠Patients	≠CDFS*	(%)	≠ANED**	(%)
T-10	15	10	(67)	11	(73)
T-12	5	5	(100)	5	(100)
Total	20	15	(75)	16	(80)

*CDFS Continuous disease free survival

**ANED Alive with no evidence of disease

DISCUSSION

At the time of this writing, the utility of adjuvant chemotherapy for the treatment of osteogenic sarcoma has been unequivocally documented.[8,11,12] Many investigators involved in the treatment of this disease had no question in their mind that the malignant nature of osteogenic sarcoma has not changed in recent years. This was finally confronted and confirmed by the recent POG study where only 5 of 19 patients not offered adjuvant chemotherapy did not relapse.[11] It is unfortunate for those patients that the controversy about chemotherapy (created by groups not utilizing the optimal drugs and drug dosages that had been reported in our pilot studies) caused the medical community to mount this prospective randomized POG study. Fortunately, the investigators recognized the early significance which developed between the treated group and the untreated group and terminated that study, having answered the question about the utility of adjuvant chemotherapy in osteogenic sarcoma once and for all.

Preoperative chemotherapy although popularized in our early treatment of patients with osteogenic sarcoma, has now become the state-of-the-art standard for many malignancies. It offers the advantage of early systemic treatment for both gross and microscopic metastatic disease in an attempt to eradicate that disease prior to surgical intervention for the primary tumor.

The true concept of neoadjuvant chemotherapy as defined in patients with osteogenic sarcoma also should take into account that the response of the primary tumor can act as a prognostic indicator of the usefulness of primary preoperative chemotherapy. Patients not having a complete response to preoperative chemotherapy might do better with other alternative chemotherapy. The addition of alternative or second line chemotherapy should be instituted immediately postoperatively in those patients who do not respond well to the preoperative chemotherapy. This gives the patient with a high risk of relapsing a better chance at cure since chemotherapy is most effective before the patient relapses. The knowledge of the limited utility of one form of chemotherapy in a patient obtained through observation of the effect of preoperative chemotherapy should alert the physician to the possible need for more aggressive therapy postoperatively.

Finally the use of preoperative chemotherapy in osteogenic sarcoma has allowed us to use the good response of the primary tumor to define an "end point" of chemotherapy, allowing us to shorten the course of therapy in approximately 50% of good responding patients treated on the T-12 protocol. This approach will greatly reduce the morbidity, cost and potential long term side effects in approximately 50% of patients, who can be identified through the use of preoperative chemotherapy. It is suggested that this approach be tried in other malignancies where preoperative chemotherapy can give rise to a substantial complete response rate.

A final note of caution concerns the fact that chemotherapy still cannot replace adequate surgery for the primary tumor. With the recent enthusiasm for limb salvage surgery for osteogenic sarcoma, that procedure might possibly be offered to patients who would do better with amputation. Although limb salvage seems perfectly safe in the upper extremity, there were 8 documented local recurrences in lower extremity lesions and one death secondary to limb salvage surgery. An additional patient who relapsed and died of disease, had a delayed amputation after initial limb salvage surgery resulted in a resection with positive microscopic margins. Our experience and that of others[12] indicates that amputated patients actually have a better survival than those patients having limb salvage surgery for lower extremity lesions even though the latter patients usually have smaller lesions at diagnosis. The current enthusiasm for limb salvage surgery should not overlook the fact that there is still a place for amputation in the treatment of some patients with osteogenic sarcoma. However, these few patients can still profit from preoperative chemotherapy.

1. Edmonson, JH, Green, SJ, Ivins, JC, Gilchrist, GS, Creagan, ET, Pritchard, DJ, Smithson, WA, Dahlin, DC, Taylor, WF. A controlled pilot study of high dose methotrexate as postsurgical adjuvant treatment for primary osteosarcoma. Journal of Clinical Oncology, Vol 2, No 3 pp 152-156 (March) 1984.
2. Carter, SK. Adjuvant chemotherapy in osteogenic sarcoma: The triumph that isn't? Journal of Clinical Oncology, Vol 2, No 3, pp 147-148 (March) 1984.
3. Marcove, RC, Mike V, Hajek JV, et al: Osteogenic sarcoma under the age of 21. A review of 145 operative cases. Journal of Bone and Joint Surgery. 52A:411-423, 1970.
4. Sutow, WW,, Sullivan, MP, Wilbur, JR, Cangir, A. A study of adjuvant chemotherapy in osteogenic sarcoma. Journal of Clinical Phamacol 1975; 7:530-533.
5. Cortes, EP, Necheles, TF, Holland, JF, Glidewell, O. Adriamycin (ADR) alone vs. ADR and high dose methotrexate-citrovorum factor rescue (HDM-CFR) as ajuvant to operable primary osteosarcoma. A randomized study by Cancer and Leukemic Group B (CALGB). Proc AM Assoc Cancer Res 1979; 20:412.
6. Pratt, CB, Shanks, EC, Hustu, HO, et al. Adjuvant multiple drug chemotherapy for osteogenic sarcoma of the extremity. Cancer 1977, 39:51-57.

7. Rosen, G, Marcove, RC, Caparros B, et al: Primary osteogenic sarcoma. The rationale for preoperative chemotherapy and delayed surgery. Cancer 43:2163-3177, 1979.
8. Rosen, G, Caparros, B, Huvos, AG, Kosloff, C, Nirenberg, A, Cacavio, A, Marcove, RC, Lane, JM, Mehta, B, Urban, C. Preoperative chemotherapy for osteogenic sarcoma: Selection of postoperative adjuvant chemotherapy based on the response of the primary tumor to preoperative chemotherapy. Cancer 49: 1221-1230, 1982.
9. Rosen, G, Nirenberg, A. Chemotherapy for osteogenic sarcoma: An investigative method, not a recipe. Cancer Treat. Rep. 66:1687-1697, 1982.
10. Mosende C, Guttierez, M, Caparros, B, Rosen, G: Combination chemotherapy with bleomycin, cyclophosphamide and dactinomycin for the treatment of osteogenic sarcoma. Cancer 40:2779-2786, 1977
11. Link, MP. The role of adjuvant chemotherapy in the treatment of osteosarcoma of the extremity: Preliminary results of the multi-institutional osteosarcoma study. In Proceedings of National Institutes of Health Consensus Development Conference on "Limb Sparing Treatment: Adult

soft tissue and osteogenic sarcomas". pp 74-78, Dec. 3-5, 1984.

12. Winkler, K, Beron, G, Kotz, R, Salzer-Kuntschik, M, Beck, WB, Ebell, W, Erttmann, R, Gobel, U, Havers, W, Henze, G, Hinderfeld, HL, Hocker, P, Jobke, A, Jurgens, H, Kabisch, h, Preusser, P, Prindull, G, Ramach, W, Ritter, J, Sekera, J, Treuner, J, Wust, G, Landbeck, G. Neoadjuvant chemotherapy for osteogenic sarcoma: Results of a cooperative German-Austrain Study. Journal of Clinical Oncology, Vol 2, No 6, pp 617-623, 1984.

13. Rosen, G, Murphy, ML, Huvos, AG, et al. Chemotherapy, en block resection and prosthetic bone replacement in the treatment of osteogenic sarcoma. Cancer 1976; 37:1-11.

14. Rosen, G. High-dose methotrexate with leucovorin rescue: Treatment of osteogenic sarcoma and guidelines for clinical use. In Pharmanual: A comprehensive guide to the therapeutic use of methotrexate in osteogenic sarcoma. Editor G. Rosen pp 47-83, 1984.

Primary Chemotherapy in Cancer Medicine, pages 53–57
© 1985 Alan R. Liss, Inc.

COMBINATION CHEMOTHERAPY PRECEDING
SURGERY IN OSTEOGENIC SARCOMA

A.T. van Oosterom [*], P.A.Voûte [**],
A.H.M.Taminiau [*] and J.W. van der Eijken [***]

[*] Univerisity Hospital, Leiden
[**] Emma Kinderziekenhuis, Amsterdam
[***] Onze Lieve Vrouwe Gasthuis, Amsterdam
The Netherlands

SUMMARY

In 19 unselected subsequently entered non-metastatic
patients with a normal osteogenic sarcoma two different
just tolerable chemotherapy combinations were applied pre-
and postoperatively. The median follow-up time after discontinuation of chemotherapy is 26+ months. Nine patients
have failed, all showing pulmonary metastases, six have
died despite several heavy salvage regimens. So the disease free survival rate is 53%. Longer follow-up in this
group and the European Osteosarcoma Intergroup Study will
be needed to clarify the value of neoadjuvant chemotherapy
in this disease.

INTRODUCTION

Until the early seventies the overall survival rate
of patients with osteogenic sarcoma treated with adequate
local treatment was dismal. Less than 25% of the patients
survived (4). Thereafter many reports were published
claiming improved survival with the application of postoperative adjuvant treatment. Still the 5-year survival
rate seldomly exceeded 40%. In randomized series, however,
the survival gain of the groups who had adjuvant treatment,
being it radiotherapy to the lungs or chemotherapy, could
not be confirmed. There are many reasons to which this
reported survival gain in non-randomized series can be attributed. The main reasons are: variation in histological
types of osteosarcoma, non-uniform staging criteria, em-
ployment of different regimens, variation in drug-

doses, frequency of adminstration and duration of treatment,
but most importantly the early reporting of results at a
time when many patients were still either on treatment or
at least at high risk for recurrence. While reviewing the
published non-randomized series it is obvious that the best
projected survival rates were observed in the series with
the shortest median follow-up.

In the Netherlands most centres were participating in
the EORTC-osteosarcoma studies. In the last study as reported
by Burgers et al (1) the survival remained disappointing
notwithstanding the application of postoperative radiotherapy
and chemotherapy.
The reports of Rosen (3 , 4) and the confirmation by Winkler
(5) of better results obtained in patients with osteosarcoma
if the local treatment was preceeded by agressive chemotherapy led us into investigations piloting this option.

MATERIAL AND METHODS

In Amsterdam and Leiden starting january 1982 all subsequent patients with histologically proven normal osteogenic sarcoma were entered into these pilot studies. The
pretreatment work-up consisted of full blood counts,
biochemistry profiles revealing normal liver and kidney
functions,chest-X-ray, full lung tomography, CT scan of the
lungs and the affected bone, Tc bone scan, X-rays of the
affected bone with an angiography. Histological specimens of
all patients were reviewed   by the Netherlands Bone Tumor
Registry Panel of the Netherland Cancer Foundation.
Excluded were patients with a paraosteal,periosteal, pagetoid
and postirradiation osteosarcoma.
Patients who had prior chemotherapy, prior radiotherapy,
prior surgery exceeding a biopsy and patients who had signs
of metastatic spread at entry were also excluded. Two patients
who had already been treated prior to the official start
of the protocol but had the same treatment are included in
this report.

Two treatment regimens were applied: one regimen (A)
consisted of Vincristine 1.5 mg/m^2 day 1, Methotrexate
7.5 g/m^2 with Citrovorum factor rescue day 2 and Adriamycin
45 mg/m^2 days 12, 13; the whole cycle was repeated on day 25
after which the operation was scheduled on day 49. Postoperatively one more cycle with the same drugs was given.
The other regimen (B) consisted of Adriamycin 25 mg/m^2
days 1, 2 and 3 and Cisplatin 100 mg/m^2 day 1 as a 24-hours
continuous infusion. This regimen was repeated every three

weeks. After three cycles the operation was performed followed by again three cycles.
All patients were thereafter followed six-weekly for the
first 18 months, bimonthly from one and a half to three years
and thereafter every three months. Follow-up investigations
included physical examination, alkaline phosphatase,
creatinine, serum lactic dehydrogenase, chest X-ray, X-ray
of the affected bone if a reconstruction had been performed.
Further investigations were only performed if indicated.

RESULTS

Until september 1984 a total of 38 patients were
eligible in both hospitals. The group consisted of 17 males
and 21 females with a median age of 15.7 years (range 6-26).
Of these patients 19 entered into the EORTC Osteosarcoma
Intergroup Study, which started july 1983. Their follow-up
after the end of chemotherapy is less than one year and
they will therefore not be included in this report.
The remaining group of 19 patients consists of 9 males and
10 females. The age ranges from 6-20 years (median 14). The
affected bone was femur in 12, fibula in 2, humerus in 3,
tibia in 1 and pelvis in 1. The follow-up after cessation
of chemotherapy ranges from 14-49+ months (median 26+ months).
Nine patients have failed,all with recurrences in the lungs.
They recurred after 5,6, 8,9,9,10, 11, 15 and 16 months
respectively, median 9 months. All but one had metastatec-
tomies followed by chemotherapy with several heavy regimens
including experimental drugs. Six patients have already
died, three are still on treatment.
The toxicity of the regimens applied consisted of the non-
haematological   toxicities: alopecia, nausea, vomiting
and diarrhoea for both regimens in all patients and a modest
(less than 25%) drop in creatinine clearance for the patients
with regimen B. The haematological toxicity observed was
less heavy with the regimen A where Adriamycin only had to
be modified to 80% in the last cycle. However, with regimen
B leuko- and thrombocytopenia grade 4 (WHO,6) was observed
in most patients after the fourth or fifth cycle necessit-
ating dose modification of Adriamycin to 80% for the last
one or two cycles. No toxic deaths or severe infections
were encountered.

DISCUSSION

The survival of patients with an osteogenic sarcoma in who after optimal local treatment postoperative adjuvant chemotherapy was applied remained disappointing in randomized series. Also in non-randomized series with a median follow-up of over two years after the cessation of all treatment the survival remained dismal, generally less than 40%. With the application of aggressive preoperative chemotherapy preceding surgery (neoadjuvant chemotherapy) three year survival rates exceeding 60% were reported (2,3,5). In this report our 26+ months survival is 53% (10/19) without any evidence of disease during careful follow-up. The data are small and longer follow-up is needed to obtain the precise figure. The toxicities encountered are heavy but tolerable, but we don't feel that the application of heavier regimens is justified. The data obtained, however, have encouraged our participation in the large ongoing EORTC/MRC neoadjuvant pilot study. In this study Regimen B and an High-dose Methotrexate + Regimen B combination are being compared. Over 120 patients have been accrued in this study within one year. Data of this and other studies have to be awaitened before the application of this type of treatment policy can be advocated for use outside the frame work of clinical trials.

REFERENCES

1. Burgers JMV, Voûte PA and van Glabbeke M (1983). Adjuvant therapy for osteosarcoma of the limbs. Proceedings 2nd European Conference on Clinical Oncology, Amsterdam: 136.
2. Rosen G, Nirenberg A, Caparros B et al. (1981). Osteogenic Sarcoma: eighty percent, three year disease-free survival with Combination Chemotherapy. Nath.Cancer Inst. Monogr. 56: 213-220.
3. Rosen G, Caparros B, Huvos AG et al. (1982). Preoperative Chemotherapy for osteogenic sarcoma, selection of postoperative adjuvant chemotherapy based on the response of the primary tumor to preoperative chemotherapy. Cancer 49: 1221-1230.
4. v.Rijssel ThG (1980). Classification and Prognosis of Osteosarcoma, in: Therapeutic Progress in Ovarian Cancer, Testicular Cancer and the Sarcoma. Editors van Oosterom AT et al.,Martinus Nijhoff Publ. London: 285-299.
5. Winkler K, Beron G, Brandeis H et al. (1983). Neoadjuvant chemotherapy for osteogenic sarcoma: Results of a

cooperative German/Austrian Study (COSS-80), Proceedings Am.Soc.Clin.Oncol. 2: 233.
6. WHO Handbook for Reporting Results of Cancer Treatment. (1979). WHO offset publication, World Health Organization Geneva.

Primary Chemotherapy in Cancer Medicine, pages 59–74
© 1985 Alan R. Liss, Inc.

HIGH-GRADE SOFT-TISSUE SARCOMAS OF THE EXTREMITY: UCLA EXPERIENCE WITH LIMB SALVAGE

Frederick R. Eilber, M.D., Armando E. Guiliano, M.D., James Huth, M.D., Joseph Mirra, M.D., and Donald L. Morton, M.D.
Division of Surgical Oncology, John Wayne Clinic, Jonsson Comprehensive Cancer Center; and Department of Pathology, UCLA School of Medicine, Los Angeles, CA 90024

Malignant soft tissue sarcomas of the extremity continue to present clinical challenges in terms of eradication of local tumor, preservation of the limbs and systemic disease control. Treatment methods for these tumors have evolved over the years from local excision, radical local excision, amputation, excision plus radiation therapy and finally multi-modality therapy. As local tumor control has improved, so too has overall patient survival rate in the past 10 years. This diversity of therapies for the primary tumor presupposes several options for treatment. In order to determine the best treatment approach, it is important to evaluate local tumor control, the complications of therapy, the ability to salvage a functionally useful limb, and, finally, the overall patient survival. To this end, we reviewed our experience with treatment of high-grade soft-tissue sarcomas at the UCLA School of Medicine over the past 12 years.

PATIENTS AND METHODS

From 1972 to 1984, the Division of Surgical Oncology, UCLA School of Medicine, evaluated and treated 237 patients with Grade 2 or Grade 3 soft-tissue sarcomas of the extremity. This patient group ranged in age from 3 to 92 years (median 46 years) and contained 126 males and 111 females. Primary tumor locations are given in Table 1, the most common site being the thigh in 98 patients (46%). Histologic type of the primary tumors is listed in Table 2. Liposarcomas were the most common histologic type. Fifty-seven patients had histologic Grade 2 tumors and 180 Grade 3 (Russell et al. 1977). By Ennenking stage, 14 were 1-A; 39 1-B; 50 2-A; and 133 2-B (Enneking et al. 1980). One-hundred

---

Table 1 — SOFT-TISSUE SARCOMA

Type	#	%
Thigh	110	46
Arm	21	9
Calf	19	8
Foot	18	8
Forearm	15	6
Buttock	16	6
Periscapular	8	3
Popliteal	7	
Groin	7	
Shoulder	6	
Axilla	4	
Wrist, Hand	4	
	237	

---

eighty-seven patients received their primary tumor treatment at UCLA, i.e., they were clinical Stage 1, and 50 patients presented for treatment with locally recurrent Stage 2 disease.

Three sequential treatment programs were employed. The first, a historical control group, consisted of 55 patients who were treated from 1972 to 1976. These patients received what was at that time thought to be the standard surgical therapy, which included amputation for 19 patients, wide excision only for 11 patients, and wide excision followed by 5000 to 6000 rads of radiation for 25 patients. Radiation therapy was given at 200 rad fractions for 5 days for 5 to 6 weeks.

A first prospective study group (3500 rads), begun in 1974, was based on a preoperative treatment regimen of intraarterial adriamycin, 30 mg/day for each of 3 consecutive days, delivered by an indwelling intraarterial catheter, for a 24-hour infusion. The catheter was placed in a high-flow vessel such as the common femoral or axillary artery. Following this treatment, patients received radiation therapy of 350 rad fractions times 10 (3500

Table 2 — SOFT-TISSUE SARCOMA — HISTOLOGY

Type	#	%
Liposarcoma	50	21
Malignant Fibrous Histiocytoma	38	16
Synovial	34	14
Rhabdomyosarcoma	23	10
Undifferentiated	23	10
Fibrosarcoma	21	9
Neurofibrosarcoma	9	
Leiomyosarcoma	8	
Extra osseous		
Osteosarcoma	6	
Chondrosarcoma	5	
Ewings sarcoma	3	
Lymphangiosarcoma	6	
Epitheloid	4	
Mesenchymal	3	
Giant-cell	2	
Clear-cell	2	
	237	

rads) (Eilber et al. 1980). The entire region of the tumor, i.e., thigh or arm, was treated, sparing only a strip of skin opposite the primary biopsy site. Approximately 1 to 2 weeks after the radiation therapy, the tumor was widely excised through normal uninvolved tissue planes, with pathologic confirmation of tumor-free margins at the time of operation. In some instances, the tumor margin was less than a millimeter, most often when the primary tumor was adjacent to an artery, vein or bone, in which case adventia, perineurium or periosteum was removed.

A second group (1750 rads) included 105 patients again treated with the identical chemotherapy regimen of intraarterial adriamycin, 30 mg/day times 3, followed by radiation therapy of 350 rad fractions times 5, followed by the identical surgical procedure.

Postoperative follow-up included physical examination and chest x-ray once a month for the first year, once every 2 months for the second year, and once every 3 months for the fourth, fifth and sixth years. Whole lung tomograms or CAT-scans of the chest were done at 6-month intervals.

Postoperative adjuvant chemotherapy was given to a proportion of the patients with Grade 3 sarcomas. Of 180 patients, 27 received the combination for adriamycin, 40 mg/m^2 given intravenously for each of 2 consecutive days, followed by high-dose methotrexate at 200 mg/kg of body weight and 80 did not receive any postoperative adjuvant chemotherapy. These two groups were treated from 1972 to 1981 and were not part of a randomized prospective trial.

Since 1981, a randomized prospective study compared no postoperative adjuvant chemotherapy (control 38 patients) with adjuvant chemotherapy of adriamycin as a single agent given at 45 mg/m^2 intravenously on each of 2 consecutive days once a month times 5 following the operative procedure (35 patients).

Statistical evaluation of the overall survival and recurrence rates was done by the lifetable method of analysis using the Mantel-Cox and Breslow-Gehan statistical methods.

Pathologic evaluation of resected tumor specimens was performed by one of the authors without prior knowledge of treatment. Ten to 20 sections were taken from different portions of the tumor and at least 10 high-power fields for each slide were examined. Necrosis was evaluated on the basis of lack of nuclei.

RESULTS

In the original treatment group (control) consisting of 55 patients treated by standard methods of amputation, wide excision or wide excision and postoperative radiation therapy, it was necessary to perform amputative procedures in 19 (35%). Complications of treatment in this group, 4/55 (7%), were wound slough, edema and neuritis. Fourteen of the 55 (25%) had local disease recurrence (Table 3). Three of the 19 (16%) who had amputation had local recurrences, as did 4/11 (36%) treated by wide excision alone and 7/25 (28%) treated by wide excision and

Table 3 — SOFT-TISSUE SARCOMA — NON-PROTOCOL

Grade	# Patients	Local Recurrences			
		Amputation	WE	WE + XRT	Total
2	18	0/1	1/6	3/11	4 (22%)
3	37	3/18	3/5	4/14	10 (27%)
	TOTAL	3/19 (16%)	4/11 (36%)	7/25 (28%)	14/55 (25%)

(11/3/84)

radiation therapy. Because of the necessity for amputative procedures in 35% of these patients and because of the disappointing 25% local tumor recurrence, efforts were directed to new methods of therapy in 1974 that consisted of preoperative treatment with intraarterial adriamycin and radiation therapy.

Treatment Group 1 (3500 rads)

Seventy-seven patients were treated with this regimen, 12 of whom had Grade 2 tumors and 65 with Grade 3. In 60 patients, this was the first treatment of their primary tumor and in 17 it was treatment for local recurrence (Table 4). Of these 77 patients, three (4%) required amputation and local tumor recurrence was noted in three (4%). Median follow-up in this group of patients is now 5 years. Complications as a result of treatment occurred in 27 (35%) and in 13 (17% of the total group) a second operation was required to treat the complication. The most commonly encountered complication was wound slough in 15 patients. Fracture of adjacent long bone occurred in 6 (11%) and required open intramedullary fixation. In all instances, pathologic evaluation showed no evidence of recurrent tumor.

Table 4 — 3500 R

Grade	Total	Stage I	II	Amp.	Local Recur.	Comp.	NED	Exp.
2	12	6	6	0	0		11/12	1
3	65	54	11	3	3		38	27
TOTAL	77	60	17	3 (4%)	3 (4%)	27 (35%)	49 (64%)	28 (36%)
						13 (17%)		

Because of this relatively high complication rate, the treatment program was altered in 1981 to reduce the radiation dose by one-half from 3500 rads to 1750 rads.

Treatment Group 2 (1750 rads)

Of the 105 patients treated, 27 had Grade 2 tumors and 78 had Grade 3 (Table 5). For 90 patients, the preoperative therapy was their first treatment, whereas 15 patients presented with local recurrences after prior therapy. Three (3%) patients required primary amputation and nine (8%) have had local disease recurrences. The median follow-up for this group is now 24 months. Complications occurred in 26 patients, and six patients required reoperation for treatment of their complication (Table 6). Only one patient had fracture of an adjacent long bone.

Complications of therapy were also evaluated for any relationship to tumor size (Fig. 1), and we found that the complication rate was directly proportional and statistically related to the primary tumor size. Of patients with tumors less than 5 cm, only 18% developed complications, whereas patients with tumors greater than 20 cm in diameter had an approximate incidence of 70% complications. The reduction in dose of radiation appeared to reduce the complications in patients with intermediate size tumors between 10 and 20 cm (Fig. 2). There was no change

Table 5 — 1750 R

Grade	Total	Stage I	II	Amp.	Local Recur.	Comp.	NED	Exp.
2	27	18	9	0	1		27	0
3	78	72	6	3	8		73	5
TOTAL	105	90	15	3 (3%)	9 (8%)	26 (24%)	100 (95%)	5 (5%)
						6 (6%)		

Table 6 — COMPLICATIONS OF THERAPY

	Control N = 6 # (%)	3500 R N = 26 # (%)	1750 R N = 26 # (%)
Fracture	–	6 (11)	1
Infection	1	2	1
Edema	1	3	1
Neuritis	2	–	–
Wound Slough	3 (5)	15 (27)	17 (16)
Seroma	3	4	2
Amputation	0	1	0
Reoperation	4/55 (7%)	14/77 (18%)	6 (6%)

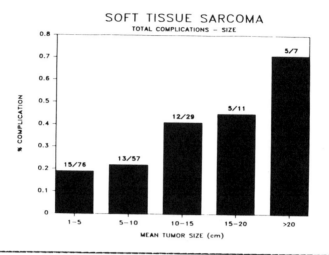

Fig. 1. Total complications compared to tumor size.

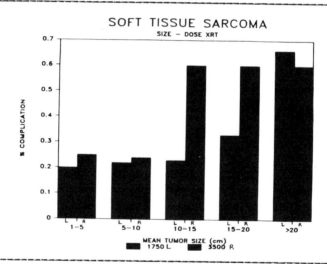

Fig. 2. Size of primary tumor vs. radiation dose complications of treatment. L = 1750; R = 3500.

in the incidence of complications in patients with tumors less than 5 cm or greater than 20 cm.

Tumor-cell necrosis was evaluated by the surgical pathologist for the two prospective treatment groups. Necrosis appears to be a grade-related phenomenon in that patients with Grade 2 tumors have less tumor-cell necrosis compared to those patients with Grade 3 tumors. In the 3500 rad-treated group, median tumor-cell necrosis for Grade 3 tumors was 80%. With the reduced dose of radiation, the median tumor-cell necrosis decreased to 55% (Table 7).

LOCAL TUMOR CONTROL

Table 8 shows the overall local tumor control for the three groups of patients. Local disease recurrences were noted in 25% of the non-protocol patients, 4% of the 3500 rad-treated group, and 8% of the 1750 rad-treated group. Although overall follow-up is only 24 months in the last group of patients, it appears that this is a reasonable estimate of the local tumor failure rate. Although failure is higher with reduced radiation, it is not statistically significant at this time. Of those patients who developed a local recurrence, the median time to recurrence in the control group was 11.5 months; for the 3500 rad-treated group it was 15 months, and for the 1750 rad-treated group it was 14 months. For approximately 50% of these patients, the only manifestation of recurrent disease was local, and for the others it was both systemic and local. Treatment of recurrent disease required amputation in seven patients, four of the control group and three of the 1750-rad group. No patient in the 3500-rad group required amputation to control locally recurrent disease.

Local tumor recurrence was not related to tumor size (Fig. 3). When the 3500-rad group was compared to the 1750-rad group, the local recurrences occurred from all tumor sizes, the highest actually from those tumors less than 5 cm in diameter in the 1750-rad group. Four of these five patients had tumors located either in the foot or distally in the forearm.

Overall patient survival is shown in Figure 4. Of those patients with Grade 2 sarcomas, 90% remain alive free of disease at a median follow-up of 6 years. Overall, of those patients with Grade 3 sarcomas, 65% remain alive free of disease at a median follow-up of 5 years.

Table 7 — PATHOLOGIC EVALUATION
OF TUMOR-CELL NECROSIS

% Necrosis	3500 R Grade 2	Grade 3		1750 R Grade 2	Grade 3	
0-10	2*	–		2	2	
10-20	2	5		3	8	
20-30	1	3		5	5	
30-40	–	3		1	5	
40-50	–	1		–	2	
50-60	–	7		1	5	Median
60-70	3	–		–	2	
70-80	–	2	Median	–	6	
80-90	1	5		1	6	
90-99	–	13		–	8	
100	–	8		–	2	
TOTAL	9	47		13	51	

*# patients with specimens showing % necrosis

Table 8 — SOFT-TISSUE SARCOMA — GRADES 2 AND 3

Study	# Pts.	# Amp.	Local Recur.	Comp.
Non-Protocol	55	19 (35%)	14/55 (25%)	4/55 (7%)
3500 R	77	3 (4%)	3/77 (4%)	14/77 (18%)
1750 R	105	3 (3%)	9/105 (8%)	6/105 (6%)
IA-IV Adriamycin 1750 R	40			

(11/3/84)

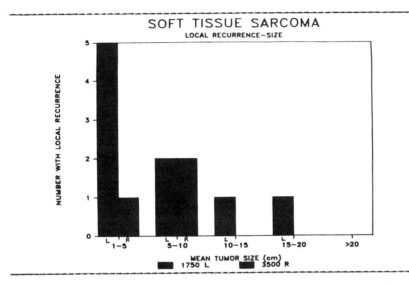

Fig. 3. Local recurrence vs. size of primary tumor and radiation dose. L = 1750; R = 3500.

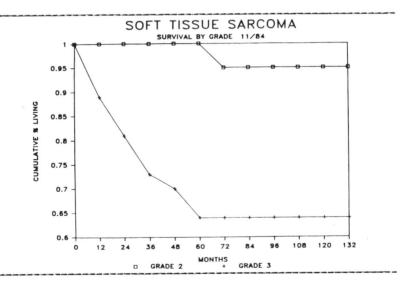

Fig. 4. Survival vs. tumor grade.

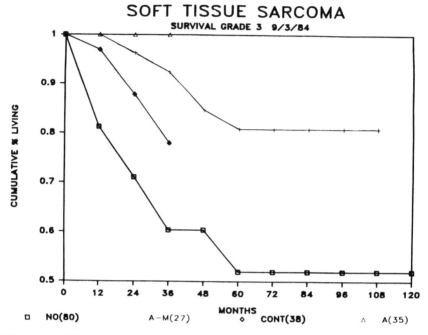

Fig. 5. Lifetable analysis of survival for patients with Grade 3 soft-tissue sarcomas. A-M = adriamycin/methotrexate; no = no treatment. Prospective randomize A = adriamycin; cont = no chemotherapy.

An evaluation of overall survival of patients with Grade 3 sarcomas, (180 patients; Fig. 5) was performed by lifetable analysis according to whether or not they received adjuvant chemotherapy. Of the 80 patients who did not receive adjuvant chemotherapy in a non-random fashion, 52% remain alive free of disease at a median follow-up of 60 months, compared to 27 patients who received adriamycin and methotrexate with an overall survival of 82% for the same period. These two curves are statistically significant to the p<.001 level, although this was not a randomized trial. Of those patients treated on a randomized prospective basis who received adriamycin or no adjuvant therapy, to date 35 patients (100%) are living, at a median follow-up of 24 months, compared to 75% of those who did not receive adjuvant therapy. At the present time these curves are not statistically significant.

DISCUSSION

The overall results of standard therapy for extremity soft-tissue sarcomas in our control series are similar to those reported by others. The necessity for amputation in 35% of these patients appears to be relatively constant. In addition, the 25% incidence of local disease recurrences also appears to be common to many reported series (Enneking et al. 1981; Brennhoud 1966; Gerner et al. 1975; Shui et al. 1975; Markhede et al. 1981).

The protocol of intra-arterial adriamycin and 3500 rads of radiation therapy was very successful in that it allowed non-amputative treatment for 95% of the patients. The local recurrence rate of 4% was superior to that of the standard methods of therapy (Lindberg et al. 1981; Lattuada, Kenda 1981; Suit et al. 1982; Lindberg 1973; Suit 1981). However, the complication rate of 35%, and reoperation rate of 17% appeared to us to be too high. The reduction in radiation dose to 1750 rads in the second treatment protocol did, in fact, reduce the serious complication rate to 6%. Again, though, the local recurrence rate of 8%, although not yet statistically different from the 3500-rad group, is of concern. Thus far, this increased local recurrence rate has not translated into decreased survival.

There does appear to be a dose response to radiation therapy in the extremity soft-tissue sarcomas. Median tumor cell necrosis with reduced radiation dropped a median of 20% and was reflected in the higher local recurrence rate. Complications of therapy could be related not only to the radiation dose but also to tumor size. Patients with larger tumors had a higher complication rate regardless of the radiation dose reduction. The radiation dose did appear to reduce the complications of the intermediate-size tumors between 10 and 20 cm.

From our data, it is not possible at the present time to determine the value of adjuvant chemotherapy in terms of overall patient survival. In a non-randomized study, it appeared that there was a survival advantage for patients receiving chemotherapy of adriamycin and high-dose methotrexate. This finding was statistically significant, but because it was not done in a randomized, prospective fashion it may well have reflected patient selection bias. Although an analysis of prognostic variables was done and the groups appeared to be equal, we cannot recommend adriamycin and methotrexate as adjuvant therapy.

Preliminary results of the randomized trial comparing adriamycin to no adjuvant chemotherapy in a randomized prospective fashion appear to be encouraging, and there does appear to be a survival advantage for those patients who received adriamycin. However, the follow-up period is not long enough for statistical significance. Overall survival from soft-tissue sarcomas is definitely related to tumor grade, and in our experience for patients with Grade 2 tumors is greater than 85%. For patients with Grade 3 soft-tissue sarcomas, the overall survival is related to tumor size regardless of primary therapy. Those patients with tumors less than 5 cm have a 5-year survival rate of approximately 87%, whereas those patients with tumors greater than 20 cm have a 62% survival rate.

From these studies it would appear that both preoperative protocols, adriamycin and radiation therapy of either 3500 or 1750 rads, allowed us to treat a very high percentage of patients by non-amputative surgery compared to non-preoperatively treated patients. In addition, the local control rate is superior to the control group in both instances. The complication rate was high in both protocol treatment groups and in the standard treatment group, although it has been reduced with the reduction in radiation dose. The local recurrence rate appears to be slightly increased with the reduced radiation but has not yet translated into decreased patient survival. Complications of therapy are clearly related to tumor size as well as to radiation dose. Overall patient survival is a multifaceted problem. From our data, we cannot support or condemn adjuvant chemotherapy (Rosenberg et al. 1983; Antman et al. 1983). Overall patient survival is directly related to the tumor grade and size in that patients with larger Grade 3 tumors have a worse prognosis than those with smaller Grade 3 tumors.

The concepts of preoperative therapy have been advocated and described by many. Treatment of a tumor prior to operation allows a clearer definition of operative margins and the surgical approach. The preoperative treatment with chemotherapy and radiation more clearly defines the tumor limits at the time of operation and allows the pathologist to evaluate the treatment effect on the resected specimen. Furthermore, all of the protocols are feasible in that 98% of the patients who were candidates for these protocols did, in fact, complete the treatment.

It would appear to us that the patient with extremity soft-tissue sarcoma is an ideal model system for sequentially testing various treatment alterations. With the preoperative therapy, evaluation can be made of local tumor control and patient survival as well as pathologic assessment of the treatment effect on the primary tumor. Thus, preoperative therapy may be an ideal scientific approach that would more fully test the effects in the patient.

REFERENCES

Russell WO, Cohen J, Enzinger F, et al. (1977). A clinical and pathologic staging system for soft tissue sarcomas. Cancer 40:1562.

Enneking WF, Spanier SS, Goodman MM (1980). Current Concepts Review: The surgical staging of musculo-skeletal sarcoma. J Bone Joint Surg 62A:1027.

Eilber FR, Mirra JJ, Grant TT, Weisenburger T, Morton DL (1980). Is amputation necessary for sarcomas? - A 7-year experience. Ann Surg 192:431.

Enneking WF, Spanier SS, Malawar MM (1981). The effect of anatomic setting on the results of surgical procedures for soft parts sarcoma of the thigh. Cancer 47:1005.

Brennhoud IO (1966). The treatment of soft tissue sarcomas — A plea for a more urgent and aggressive approach. Acta Chir Scand 131:438.

Gerner RE, Moore GE, Pickren JW (1975). Soft tissue sarcomas. Ann Surg 181:803.

Shui MH, Castro EB, Hajdu SI (1975). Surgical treatment of 297 soft tissue sarcomas of the extremity. Ann Surg 182:597.

Markhede G, Angervall L, Stenner B (1981). A multivariant analysis of the prognosis after surgical treatment of malignant soft tissue tumors. Cancer 49:1721.

Lindberg R, Martin R, Ramsdahl M, Barkley T (1981). Conservative surgery and postoperative radiotherapy in 300 adults with soft tissue sarcomas. Cancer 47:2391.

Lattuada A, Kenda R (1981). Postoperative radiotherapy of soft tissue sarcoma. Tumori 67 (Suppl A):191.

Suit HD, Proppe KH, Mankin HJ, Wood WC (1982). Radiation therapy and conservative surgery for sarcoma of soft tissue. Prog Clin Cancer 8:311.

Lindberg RD (1973). The role of radiation therapy in the treatment of soft tissue sarcoma in adults. Proc 7th Natl Cancer Congress (Philadelphia, Lippincott), p 883.

Suit HD, Proppe KH, Mankin HJ, Woods WC (1981). Preoperative radiation therapy for sarcomas of the soft tissue. Cancer 47:2269.

Rosenberg SA, Tepper J, Glatstein E, et al. (1983). Prospective randomized evaluation of adjuvant chemotherapy in adults with soft tissue sarcomas of the extremity. Cancer 52:424.

Antman KH, Blum RH, Wilson RE (1983). Survival of patients with localized high-grade soft tissue sarcoma with multimodality therapy. Cancer 51:396.

This work was supported by Grant CA29605, awarded by the National Cancer Institute, DHEW.

SECTION III
BREAST CANCER

Primary Chemotherapy in Cancer Medicine, pages 77–87
© 1985 Alan R. Liss, Inc.

NEOADJUVANT - PREOPERATIVE - CHEMOTHERAPY FOR BREAST CANCER
- PRELIMINARY REPORT OF THE VANCOUVER TRIAL

Ragaz J., Baird R., Rebbeck P., Coldman A.,
Goldie J.
Division of Medical Oncology, Cancer Control
Agency of B.C., 600 West 10,
Vancouver, B.C. V5Z 4E6, Canada

Introduction

The results of treatment with the conventional postoperative adjuvant chemotherapy show an increase in overall
survival for subgroups of patients with breast cancer (1).
Despite this improvement, however, the numbers of treatment
failure are still high. In the absence of more effective
drugs, changes in the scheduling of conventional regimens
are needed. In order to increase cure, it appears that alterations in drug scheduling are the only practical applicable option left to clinicians. As seen in several animal experiments (2, 3), preoperative - neoadjuvant - chemotherapy,
example of such an approach, is more effective than a more
delayed postoperative treatment. There are also theoretical
data available in the recent literature, indicating the
possible superiority of preoperative treatment (4).

The neoadjuvant protocol for breast cancer was started
at the Vancouver Cancer Control Agency of British Columbia
in 1981 (5). Since then, 43 patients were treated in the
phase II study with one preoperative cycle of CMF (Table 1).
Having documented the safety of such treatment, a phase III
study, randomizing premenopausal patients with newly diagnosed breast cancer into preoperative and postoperative
treatment groups, was started. In this presentation, several
theroretical and clinical aspects of our study are reported.

Background

As summarized in our recent review (6), there are several aspects in tumor biology which point towards a sound
scientific rationale for the systemic treatment timed before

the definitive locoregional therapy. Changes in the tumor genotype, leading towards resistance to multiple drugs (4) and kinetic phenomena in connection with noncurative surgery (7-10) were of major interest to our group, as their analysis has consistently indicated that a benefit of early treatment can be expected.

The changes in connection with the practical application of the preoperative treatment, however, substantially alter the conventional approach towards the management of breast cancer. Hence, before the neoadjuvant chemotherapy can be recommended to all practitioners, results of randomized or well conducted nonrandomized studies will be needed. Table 2 summarizes the main theoretical aspects of neoadjuvant treatment.

The next sections describe the main clinical features of our study.

TABLE 1

Phase II Study of Preoperative Adjuvant Chemotherapy for Breast Cancer

Diagnosis   (Fine Needle Aspiration or Open Biopsy)
    ↓
Investigations
    ↓
Chemotherapy: Cyclophosphamide 600 mg/m² i.v.
               Methotrexate   40 mg/m² i.v.
               5-FU   600 mg/m² i.v.

Definitive Surgery (Modified Radical or Partial Mastectomy,
                    with Axillary Exploration)

                          Node +VE Patients: Postoperative
                                              Chemotherapy with
                                              CMF x 6 Months

Node -VE Patients: No Further Chemotherapy

TABLE 2

Phenomena in Tumor Biology & in Clinical Management	Consequence Relevant to Neoadjuvant Chemotherapy	Reference
Unstable genotype of tumor-increased mutations	Even within short time, absolute quantum of resistant mutants increase rapidly	Goldie J, 4
Non-curative cytoreduction	Increased proliferation of the remaining cell burden	Tyzzer EE, 7 DeWyss WD, 8 Gorelik E, 9 Fisher B, 3 Simpson-Herren L, 10
Increased proliferation within tumor mass and in overall tumor cell burden	1. Increased detachment of individual malignant cells = enhanced formation of micrometastases 2. Increased repopulation of CT sanctuaries 3. Increased chance of alterations of genetic apparatus involved in cell division	Weiss L, 38 Ragaz J, 6 *
Preoperative chemotherapy	Will result in a decrease of tumor cell burden at the time of surgery; adverse effects in connection with a) non-curative surgery and b) delay with starting adjuvant chemotherapy will affect lower residual tumor cell burden	*

TABLE 2
(continuation)

Phenomena in Tumor Biology & in Clinical Management	Consequence Relevant to Neoadjuvant Chemo-therapy	Reference
Fine needle aspiration	High diagnostic accuracy in the hands of experienced cytologist	Zajicek J, 18 Rosen R, 19 Rimsten A,20 Kline RS,21
Fine needle aspiration as a primary diagnostic method	Reduction of adverse effects in connection with non-curative cytoreduction (open biopsy)	*

* Suspected but not documented in the literature

Fine Needle Aspiration for Breast Cancer

Fine needle aspiration (FNA) as the only diagnostic method for breast cancer was introduced in our region as a part of the preoperative adjuvant programme. In addition to alleviating anxiety in newly diagnosed patients by reducing the time interval between the presentation and the defini-tive diagnosis, its main advantage over the conventionally performed two stage open biopsy is thought to be a decreased tissue trauma and absence of general anaesthesia. Both are suspected to adversly affect the disease, as suggested from animal experiments examining the biological phenomena after noncurative cytoreduction (7-10). FNA also enables the most effective organization of preoperative chemotherapy. Despite its advantages, it may not be presently possible to adopt the fine needle aspiration by all the practitioners uniform-ly as many peripheral hospitals lack experienced cytologists.

Node Negative Patients

With preoperative chemotherapy, all newly diagnosed patients including those with negative axillary lymph nodes, will have received their first treatment prior to the patho-logical staging of the axilla. Since most centres do not routinely recommend adjuvant chemotherapy for low risk subgroups of patients, the following points are pertinent:

i) Animal experiments indicate that the benefit of adjuvant treatments is most readily detected in subjects with
the lowest systemic tumor cell burden (node negative patients (11).

ii) Several clinical studies show improved survival in
subgroups of breast cancer patients with node negative
glands, treated with adjuvant chemotherapy (12, 13).

iii) Preoperative adjuvant chemotherapy, limited to only
one cycle of CMF, is safe.

Clinical Aspects of the CABC Preoperative Study

i) Pilot Study

Materials and Methods

In the pilot study, a total of 43 patients received
one cycle of chemotherapy with CMF before the definitive
surgery (Table 1). Of those,15 had FNA as the only diagnostic method. As soon as possible after the diagnosis, investigations were ordered. These included blood work, bone
scan, chest x-ray and contralateral mammogramm. Afterwards,
the first course of preoperative adjuvant chemotherapy was
given. The surgery, which followed several days later, was
either a modified radical mastectomy (34 cases) or partial
mastectomy (9 patients). Twenty one days after their preoperative cycle, patients with positive axillary lymph
nodes started to receive 8 more cycles of adjuvant CMF. Patients with negative axillary lymph nodes received no further postoperative chemotherapy. Patients' ages ranged from
29-70; twenty nine were less than 50 years old. Twenty four
patients had positive axillary lymph nodes and the size of
tumor varied from 0.5 to 6 cm.

Results

Bone marrow suppression after the preoperative course
of CMF given on day 1 was assessed on day 21. Three out of
43 patients had WBC less than 2,300/cumm, with no case of
either septicaemia or prolonged fever. Three patients had a
decrease of platelet counts below 100,000/cumm, with none of
them developing postoperative bleeding and wound hematoma.
There was no case of prolonged fever and no patient developed wound abscess. Nausea, vomiting, diarrhoea and mucositis were not different from the 420 patients treated at
our centre with conventional postoperative adjuvant CMF.

The median delay between the diagnosis and the day of

the first cycle of preoperative chemotherapy was two days.
The median delay between the diagnosis and definitive surgery was 7 days.

Analysis of the first 30 premenopausal patients showed
a two year disease free survival of 86%, with 5 patients re-
curring at 6, 10, 21, 22 and 25 months. Of those, one patient died at 8 months, resulting in an overall 2 year survival of 96.7%.

ii) Preoperative Chemotherapy - Randomized Study

Since 1983, a randomization of the premenopausal patients with newly diagnosed breast cancer between preoperative and postoperative adjuvant chemotherapy with CMF, was
started. In most instances, both the randomization as well
as the preoperative chemotherapy were conducted by the surgeon performing the biopsy. In several cases, randomization
and the treatment were organized by the internists - oncologists, working in conjunction with the surgeon. As of December 1984, 52 patients were randomized. While only two
surgeons were involved in the phase II study, as a result
of educational sessions on the rationale of preoperative
adjuvant chemotherapy, organized by the investigators, 60%
of the randomized patients were referred by 16 additional
community surgeons, practising outside the oncological
centre. Presently, results on survival of the patients from
the two randomized groups are not yet available, however,
the good tolerance of the preoperative chemotherapy, as
discussed in the results of the pilot study, has been confirmed.

Discussion

Despite the evidence indicating a beneficial impact of
the conventional postoperative adjuvant chemotherapy on the
natural history of breast cancer (1, 12), the still frequent
treatment failures and the lack of new chemotherapy agents
result in development of a certain skepticism towards the
curability of breast cancer and an atmosphere of profession-
al nihilism in regards to adjuvant chemotherapy in general.
A very relevant point, not frequently discussed in the literature is the fact, that majority of the conventional postoperative chemotherapy combinations used for the adjuvant
treatment of breast cancer,consist of regimens which are of
only minimal to medium intensity in regards to the selection of individual agents or their dose. The intensity of
the treatment is shown in animal experiments to be of pri-

mary importance and the recent review of the results with
chemotherapy treatments for metastatic stage IV breast cancer, using regimens of varied intensity (34), points towards
the same direction. Therefore, it is expected that intensification of the presently used regimens may bring substantial improvements.
In addition to dose intensification, animal experiments further indicate that a relatively simple manipulation of
treatment scheduling, like shifting the systemic adjuvant
treatment into the preoperative period, may bring further
improvements in cure rate. It will be, therefore,important
to reproduce similar results in clinical studies, particularly in view of the conflicting data on the impact of the
delays with starting the first course of adjuvant chemotherapy, given in a conventional postoperative setting (14-18).

We have shown in our study, that the preoperative administration of one cycle of chemotherapy with the CMF regimen is safe. Taking information on safety of even more intensive, Adriamycin containing preoperative regimens used in
locally advanced primarily inoperable breast cancer (35-37),
we are concluding, that adverse effects of the preoperative
as opposed to postoperative administration of adjuvant chemotherapy in patients with stages I and II breast cancer, although in all likelihood not entirely absent, are clinically
acceptable.

The timing of the systemic therapy before the locoregional surgical treatment, although of main importance, is
not the only element of the neoadjuvant approach. Taking
into consideration the more recent observations on kinetic
aspects of tumor behavior after noncurative surgery, it is
proposed that repeated and prolonged surgical interventions,
like incisional two stage open biopsies with general anaesthesia and radical mastectomies, should be minimized.
Instead, fine needle aspiration, used for the primary diagnosis of breast cancer, as well as a more uniform adoption
of conservative mastectomy after a course of preoperative
chemotherapy, are to be considered. The reports on the accuracy of fine needle aspiration in obtaining a diagnosis
of breast cancer are very encouraging, especially when
mammography and clinical examinations are closely correlated
with the report of experienced cytologist (18-21). Of additional importance are data on the potential of fine needle
aspiration to obtain adequate specimens for Estrogen receptor determination, using either histochemistry (22-24) or
monoclonal antibody techniques (25-26). As well, FNA can be
used to obtain samples for the flow cytometry determination

of the pre-treatment cell cycles and DNA status of the newly diagnosed tumor. These indices, as shown in recent reviews (27-29), correlate well with subsequent survival.
Hence, the flow cytometry parameters could be used before
the preoperative chemotherapy is administered to select the
high and low risk subgroups of patients. This information,
as well as data on other prognostic factors, will be necessary for the neoadjuvant staging, important particularly
as one course or multiple treatments of preoperative chemotherapy may render the conventional histological examination of the axillary lymph glands uninterpretable. Additional presently recognizable prognostic factors to be used for
the neoadjuvant staging, will include the estimates on tumor
kinetic parameters, obtained from mammography (30) and history of the tumor (31), clinical stage and results from internal mammary node lymphoscintigraphy (32, 33).

The multiple changes in the management of newly diagnosed breast cancer in connection with the introduction of
neoadjuvant chemotherapy, will affect a large proportion of
surgeons and physicians practising outside the oncological
centres. Their cooperation with the investigators of the
neoadjuvant studies is essential to the future of the preoperative chemotherapy treatments. Therefore, formation of
effective mechanisms for such collaboration is a necessary
part of the neoadjuvant approach. These may include, in addition to educational sessions for the practitioners, also
financial renumeration of referring physician, similar to
the approach taken by large collaborative groups (N.S.A.B.P.
or N.C.I.). Without a well established mechanism, which
secures workable arrangements for the implementation of a
novel approach, accrual of patients for the studies like the
preoperative adjuvant chemotherapy of breast cancer, will be
difficult.

In conclusion, we have shown that the preoperative adjuvant chemotherapy for breast cancer is safe. Because of
its sound scientific rationale, all attempts should be made
to test this new approach in well organized, multicentre
studies.

References

1.   Salmon SE, Jones SE, ed (1984). Adjuvant therapy of
cancer IV. Grune and Stratton, New York (in press).
2.   Corbett TH, Griswold DP Jr, Roberts BJ, et al (1978).
Biology and therapeutic response of a mouse mammary adenocarcinoma (16/C) and its potential as a model for surgical

adjuvant chemotherapy. Cancer Treat Rep 62:1471-1488.

3.   Fisher B, Gunduz N, Saffer EA (1983). Influence of the interval between primary tumor removal and chemotherapy on kinetics and growth of metastases. Cancer Res 43:1488-1492.

4.   Goldie JH, Coldman AJ (1979). A mathematical model for relating the drug sensitivity of tumors to their spontaneous mutation rate. Cancer Treat Rep 63:1727-1733.

5.   Ragaz J, Baird R, Goldie J, et al (1983). Neoadjuvant - preoperative (preop) adjuvant chemotherapy (CG) for breast cancer - new approach for the management of breast cancer. Proc Amer Soc Clin Oncol 2:C-434:111.

6.   Ragaz J, Coldman A, Baird R, et al (1985; in press). Neoadjuvant chemotherapy for breast cancer - review. In Diagnosis, Management and Therapeutics, Ariel I, Cleary JB (ed), McGraw-Hill, New York.

7.   Tyzzer EE (1973). Factors in the production and growth of tumor metastases. J Med Research 28:309-332.

8.   DeWyss WD (1972). Studies correlating the growth rate of a tumor and its metastases and providing evidence for tumor-related systemic growth-retarding factors. Cancer Res 32:374-379.

9.   Gorelik E, Segal S, Feldman M (1978). Growth of a local tumor exerts a specific inhibitory effect on progression of lung metastases. Int J Cancer 21:617-625.

10.   Simpson-Herren L, Sanford AH, Holmquist JP (1976). Effects of surgery on the cell kinetics of residual tumor. Cancer Treat Rep 60:1749-1760.

11.   Schabel FM, Griswold DP, Corbett TH, et al (1979). Recent studies with surgical adjuvant chemotherapy vs immunotherapy of metastatic solid tumors of mice. Adjuvant Therapy of Cancer II. Jones SE, Salmon SA (eds), Grune and Stratton, New York, pp 3-17.

12.   Nissen-Meyer R, Kjellgren K, Malmio K, et al (1978). Surgical adjuvant chemotherapy: Results with one short course with cyclophosphamide after mastectomy for breast cancer. Cancer 41:2088-2098.

13.   Brooks J, Allen S, Chase E, et al (1981). Adjuvant use of Adriamycin and cyclosphosphamide in node negative carcinoma of the breast. Adjuvant Therapy of Cancer III. In Salmon SE, Jones SE, (eds), Grune and Stratton, New York, pp. 463-471.

14.   Nissen-Meyer R (1979). One short chemotherapy course in primary breast cancer: 12-year follow-up in series 1 of the Scandinavian adjuvant chemotherapy study group; in Salmon SE and Jones SE (eds): Adjuvant Therapy of Cancer II, pp 207-221.

15. Jones SE, Brooks RJ, Takasugi BJ, et al (1984; in press). Current results of the University of Arizona adjuvant breast cancer trials (1974-1984). Adjuvant Therapy of Cancer IV.

16. Sulkes A, Brufman G, Rizel S, et al (1983). The effect of postoperative radiotherapy on the feasibility of optimal dose of adjuvant chemotherapy in stage II breast carcinoma. Int J Radiation Oncol BiolPhys 9:17-21.

17. Glucksberg H, Rivkin SE, Rasmussen S, et al (1982). Combination chemotherapy (CMFVP) versus L-phenylalanine mustard (L-PAM) for operable breast cancer with positive axillary nodes. Cancer 50:423-434.

18. Zajicek J (1974). Aspiration biopsy and cytology of supradiaphragmatic organs, in Karger S (ed): Monographs and Clinical Cytology.

19. Rosen R, Hajdu SI, Robins G (1972). Diagnosis of carcinoma of the breast by aspiration biopsy. Surg Gyne & Obs 134.

20. Rimsten A, Stenkvist B, Johanson H, et al (1975). The diagnostic accuracy of palpation and fine-needle biopsy and an evaluation of their combined use in the diagnosis of breast lesions: Report on a prospective study in 1244 women with symptoms. Ann Surg 182:1-8.

21. Kline RS (1981). Masquerades of malignancy: A review of 4,241 aspirates from the breast. Acta Cytologica 24:263-266.

22. Bennington JL (1983). Immunoperoxidase estrogen receptor assay for human breast cancer. Front Radiat Ther Onc, Karger, Basel, 17:60-68.

23. Schimizu M, Wajima O, Miura M, Katayama I (1983). PAP immunoperoxidase method demonstrating endogenous estrogen in breast carcinomas. Cancer 52:486-492.

24. Parl FF, Wetherall NT, Malter S, et al (1984). Comparison of histochemical and biochemical assays for estrogen receptor in human breast cancer cell lines. Cancer Res 44: 415-421.

25. Greene GL, Jensen EV (1982). Monoclonal antibodies as probes for estrogen receptor detection and characterization. J Steroid Biochem 16:353-359.

26. Greene GL, Fitch FW, Jensen EV (1980). Monoclonal antibodies to estrophilin probes for the study of estrogen receptors. Proc Natl Acad Sci 77:157-161.

27. Auer G, Tribukait B (1980). Comparative single cell and flow DNA analysis in aspiration biopsies from breast carcinomas. Acta Path Microbiol Scand 88A:355-358.

28. Kute TE, Muss HB, Anderson D, et al (1981). Relationship of steroid receptor, cell kinetics and clinical status in patients with breast cancer. Cancer Res 41:3524-3529.

29. Olszewski W, Darzynkiewicz Z, Rosen PP, et al (1981).

Flow cytometry of breast cancinoma: Relation of DNA ploidy level to histology and estrogen receptor. Cancer 48: 980-984.
30. Heusel L, Spratt JS, Polk HC Jr (1979). Growth rates of primary breast cancers. Cancer 43:1888-1894.
31. Boyd NF, Meakin JW, Hayward JL, et al (1981). Clinical estimation of the growth rate of breast cancer. Cancer 48: 1037-1042.
32. Ege GN (1978). Internal mammary lymphoscintigraphy: a rational adjunct to the staging and management of breast carcinoma. Clin Radiol 29:453-456.
33. Manji MF (1982). Internal mammary lymphscintigraphy in breast carcinoma: possible significance in relation to current treatment. Jour Can Assoc Radiol 33: 10-14.
34. Hryniuk W, Bush H. The importance of dose intensity in chemotherapy of metastatic breast cancer. Jour Clin Oncol.
35. Papaioannou A, Lissaios B, Vasilaros S et al (1983). Pre- and postoperative Chemoendocrine Treatment with or without Postoperative Radiotherapy for Locally Advanced Breast Cancer. Cancer 51:1284-1290.
36. Aisner J, Morris D, Elias EG et al (1982). Mastectomy as an Adjuvant to Chemotherapy for Locally Advanced or Metastatic Breast Cancer. Arch Surg 117:882-887.
37. Hagelberg RS, Jolly PC, Anderson RP (1984). Role of Surgery in the Treatment of Inflammatory Breast Carcinoma. Amer Jour Surg 148:125-131.
38. Weiss L (1980). Metastasis: Differences Between Cancer Cells in Primary and Secondary Tumors. Pathobiology Annual; Ioachim LH ed, Raven Press, New York, 10:51-75.

Primary Chemotherapy in Cancer Medicine, pages 89-94
© 1985 Alan R. Liss, Inc.

COMBINED MODALITY TREATMENT WITH INITIAL CHEMOTHERAPY IN
T_4 AND/OR N_2-N_3 PRIMARY BREAST CANCER.

G.H. Blijham, A.H. Keijser, J.D.K. Munting,
H. Stroeken, Th.Wiggers, J.Wils and L. Schouten.
Breast Cancer Group of the Comprehensive Cancer
Centre Limburg (IKL), Maastricht, The Netherlands.

According to an estimation of Henderson and Canellos (1)
patients presenting with breast cancer which appears locoregionally confined in fact have micrometastases in around
70% of cases. By definition, these patients can not be cured by locoregional treatment alone, and should potentially
benefit from systemic treatment. On the other hand, current
adjuvant trials, though in many cases showing benefits in
terms of prolongation of disease-free survival for subgroups
of patients, suggest adjuvant therapy to be of value for
only a proportion of patients so treated; the remaining and
often majority of patients are treated with toxic therapy
without experiencing appreciable benefit (2).
    Chemotherapy starting before the removal of measurable
disease, that is before locoregional treatment, may be used
as an in-vivo chemosensitivity assay; the selection of a
responding population which is treated with additional courses after surgery or irradiation may greatly improve the
cost-benefit ratio of such treatment, whereas poor prognosis
non-responding patients may be offered more experimental
treatment. Furthermore, the Goldie and Coldman model (3)
predicts that the transition from an almost exclusively or
predominantly sensitive to a predominantly resistant tumor
cell population may occur during only a few doublings of the
tumor. This makes another argument to treat micrometastatic
patients as early as possible with systemic treatment.
    One of the problems inherent to the development of trials
applying these principles, however, is a diagnostic one:
how is one to select patients with a reasonably high risk
of having micrometastases without being able to perform

prognostically important staging procedures such as an
axillary dissection or without determining other prognostic
factors such as the presence of hormone receptors.
Investigators have therefore often limited the first exploration of the principles of early chemotherapy to patients
whose prognosis is thought to be poor on clinical grounds,
such as those with inflammatory cancers or signs of inope-
rability (4, 5). One may question the value of data obtained in this patient population for the treatment of patients with more limited disease. However with controlled
treatment, good follow-up and carefull analysis some hypo-
theses regarding the relation between in-vivo chemosensitivity and prognosis may be either strengthened or made
less likely.

It is with this background in mind that we started to
develop a community-wide protocol for the treatment of
stages I-III Breast Cancer, which was started in May,1982.
In this presentation a brief outline of this protocol is
given, and preliminary results which may be relevant for
the topic of Neoadjuvant Chemotherapy are presented.

OUTLINE OF THE PROTOCOL.

In table 1 a brief overview of the treatments applied
is given.

Table 1. Outline of the IKL Breast Cancer Protocol.

Group 1	T_1, T_2, T_3, N_0	Modified Radical Mastectomy or (T_1) Lumpectomy + Breast Radio-therapy
Group 2	T_1, T_2, T_3, N_1	Modified Radical Mastectomy or (T_1) Lumpectomy + Breast Radio-therapy Adjuvant Chemotherapy Randomization to Adjuvant Hormonotherapy
Group 3	T_4 or N_2, N_3	Chemotherapy, 2 courses Assessment of Response Appropriate Locoregional Treatment Chemotherapy, 4 courses Randomization to Adjuvant Hormono-therapy

All patients with medial or central tumor receive paraster-
nal radiotherapy.

The FAC chemotherapy consisted of 5-Fluorouracil 500 mg/ m^2, Doxorubicin 40 mg/m^2 and Cyclophosphamide 500 mg/m^2, all administered on day 1. Medroxyprogesterone Acetate (MPA) was given i.m. at a dose of 500 mg/m^2 each day x 28 days, thereafter twice weekly for 5 months. This should be considered high dose, which almost always will lead to adrenal suppression due to glucocorticoid activity. In some cases oral administration was necessary in which instance serum cortisol levels were determined to control for adequate MPA levels.

In table 2 the patient accrual as of September 1984 is depicted.

Table 2. Patient Characteristics.

Group I	96 patients
Group II	250 patients
Group III	25 patients

Since the patients in group I and II, which together include the T_1 to T_3 and N_0 plus N_1 tumors, are not the subject of this Symposium, we will limit the discussion of these groups to 3 conclusions :

(i)   in the great majority of cases the first course of chemotherapy is started within 14 days after surgery, which is in contrast to many other trials, and may be of benefit if early treatment is important

(ii) quite a few patients treated with breast-conserving therapy have now received the combination of intensive radiotherapy to the breast and FAC chemotherapy without serious toxicity

(iii) virtually no patient, even if of older age (the age limit is 70) has refused or abrogated adjuvant treatment and in less then 5% of patients dose reductions were necessary.

PREOPERATIVE CHEMOTHERAPY.

Chemotherapy preceding surgery or irradiation was used in patients presenting with T_4 and/or N_2-N_3 tumors; the objectives of this part of the protocol are given in table 3.

Table 3. Objectives of the protocol
for T_4 and/or N_2, N_3 patients.

1. Which is the prognosis of an unselected population of
   T_4 and/or N_2, N_3 breast cancer patients treated with
   a combined modality approach.
2. What is the predictive value of the initial response to
   FAC chemotherapy for disease-free and overall survival?
3. Does up-front MPA treatment add anything to FAC chemotherapy, and if so is that related to estrogen receptor
   status and initial response to FAC ?

Sofar, 25 patients have been entered; characteristics are
given in table 4.

Table 4. Characteristics of group III patients.

n = 25		
T_4	20	
N_2, N_3	12	
ER	negative	10 (< 10 fmol/mg)
ER	positive	15, median 35 fmol/mg

About 40% of the patients were ER-negative; ER-negative
tumors constituted only 25% of those presenting with more
limited disease. Of the 17 patients evaluable for response
10 had a partial or complete remission after only 2 courses of FAC (59%); responses were documented by mammography.
In table 5 some very preliminary survival data are given.
If these results are holding up with larger numbers they
seem to suggest a recurrence rate of 20% during the first
and of 15% during the second year after diagnosis.

Table.5. Disease-free survival after diagnosis.

- progressive or recurrent 9/16, at a median of
  9 months (4-34)
- disease-free 7/16, at a median of 21+ months (10-25)
- no relation of survival with initial response or ER

Of course the numbers are far too small to try and relate
these survival data to patient characteristics, such an
extent of disease, receptor status and the extent of response to initial chemotherapy; for the time being no relation between the response to chemotherapy and survival
has been seen.

Survival data related to MPA treatment are depicted in table 6 and seem to indicate that treatment with MPA, to which the patients were randomized, may confer a survival benefit; this difference of course is not statistically significant due to the very small numbers.

Table 6. MPA treatment and disease-free survival.

		disease-free	progressive
with MPA	(8)	5	3
without MPA	(8)	2	6

DISCUSSION.

In this presentation our efforts are described to use early postoperative and preoperative combined hormono- and chemotherapy in breast cancer patients. It is important to stress, as a potentially important determinant of our study, that it includes all patients in our area, thereby avoiding selection bias and making the results applicable to the population at large. Obviously, the accrual period is too short and the numbers are too small to draw meaningfull conclusions. The MDAH-Group has treated 90 patients with advanced or inflammatory breast cancer with 3 courses of FAC, followed by surgery and further chemotherapy (6). They correlated the presence or absence of gross tumor in the surgery specimen with 3 years survival, and found this correlation to be highly significant. If this type of results can be confirmed, for instance in our own study, time has come to perform similar studies in patients with less advanced stages of breast cancer.

REFERENCES.

1. Henderson C, Canellos GP (1980). Cancer of the Breast. New Engl J Med 302: 17-30.
2. Bonadonna G, Valagussa P (1985). Systemic Therapy for Resectable Breast Cancer. J Clin Oncol 3: 259-275.
3. Goldie JH, Coldman AJ (1979). A mathematic model for relating the drug sensitivity of tumors to the spontaneous mutation rate. Cancer Treat Rep 63: 1727-1733.
4. DeLena M, Zucale R, Viganotti G et al. (1978). Combined chemotherapy-radiotherapy approach in locally advanced (T3b-T4) breast cancer. Cancer Chemother Pharmacol 1: 53-62.

5. Buzdar AU, Montagne ED, Barker JL, Hortobagyi GN, Blumenschein GR (1981). Management of inflammatory carcinoma of breast with combined modality approach - an update. Cancer 47: 2537-2542.
6. Feldman L, Hortobagyi G, Buzdar A, Blumenschein G. (1984). Pathologic complete remission (CR) in patients (pts) with inflammatory breast cancer (IBC) and locally advanced breast cancer (LABC). Proc.AACR 45: 781.

Primary Chemotherapy in Cancer Medicine, pages 95–104
© 1985 Alan R. Liss, Inc.

PREOPERATIVE CHEMOTHERAPY IN THE TREATMENT OF INFLAMMATORY
BREAST CANCER

R. Keiling, N. Guiochet, H. Calderoli,
P. Hurteloup, Cl. Krzisch,
Centre Hospitalier et Universitaire,
Strasbourg,
France

Preoperative chemotherapy seems a logical approach
for acute or inflammatory breast cancer, since loco-regional treatment such as surgery or radiotherapy is unable to
cure the subclinical systemic disease which is practically
always present. In fact, it is infrequently possible to
achieve even local control with this approach.

We began a pilot study in January of 1980. In this
first trial, the systemic treatment was given as early as
possible in order to test both feasibility and tolerance,
as well as the in-vivo response to drug. Forty-one patients
were entered in this study.

As a continuation of this, a randomized study was then
initiated in March of 1982, comparing two treatment regimens containing 4'-epidoxorubicin (epirubicin), an analog
of doxorubicin. The aim of this second study was to compare
the efficacy and toxicity of a one-day schedule with that
of a fractionated 6-day schedule. In addition, we wished to
examine the cardiotoxicity of epirubicin (E) by monitoring
the isotopic ventricular ejection fraction before, during
and at the end of treatment.

A clear definition of inflammatory or rapidly progressing breast cancer (with short doubling time) is difficult.
This may contribute to therapeutic results which are at
times discordant. Locally advanced breast cancer with skin
involvement can look like inflammatory cancer, although its
biological behaviour is quite different. While the doubling
times of the two tumor types are quite similar, locally
advanced breast cancer does not respond to chemotherapy as
well as rapidly progressing inflammatory cancer. In order
to effectively exclude locally advanced disease from the

trial, a short time of evolution was added to the eligibility criteria.

Materials and Methods

The eligibility criteria for the two studies were as
follows:
1. presence of clinical symptoms of inflammation such
   as warmth, erythema, oedema, tenderness and/or
   swelling of a part of or of the whole breast;
2. thermographic aspect of fast tumor growth;
3. a short clinical course before diagnosis (≤ 2
   months);
4. patients free from detectable metastatic disease;
5. no overt cardiac disease, contra-indicating
   anthracycline use;
6. age ≤ 70 years.

Pretreatment evaluation consisted of mammography,
thermography and drill-biopsy, both for histopathological
diagnosis and for hormonal receptor assay, chest X-ray,
bone scan and liver ultrasound. In the second study, isotopic ventricular ejection fraction was also monitored, before, during and at the end of treatment.

Forty-one patients meeting the above criteria entered
the pilot study between 1 January 1980 and 31 January 1982
when the trial was closed to patient accrual. At time of
analysis, the median follow-up was 30 months. The second,
randomized trial is still ongoing; as of December 1984, 37
patients had been randomized, 18 to regimen A and 19 to
regimen B. Median age was 50 years in the first trial and
51 years in the second, including arms A and B. This is
somewhat lower than the median age of the average breast
cancer patient in our country (62 years). The hormonal receptor status of all patients in both trials is listed in
Table 1.

n	Trial 1 41	Regimen A 18	Regimen B 19	Total 78
ER- PGR-	35	11	11	57
ER+ PGR-	1	3	4	8
ER+ PGR+	4	3	3	10
ER- PGR+	0	1	1	2
Receptor unknown	1			1

Table 1: Hormonal receptor status

The proportion of receptor-negative tumors was much higher than is generally reported for other types of breast cancer.

Treatment Regimens

First study:
Pre-operative chemotherapy: adriamycin (A) 20 mg/m² on day 1 and 2, vincristin (V) 1 mg/m² on day 2; cyclophosphamide (C) 300 mg/m², 5-fluorouracil (5-FU) 400 mg/m², both given on days 3 through 6. The next cycle was begun on day 29. A total of four courses was administered

Radical modified mastectomy was performed 4 weeks after completion of the fourth course.

Post-operative chemotherapy (started on the second post-operative day): A 20 mg/m² on day 1 and 2, and V 1 mg/m² on day 2; C 300 mg/m² and methotrexate (MTX) 2 x 25 mg/m², mornings and evenings, both given on days 3 and 4; and C 300 mg/m² on day 5. After a total of 8 cycles had been given, one each month for 8 months, the course of therapy was completed with 20 mg/m² melphalan given once per month for three months.

Second study:
Patients were randomized for assignment to either regimen A or B.

Regimen A: E 30 mg/m² on day 1 and 2 and V 1 mg/m² on day 2; C 300 mg/m² and 5-FU 500 mg/m², both given daily from day 3 until and including day 6. The following cycle was begun on day 29.

Regimen B: E 60 mg/m², V 1 mg/m², 5-FU 500 mg/m² and C 500 mg/m² on day 1. The following cycle was begun on day 21. The dose of E was equal to that in regimen A. However, the doses of the other three drugs were lower and the interval between cycles was shorter.

Six cycles of either A or B were given pre-operatively, followed by modified radical mastectomy performed 4 weeks after the sixth cycle. An additional five cycles were given post-operatively. The cumulative dose of E given in 11 cycles of either A or B was 660 mg/m². The total course was completed with 6 cycles of "maintenance chemotherapy", consisting of vindesine 3 mg/m² on day 1; MTX 15 mg/m² and thiotepa 10 mg/m², both given on days 2 and 3. The next cycle was begun on day 29.

Results

Evaluation of the results consisted of histopathologi-

cal study of the operative specimens, the analysis of fail-
ures as a function of previous response, the period of dis-
ease-free survival, and overall survival.
Histopathologically, the post-chemotherapy status was
classified according to three categories or grades:
Grade 1: complete sterilization with no indication of
         invasive cancer;
Grade 2: major regression including necrosis and
         fibrosis. Minimal viable tumor presence;
Grade 3: only minor change in tumor status.

First study:

After a median follow-up period of 30 months, 24 of a
total of 41 patients are presently alive and disease-free
for a median period of 44 months (range 36-58 months).
Actuarial disease-free survival is thus 54% at 58 months;
overall survival is 63% (Fig. 1).

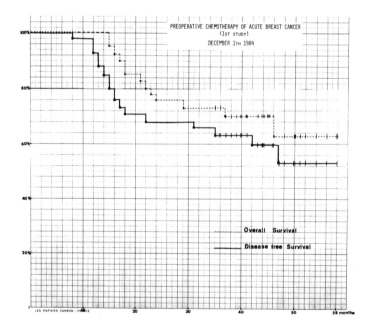

Fig. 1: First study: actuarial disease-free survival (———)
        is 54% and overall survival (----) is 63% at 58
        months.

Among the 10 patients classified as grade 1, only one failure was noted. Among grade 2 patients, 11/20 failed, and 5/11 of the grade 3 patients (Table 2).

POST CHEMOTHERAPY HISTOLOGICAL FEATURES

	T		N	RELAPSES	
Grade 1	10	N−	8	1	} 1
		N+	2	0	
Grade 2	20	N−	6	4	} 11
		N+	14	7	
Grade 3	11	N−	3	1	} 5
		N+	8	4	
TOTAL	41			17 (42%)	

Table 2: First study: Post-chemotherapy histological study of operative specimen and relapses.

The sites of relapse are listed in Table 3. The two patients listed as loco-regional relapses are now disease-free following radiotherapy.

METASTASES	8
LOCO-REGIONAL + METASTASES	7
LOCO-REGIONAL ALONE	2
TOTAL	17

Table 3: First study: Sites of relapse

Second Study (Regimen A vs B):

At this point in time, disease-free survival is significantly better for regimen A (86%) than for regimen B (58%;

p = 0.03), Fig. 2.

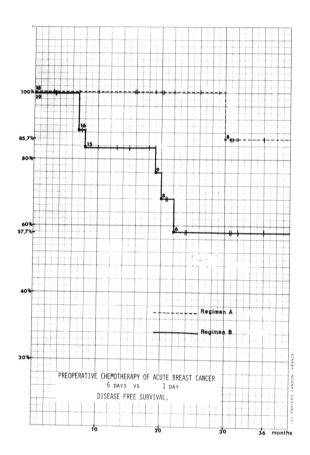

Fig. 2 : Regimen A vs B   : Actuarial DFS at 36 months:
Regimen A (----) 86%; Regimen B (———) 58%;
p = 0.03.

At this point in the trial, there are no significant differences in overall survival between regimen A and B (86%
and 77%, respectively; n.s.), Fig. 3. After a median follow
up period of 16 months, 1 failure has occurred among patients treated with the A regimen and 6 failures among
patients treated with the B regimen. All fail-

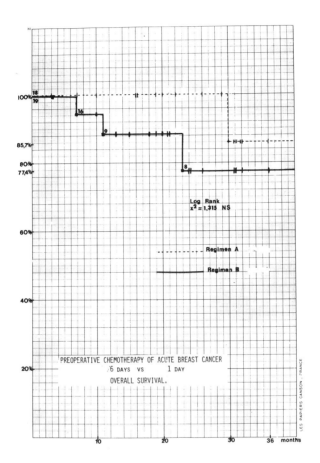

Fig. 3: Regimen A vs B: Actuarial overall survival at
36 months: Regimen A (----) 86%; Regimen B (———)
77%; n.s.

ures had been categorized as grade 3 responders.
Table 4 describes the sites of relapse of these patients.
These data are preliminary as the trial is still ongoing.

	REGIMEN A	REGIMEN B
METASTASES	1	2
LOCO-REGIONAL + METASTASES	0	3
LOCO-REGIONAL ALONE	0	1

Table 4: Regimen A vs B: Sites of relapse

TOXICITY

Treatment tolerance in both studies was good. Side effects which were encountered included nausea, vomiting and alopecia. Severe bone marrow toxicity was not observed. In instances where neutrophils fell below 2000 and/or platelets below 100.000, treatment was postponed one week. In the randomized study, the isotopic ventricular ejection fraction (VEF) was monitored before, during and at the end of treatment, as a control for possible cardiac toxicity. It should be noted, however, that despite the high doses of epirubicin given (25 patients have currently received a total dosage of 660 mg/m^2), the VEF measured at the end of treatment never fell below the normal value (0.50). In fact, no cardiac dysfunction was noted in any patient, Fig. 4.

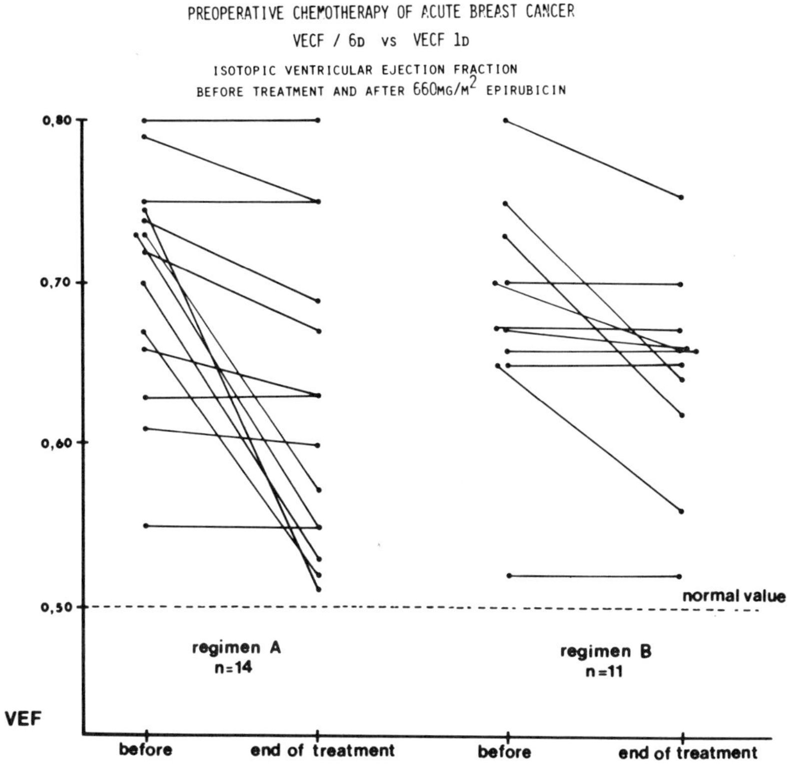

PREOPERATIVE CHEMOTHERAPY OF ACUTE BREAST CANCER
VECF / 6D vs VECF 1D
ISOTOPIC VENTRICULAR EJECTION FRACTION
BEFORE TREATMENT AND AFTER 660MG/M^2 EPIRUBICIN

Fig. 4: Regimen A vs B: Isotopic ventricular ejection
fraction before and at the end of treatment
(cumulative dose of Epirubicin = 660 mg/m^2)

COMMENTS

It appears that both pre- and post-operative chemotherapy are effective in treatment of inflammatory breast cancer. Although the second study of pre-operative chemotherapy is not yet complete, it appears that the fractionated, 6-day schedule (A) results in a longer period of disease-free survival than does the 1-day schedule (B).

Despite these promising results, some questions remain:

1) Is there a need for second-line chemotherapy for non- or poor responders?

2) Is the maintenance chemotherapy (vindesine, MTX, thiotepa) useful?

3) Is loco-regional, post-operative radiotherapy indicated, in view of the number of loco-regional relapses seen (9/14 patients in the first study and 4/37 in the second). There seems to be no justification for irradiation in Grade 1 responders. However, irradiation might result in better local control in poor (Grade 2 and Grade 3) responders.

Primary Chemotherapy in Cancer Medicine, pages 105–116
© 1985 Alan R. Liss, Inc.

INDUCTION CHEMOTHERAPY OF BREAST CANCER

G.N. Hortobagyi, A.U. Buzdar, F.C. Ames, G.R.
Blumenschein, and E.D. Montague
Departments of Medical Oncology (GNH, AUB, GRB),
Surgery (FCA) and Radiotherapy (EDM), University
of Texas M.D. Anderson Hospital, Houston, Texas
77030

INTRODUCTION

Patients with unresectable primary breast cancer (T3-B,
T4, or N3), even in the absence of distant metastases, had a
very poor prognosis when treated with local therapies alone
(Atkins, 1961; Baclesse, 1949). Some patients with unresectable, locally advanced breast cancer, were not candidates for local therapies so hormonal therapy was administered (Rubens, 1977). Of those patients who responded to
endocrine treatment, some had a substantial decrease in
tumor burden resulting in operable lesions. However, only
20-30% of patients responded to endocrine therapy and only
a fraction of these had objective regressions sufficient to
transform a previously unresectable lesion in an operable
tumor. Consequently, this type of multimodal therapy was
not commonly employed. In the early 70's it became evident
that combination chemotherapy was effective in producing
objective regressions in more than half of patients with
metastatic breast carcinoma (Carter, 1972). This was especially true in soft tissue lesions so combination chemotherapy was incorporated with more and more frequency into
the primary and preoperative treatment of locally advanced,
non-metastatic breast cancer, including inflammatory carcinoma. Over the past 15 years, it has been demonstrated
that the combination of systemic and local therapies is the
treatment of choice for locally advanced breast cancer and
that this treatment strategy has resulted in improved survival for patients who present at this stage of the disease.

In this paper we will present the experience acquired at the M.D. Anderson Hospital and Tumor Institute with induction chemotherapy as part of a multimodal treatment approach in primary breast carcinoma since 1973.

MATERIALS AND METHODS

Between 1973 and 1981, 156 patients with locally advanced primary breast carcinoma without evidence of distant metastases were treated with induction combination chemotherapy. Sixty-three of these patients had inflammatory breast carcinoma. Chemotherapy consisted of 5-FU 500 mg/m^2 IV on days 1 and 8, Doxorubicin (adriamycin) 50 mg/m^2 IV on day 1 and cyclophosphamide 500 mg/m^2 IV on day 1 (FAC) (Hortobagyi, 1979) (Table 1). Identical cycles of chemotherapy were repeated every 3 weeks with appropriate dosage modifications as required by hematologic and other toxicity. In general, 3 cycles of chemotherapy were administered during the induction phase. The response to the initial 3 cycles of chemotherapy was then assessed by clinical and radiographic means before the institution of local therapy. From 1973 to 1978, local therapy for patients with inflammatory breast carcinoma consisted exclusively of radiation therapy to the breast and regional lymphatics, as described elsewhere (Buzdar, 1981). Between 1978 and 1981, local therapy for patients with inflammatory breast carcinoma included a total mastectomy with axillary dissection following induction chemotherapy, and radiation therapy consolidation at the conclusion of all planned chemotherapy (Fastenberg, 1985). Patients with locally advanced, noninflammatory breast carcinoma, were treated with radiation therapy alone following induction chemotherapy if response to systemic treatment was good and only minimal residual disease (<2 cm in largest diameters) remained. Patients with a modest or no response to induction chemotherapy underwent a total mastectomy with axillary dissection followed by comprehensive radiation therapy and additional chemotherapy for a total duration of 2 years (Hortobagyi, 1983). Between 1978 and 1981, all patients with locally advanced, non-inflammatory breast cancer were treated with a modified radical mastectomy (or extended simple) between cycles 3 and 4 of chemotherapy, and consolidation radiation therapy at the conclusion of all planned chemotherapy (2 years) (Kantarjian, 1984).

Postoperatively (or after completion of radiation therapy if that was the first modality of local treatment) FAC was continued until reaching a total cumulative dose of adriamycin of 450 mg/m^2. At that time, chemotherapy was continued with a CMF combination as shown in Table 1. Following completion of the entire treatment program, patients were followed at 3-4 month intervals for the first 3 years and every 6-12 months thereafter. During follow-up examination, biochemical survey, carcinoembryonic antigen, chest x-ray, bone and liver scans and yearly mammograms were performed (Buzdar, 1981; Hortobagyi, 1983).

Disease-free and overall survival curves were constructed utilizing the Kaplan and Meier method, and differences between curves were determined by the generalized Wilcoxon test.

TABLE 1. Multimodal Treatment for Advanced Non-Metastatic Breast Cancer

---

Induction regimen:
Fluorouracil	500 mg/m^2	IV, days 1 + 8
Adriamycin	50 mg/m^2	IV, day 1
Cyclophosphamide	500 mg/m^2	IV, day 1

After reaching 450 mg/m^2 of adriamycin chemotherapy was continued as follows:
Fluorouracil	500 mg/m^2	PO, days 1 + 8
Methotrexate	30 mg/m^2	IM, days 1 + 8
Cyclophosphamide	500 mg/m^2	PO, day 2

Chemotherapy cycles were repeated every 21 days. Immunotherapy with BCG by scarification was administered on days 9, 13 and 17 of each cycle of FAC and CMF for patients entered between 1973 and 1978.

Treatment sequence used between 1973 - 1978
FAC x 3 $\longrightarrow$ Surgery +/or Radiotherapy $\longrightarrow$ FAC x 6 $\longrightarrow$ CMF x 20

Treatment sequence used between 1978 - 1981
FAC x 3 $\longrightarrow$ Surgery $\longrightarrow$ FAC x 6 $\longrightarrow$ CMF x 20 $\longrightarrow$ Radiotherapy

RESULTS

Ninety-three patients with locally advanced (LABC),
non-inflammatory breast carcinoma and 63 patients with inflammatory breast carcinoma (IBC) were included in this review. The patient characteristics at presentation are depicted on Table 2. Most patients included in this analysis
had very advanced disease, reflecting the referral pattern
during the years these patients were accrued. For most
patients information about estrogen receptor status was not
available since this assay became routine only towards the
end of the patients' accrual. The overall response rate
after induction chemotherapy was 86% for the locally advanced, non-inflammatory breast cancer patient and 68% for
patients with inflammatory breast cancer (Table 3). The
distribution of local therapies administered to these two
groups of patients is shown in Table 4. Eighteen percent
of patients did not receive radiotherapy because progressive
or recurrent disease developed well before radiotherapy was
planned to be given or had other medical reasons to omit
radiotherapy. In addition, 2 patients with progressive
disease during the induction chemotherapy phase were not
candidates for local or regional therapy. 96% of the 93
patients with LABC and 92% of the 63 patients with IBC were
rendered free of disease after induction chemotherapy and
the first local therapy. The disease-free survival and
overall survivals of these two groups of patients are shown
in Figures 1 and 2, respectively. The median disease-free
survival for LABC was 30 months, while it was 24 months for
IBC patients. The median survival for patients with LABC
is expected to exceed 66 months, while it was 43 months for
patients with IBC. While the disease-free survival observations are completed, the overall survival figures are pro-
jections. Thirty percent of patients with IBC and 36% of
patients with LABC were relapse-free at 5 years. The cor-
responding survival figures are projected to be 38% and 50%
for IBC and LABC, respectively. The median relapse-free
survival for the 9 patients with stage IIIa disease is projected to exceed 45 months.

TABLE 2. Pretreatment Patient Characteristics

	Inflammatory	Non-Inflammatory	Total
No. of Patients	63	93	156
Median Age in Years	51	56	54
(Range)	(27-78)	(28-79)	(27-79)
Race			
Caucasian	50	77	127
Other	13	16	29
Menopausal Status			
Premenopausal	23	34	57
Postmenopausal	40	59	99
Clinical Stage (TNM)			
IIIa $T_{(2-3)}N_{(1-2)}$	–	9	9
IIIb	63	84	147
$T_{1-3}N_3$	–	10	10
T_4N_{0-2}	47	55	102
T_4N_3	16	19	35
Estrogen Receptor Status			
Positive	–	25	25
Negative	–	22	22
Unknown	63	46	109

TABLE 3. Response Rate

| | No. of Patients (%) | | |
	Inflammatory	Non-Inflammatory	Total
After Induction Chemotherapy			
Complete Remission	9	17	26(17)
Partial Remission	34	63	97(62)
No Change	17	12	29(19)
Progressive Disease	3	1	4(2)
After FAC and Local Therapy			
Disease-Free	57	89	146(94)
Residual or Metastatic Disease	6	4	10(6)

TABLE 4. Local Therapy and Recurrence

| | No. of Patients (%) | | |
	Inflammatory	Non-Inflammatory	Total
Local Therapy			
Surgery	7	18	25(16)
Radiotherapy	41	22	63(40)
Both	14	52	66(42)
None	1	1	2(1)
Local Recurrence			
Chest Wall/ Lymphatics	9	17	26(17)

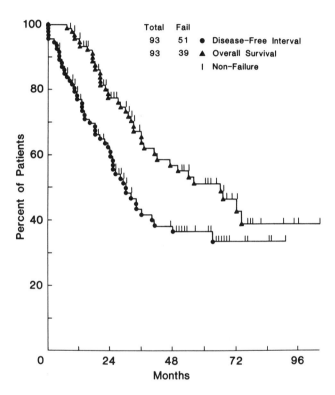

Figure 1. Disease-free interval (DFI) and survival of
patients with locally advanced breast cancer treated with
the combined modality approach. Reproduced with permission
from Kantarjian et al, 1984.

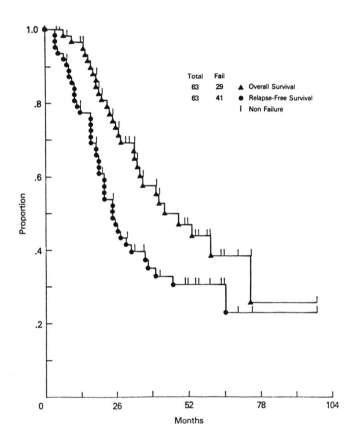

Figure 2. Disease-free survival and overall survival of patients with inflammatory breast cancer. Reproduced with permission from Fastenberg et al, 1985.

In patients with LABC, distant metastases occurred in 33 patients (37%), while local regional failure was observed in 17 patients (18%). Local regional recurrence rate was 14% for patients with IBC, while 48% developed distant metastases. No difference in prognosis according to menopausal status was observed in patients with LABC, while postmenopausal patients did substantially better than premenopausal patients among the group of IBC. The relapse-free survival for patients with IBC $\geq$50 years was 36 months compared with 19 months for those <50 years (p=.05).

Since clinical assessment of response to induction chemotherapy was not always accurate, we evaluated the subgroup of patients with both IBC and LABC who underwent a total mastectomy and axillary dissection immediately following induction chemotherapy. Of the 156 patients included in this study, 90 (21 with IBC and 69 with LABC) had induction chemotherapy followed immediately by a surgical procedure. Review of the pathological evaluation of the mastectomy specimen revealed that 15 (17%) had no macroscopic evidence of residual malignancy (Group A) and, in fact, 6 of these 15 had no residual disease at all. The other 75 patients (83%) had macroscopic residual tumor in the mastectomy specimen (Group B). Group A patients consisted of 4 patients with IBC and 11 with LABC. The disease-free survival of patients in Group A was projected to be in excess of 60 months, while it was only 29 months for patients in Group B (p<0.01). All 4 patients with IBC in Group A remain free of disease, and 8 of the 11 patients with LABC in Group A also remain disease-free.

This multimodal treatment program was well tolerated. Nausea, vomiting and alopecia were experienced by most patients but were completely reversible. Myelosuppression was moderately severe, but infectious complications were few. Toxicity related to radiotherapy was minor. Only one treatment related death was observed in a patient who developed doxorubicin-cardiomyopathy. Compliance was excellent in the group of patients with IBC; however, patients with LABC had a high rate of protocol deviations that delayed or prevented the completion of planned therapy. We noted in this analysis that the response to induction chemotherapy correlated well with long term prognosis; thus the median survival of patients who achieved an objective clinical remission was twice as long as one observed in the group of patients without a response (p=0.05).

DISCUSSION

This experience demonstrates that the combined use of chemotherapy, surgery, and radiation therapy results in an increased rate of complete remission for patients who present with a locally advanced breast cancer (both in-flammatory and non-inflammatory in character). In addition, this is made possible with less radical local treatment pro-cedures. In consequence, 40% of patients so treated con-served their breast while receiving a most appropriate treatment. The outcome of these patients was no different from the outcome of patients who did receive a mastectomy.

While it has not been clearly established that the treatment sequences described in this paper are the optimal way of combining these three treatment modalities, the use of induction chemotherapy offers several advantages. First of all, the use of chemotherapy as the first modality of treatment allows a clear evaluation of the effectiveness of this treatment. This, of course, would not be possible after a mastectomy, when no measurable disease remains. Consequently, for the 20-40% of patients who do not re-spond to induction chemotherapy, postoperative therapy with the same combination can be avoided while other, more ef-fective combinations could be used. Second, it seems that the response to induction chemotherapy, whether measured clinically or, preferably, pathologically, provides the best correlation with long-term disease-free and overall sur-vival. This would be expected since combination chemo-therapy would influence not only local control but distant metastasis as well.

The experience described in this paper was obtained in patients with markedly advanced and mostly inoperable breast cancer. In view of the effectiveness and the good toler-ance to this multimodal approach, we have employed this treatment modality in earlier stages of disease. Since 1981, a number of patients with stage IIIa breast cancer have been treated according to this treatment strategy. However, their follow-up is too early to be reported at this time. Postoperative adjuvant chemotherapy has been shown to improve disease-free and overall survival of patients with breast cancer at high risk or systemic dis-semination (Buzdar, 1979; Fisher, 1977). The use of preoperative, or neoadjuvant, or induction chemotherapy would represent a refinement of adjuvant treatment and should be carefully evaluated in prospective trials in patients with early breast cancer.

REFERENCES

Atkins HL, Horrigan WD (1961). Treatment of locally advanced carcinoma of the breast with roentgen therapy and simple mastectomy. Am J Roentgenol Radium Ther Nucl Med 85:860-864.

Baclesse F (1949). Roentgen therapy as sole method of treatment of cancer of breast. Am J Roentgenol Radium Ther Nucl Med 62:331-349.

Buzdar AU, Blumenschein GR, Gutterman JU, et al (1979). Postoperative adjuvant chemotherapy with fluorouracil, doxorubicin, cyclophosphamide and BCG vaccine - a follow-up report. JAMA 242:1509-1513.

Buzdar AU, Montague E, Barker J, et al (1981). Management of inflammatory carcinoma of the breast with a combined modality approach - an update. Cancer 47:2537-2542.

Carter SK (1972). Single and combination nonhormonal chemotherapy in breast cancer. Cancer 30:1543-1555.

Fastenberg NA, Buzdar AU, Montague ED, et al (1985). Management of inflammatory carcinoma of the breast: a combined modality approach. Am J Clin Oncol (in press).

Fisher B, Glass A, Redmond C, et al (1977). L-phenylalanine mustard (L-PAM) in the management of primary breast cancer: an update of earlier findings and a comparison with those utilizing L-PAM plus 5-fluorouracil (5-FU). Cancer 39:2883-2903.

Hortobagyi GN, Gutterman JU, Blumenschein GR, et al (1979). Combination chemoimmunotherapy of metastatic breast cancer with 5-fluorouracil, adriamycin, cyclophosphamide, and BCG. Cancer 43:1225-1233.

Hortobagyi GN, Spanos W, Montague ED, et al (1983). Treatment of locoregionally advanced breast cancer with surgery, radiotherapy, and combination chemotherapy. Intl J Radiat Oncol Biol Phys 9:643-650.

Kantarjian HM, Hortobagyi GN, Smith TL, et al (1984). The management of locally advanced breast cancer: a combined modality approach. Eur J Cancer Clin Oncol 20(11):1353-1361.

Rubens RD, Armitage P, Winter PJ, Tong D, Hayward JL (1977). Prognosis in inoperable stage III carcinoma of the breast. Europ J Cancer 13:805-811.

SECTION IV
LUNG CANCER

Primary Chemotherapy in Cancer Medicine, pages 119-126
© 1985 Alan R. Liss, Inc.

CHEMOTHERAPY FOR LOCALLY ADVANCED LUNG CANCER: RATIONALE
AND ISSUES

Franco M. Muggia, M.D., Ronald H. Blum, M.D.,
Jay S. Cooper, M.D., Dorothy McCauley, M.D.
Rita & Stanley H. Kaplan Cancer Center
NYU Medical Center
New York, NY 10016

While systemic therapy has become the major ingredient
in the treatment of small cell lung cancer (SCLC), it has
usually been relegated for use in the most advanced stages
of other types of lung cancer. We review here the rationale
and issues for chemotherapy given to localized stages of
non-small cell lung cancer (NSCLC).

I. Rationale

Studies from past surgical series have amply confirmed the great likelihood of having distant metastases already present at the time of surgery for lung
cancer. Although cure rates from local therapies are
superior in NSCLC than in SCLC, until recently survival
at 5 years were below 50% for all histologies. Past
series emphasized the importance of histology, size,
location of primary tumors, and presence or absence of
regional lymph node involvement in determining prognosis. Data from Johns Hopkins surgical pathology (1964-
1973) may be considered representative (1). Resections
were carried out in 177 of 435 patients (40%) and the
minimum follow up was 2 years; prognostic factors were
analyzed as independent variables. The histologies of
resected patients were 16 small cell and 63, 59, and
39 squamous, adeno, and large cell respectively. Negative lymph nodes were present in 3, 36, 34 and 22 patients respectively and the 5 year survival rates in
these most favorable node negative patients were 33%
(1 pt), 44%, 35% and 41% respectively. With primaries
< 3 cm only a small subset of 12 patients with large

cell carcinomas had a greater than 50% 5 year survival rate. With tumor > 3 cm the 5 year survival rates
were 0, 28, 24 and 17% respectively for small, squamous, adeno and large cell. Although early disease
dissemination was mounted as a powerful argument for
chemotherapy in SCLC, surgival results in NSCLC are
hardly cause for complacency.

Comparable data from current trials with prospective staging suggests a considerable better outlook
particularly for properly staged T_1N_0 lesions (2).
Five year survival rates of 85% for T_1N_0 and 55% for
T_1N_1 and T_2N_0 have been reported (3). In part computerized tomography and better surgical staging are
changing the population included in such statistics.
It is worth reviewing recent studies for analysis of
prognostic factors using current diagnostic and therapeutic methods and multivariate analysis.

The pattern of recurrence from resected Stage I
patients included in the Lung Cancer Study Group trial
has now been analyzed in detail (4). These include 134
recurrences (34%) from a total of 390 eligible patients
(211 on BCG + Isoniazid and 189 on placebo) at a mean
follow-up of 3.4 year. Central pathology review classified patients as 171 squamous, 191 adeno, 12 large cell
and 10 adenosquamous (6 patients were not reviewed).
Of all patients only 32 of the patients were staged as
T_1N_1. Squamous cell histologies included 65 T_1N_0 and
86 T_2N_0 patients; a similar subdivision for adenocarcinoma was 86 and 93, respectively. First recurrences were
subdivided as "local only", "brain only" and "other"
and were documented by x-ray or scan in 80% and by
autopsy in 15% when lesions involved brain, bone or
liver; other recurrences were usually documented histologically. The pattern indicated a total of 30% relapses locally (involved lung and/or mediastinum) 23%
in brain and 47% in various sites which include bone
and contralateral lung accounting for more than half
of these. Brain relapses were more common with increasing TN status and with non squamous histologies but
otherwise recurrence patterns were quite similar across
all Stage I patient subsets. These recent findings re-
enforce the need for systemic therapy in the treatment
strategy for all lung cancer with the possible excep-
tion of T_1N_0 lesions.

Gail has analyzed further in these patients those
prognostic factors which correlate with recurrence and

those which correlate with deaths (5). A multivariate
model of recurrence classifies patients into low,
intermediate and high risk groups based on tumor size
and location (T_1, T_2), histologic type (squamous, non-
squamous/mixed) and nodal status (N_0, N_1). These risk
groups appear in Table 1 and indicate that one can probably refine risk groups for recurrence in subsequent
trials if one utilizes surgical staging. On the other
hand all non squamous tumors and the T_2 squamous
lesions fall at least in an intermediate risk group
which may be theoretically be placed on adjuvant
trials.

TABLE 1
Risk Groups for Recurrence in Stage I+

Risk	Stage-histology	n of pts	Estimated % by relapse free	Obser- ved by RFS	Obser-* ved* by Survival
Low	T_1N_1 squamous	20	90%		
	T_1N_0 squamous	65	89%	90%	85%
Medium	T_1N_0 nonsquamous	98	66%		
	T_2N_0 squamous	87	58%	62%	73%
High	T_2N_0 nonsquamous	110	47%		
	T_1N_1 nonsquamous	12	38%	50%	40%

+ Lung Cancer Study Group data analyzed by Gail et al (5)
* Survival groupings take into consideration performance
  status and infection, e.g. T_2N_0 nonsquamous without complications becomes medium risk; with infection all categories assume next higher risk (5)

When one examines factors relating to increased
mortality, postoperative empyema, pneumonia or wound
infections carried increased risk of death, but not
recurrence. Preoperative performance status also added
to pathology and histology in predicting survival.
Monitoring for increased risk by determining a relative
hazard and a window of 170 days follow up indicates
strong association with recurrence and death with a
decline in performance status and leukocytosis (>
9100 cells/mm³) occurring six months earlier, a weak
association for increased CEA and a trend only for
persistent smoking. Initial leukocyte count and high

LDH also correlated with an overall risk of recurrence (Table 2). This data in the earliest stages of lung cancer may help refine prognostic factors in other stages.

TABLE 2
Stage I Recurrence Rate Factors+

Significant Ratios

TN code (T_1N_0 vs others)
Histology (squamous vs others)
LDH (LDH < 149 vs ≧)
Neutrophil count (< 5400 vs ≧)

+ Feld et al, 1984: Lung Cancer Study Group Data (4)

II. Issues in Primary Chemotherapy

Several questions may be posed as one considers a strategy of initial chemotherapy.

1. Which patients should be selected? Until an impact of systemic therapy can be documented on NSC lung cancer, trials have been generally included Stage III M_0 patients. Such patients may be expected to have a shorter time to recurrence and greater number of recurrences than the previously cited Stage I patients. No differences would be expected among the various histologies. One may properly raise the question of treatment of earlier stages and this awaits further confirmation of feasibility and suggested efficacy in the more advanced situation. However, it should be noted that current selection places a high demand on the efficacy of systemic therapy.

2. Do we possess effective systemic treatment? Systemic treatment of NSC lung cancer has a record of claims followed by disappointments. Suggested superior efficacy for cisplatin containing combinations is derived from various trials previously reviewed (6,7). We have been encouraged by high response rates in small number of patients with Stage III M_0 lesions utilizing a cisplatin plus vinblastine combination. In the utilization of primary chemotherapy, however, the percent of patients showing immediate progression and the possible increase in morbidity follo-

wing subsequent radiation and/or surgery become important issues. For these reasons we have preferred
to refine data on our two drug combination rather
than proceed to potentially more toxic regimens.It
is also possible that small efficacy differences in
advanced disease settings may become greater in
earlier stages. Comparative studies such as performed by the Eastern Cooperative Oncology Group are
therefore important. Comparison of treatment versus
no treatment in advanced lung cancer is of course
relevant. Again these results may not be applicable
to earlier stages and to all regimens. However,
these treatments must be carried out in the context
of trials.

3. Are there data supporting a role for adjuvant therapy? Our previous review prior to cisplatin combinations, indicated that adjuvant chemotherapy was ineffective (8) and even deleterious (9). More recently, Lung Cancer Study Group data in Stage II nonsquamous resected indicated that chemotherapy with
cyclophosphamide, adriamycin and cisplatin may improve disease free survival (10) compared to
patients receiving Levamisole. A full report is a-
waited. Skarin et al reported primary use of
cyclophosphamide, adriamycin and cisplatin followed
by radiation and then surgery in marginally resectable non-small cell lung cancer. Eleven of 12 patients were resected without gross residual disease;
eight had no evidence of disease 6+ to 13+ months
after treatment (11). The group from Rush have also
utilized this approach originally with cisplatin
and mitomycin prior to radiation (12) and more recently with cisplatin/5FU and simultaneous radiation (13). Results are preliminary but indicate the
feasibility of approaches similar to our own.

4. What are possible detrimental consequences of such
strategy? The major deterrents to utilizing adjuvant
treatment in NSCLC are lack of efficacy and actually
decreasing chances for cure. As for the latter,
current patient selection includes those in whom
cures from radiation alone are below 20%. Therefore
to embark in trials designed to improve the probability of this survival figure is justified. Current
studies suggest that some efficacy is present, and
at acceptable toxicity (10). Nevertheless, considerably greater experience must be accrued with neo-

adjuvant therapy and possible complications that may occur with radiation and with subsequent surgical resections.

5. Are these alternate strategies that need testing? The high risk of brain metastases that has already been noted in neoadjuvant therapy (11, 13) indicates a possible failure of chemotherapy to prevent CNS relapses. Prophylactic brain irradiation has to be considered as a possible option in future trials. Alternatively, systematic restaging including brain CT may be important. Local radiation given as primary modality to be followed by chemotherapy which has been a strategy utilized in the past is likely to give inferior results since it does not address the issue of systemic therapy until several weeks later and chemotherapy is more difficult to administer without complications. Because of the risk of complications from giving chemotherapy after chest irradiation we have not favored reinstituting chemotherapy after local therapy.

III. Conclusions

We have found persuasive arguments for beginning treatment of Stage III M_0 lesions with chemotherapy. The chemotherapy selected has been cisplatin with vinblastine which has a reproducible record of efficacy and tolerance in our hands. Prospective trials will be needed to determine whether such treatment will improve the survival of patients with NSC lung cancer. However, we are convinced that the rationale for its use in this disease is greater than in many other circumstances. Careful selection of an acceptable chemotherapy regimen which is preferably compatible with subsequent and/or simultaneous radiation is an important aspect of this approach. Because T_1 squamous lesions carry a distinctly better outlook, such patients would likely be excluded from all future trials. Other early lesions, however, may represent distinctly relevant targets for adjuvant trials including approaches utilizing chemotherapy prior to any local therapy.

REFERENCES

1. Katlic M, and Carter D. Prognostic implications of histology size and location of primary tumors. In: Lung Cancer: Progress in Therapeutic Research. F Muggia and M Rozencweig (Eds.). Raven Press, NY, pp. 143-150, 1979.

2. Mountain CF, Gail MH. Surgical adjuvant intrapleural BCG treatment for Stage I non-small cell lung cancer. Preliminary report of the National Cancer Institute Lung Cancer Study Group. J. Thorac Cardiovasc Surg. 28:649-657, 1981.

3. Williams DE, Pairolero PC, David CS, et al. Survival of patients surgically treated for Stage I lung cancer. J. Thorac Cardiovasc Surg. 82:70-76, 1981.

4. Feld R, Rubinstein LV, Weisenberger TH, and the Lung Cancer Study. Site of recurrence in resected Stage I non-small cell lung cancer: A guide for future studies. J. Clin Oncol. 2:1352-1358, 1984.

5. Gail MH, Eagan RT, Feld R, Ginsberg R, Goodell B, Hill, L, Holmes EC, Lukeman J, Mountain CF, Oldham RK, Pearson FG, Wright PW, Lake WHJ, and the Lung Cancer Study Group. Prognostic factors in patients with resected Stage I non-small cell lung cancer. Cancer. 54:1802-1813, 1984.

6. Muggia FM, Blum RH, and Foreman JD. Role of chemotherapy in the treatment of lung cancer: Evolving strategies for non-small cell histologies. Int J Rad Oncol Biol Phys. 10:137-145, 1984.

7. Muggia FM, and Blum RH. Treatment of non-small cell lung cancer. Cancer: Strategies with combination chemotherapy including etoposide. In: Etoposide (VP-16): Current status and new developments. BK Issell, FM Muggia, and SK Carter (Eds.). Acad Press, NY, pp. 215-223, 1984.

8. Legha SS, Muggia FM, and Carter SK. Adjuvant chemotherapy in lung cancer: Review and prospects. Cancer. 39:1415-1424, 1977.

9. Brunner KW, Martholar T, and Muller W. Adjuvant chemotherapy with cyclophosphamide for radically resected bronchogenic carcinoma: 9 year follow up. In: Lung Cancer: Progress in therapeutic research. FM Muggia and M Rozencweig (Eds.). Raven Press, pp. 418-420, 1979.

10. Holmes EC, Eagan RT and the Lung Cancer Study Group. Surgical adjuvant therapy of resectable Stage II/III

adenocarcinoma and large cell undifferentiated carcinoma of the lung. Proc Amer Soc Clin Onc. 3:220, 1984.
11. Skarin A, Veeder M, Malcolm A, et al. Chemotherapy prior to radiotherapy and surgery in marginally resectable non-small cell lung cancer. Proc Amer Soc Clin Onc. 1:143, 1982.
12. Fuller BZ, Buromi PD, Reddy SG, et al. Cisplatin and mitomycin C preceding local therapy in squamous cell bronchogenic carcinoma. Proc Amer Soc Clin Onc. 1:144, 1982.
13. Trybula M, Taylor SG IV, Bonomi P, et al. Preoperative simultaneous cisplatin/5-Fluorouracil and radiotherapy in clinical stage III bronchogenic carcinoma. Proc Amer Soc Clin Onc. 4:   , 1985.

Primary Chemotherapy in Cancer Medicine, pages 127–132
© 1985 Alan R. Liss, Inc.

CHEMOTHERAPY (CAP) PRIOR TO RADIOTHERAPY (RT) AND SURGERY
IN MARGINALLY RESECTABLE STAGE III M_0 NON-SMALL CELL LUNG
CANCER.

A. Skarin, A. Malcolm, N. Leslie,
P. Oliynyk, R. Overholt, E. Frei, III

Dana-Farber Cancer Institute
Joint Center for Radiotherapy
Harvard Medical School
Boston, Ma. 02115

The prognosis of patients with Stage III M_0 non-small
cell lung cancer (NSCLC) is poor, with only 6-15% surviving
at 5 years despite use of radiotherapy (Caldwell, et al
1968; Hellman, et al 1964; Petrovich, et al 1981). In
selected patients, aggressive surgery and radiotherapy with
or without chemotherapy (Martini, et al 1980; Takita, et al
1978) have resulted in some improvement in survival. Similarly, use of radiotherapy and chemotherapy has increased
median survival (Eagan, et al 1981). In order to improve
the prognosis, a multidisciplinary treatment program was
initiated at our Center in October 1980. The protocol was
based upon the effectiveness of platinum containing combination chemotherapy regimens (Eagan, et al 1977), and our
experience with aggressive surgery in palliative cases
(Overholt, et al 1975) and combined surgery and radiotherapy
in marginally resectable cases (Sherman, et al 1978). The
objectives were to employ initial CAP chemotherapy followed
by radiotherapy in order to render borderline resectable
cases resectable, and to improve local control and overall
survival by post-op radiotherapy and CAP chemotherapy.

MATERIALS AND METHODS

Patients with biopsy proven NSCLC were clinically
staged by physical exam, laboratory chemistries, creatinine
clearance and blood counts, chest film, chest and upper
abdominal CT scan, brain CT scan, and bone nuclide scans.
Surgical staging to confirm Stage III M_0 disease (T_3 and/or
N_2) consisted of mediastinoscopy and/or mediastinotomy

(Chamberlain procedure). Patients were eligible for treatment if no significant comorbid disease (pulmonary, cardiac, renal, or hepatic) existed, and marginally resectable lung cancer was demonstrated, defined as follows: T_3 (any N)- superior sulcus or chest wall lesion with direct local invasion, but excluding carinal primaries and pleural effusions; N_2 (T_1 or T_2)- unilateral mediastinal metastases that are freely movable (i.e. not rigid or fixed to adjacent structures such as extensive extranodal disease). N_2 (T_3) indicated nodal disease as above but also direct extension of the primary lesion into adjacent central structures. Treatment consisted of initial CAP chemotherapy as follows: cyclophosphamide 500mg/m^2 i.v., doxorubicin 50mg/m^2 i.v., and cis-platinum 50mg/m^2 i.v. given on day 1 and 21. Response to CAP was assessed by repeat chest films and in some patients CT scans with measurement of tumor masses. A partial response (PR) was defined as >50% reduction in the size of all lesions, marginal response (MR) <50% regression, stable disease (SD) no major change in size of lesions, while progressive disease (PD) signified increase in size of existing lesions or development of new metastases. After a 3-4 week recovery, the first part of a split course of radiotherapy was given (3000 rad). Clinical re-staging procedures were repeated to rule-out any early metastases, and if none were evident, thoracotomy with radical resection (including mediastinal lymph node dissection) was carried out. Following recovery from surgery, thoracic radiotherapy was completed (2500-3000 rad). After 1983, prophylactic cranial radiotherapy was administered (3600 rad in 18 fractions). Finally 4 additional copies of CAP at 3 week intervals was administered to those patients initially responding to CAP. Informed consent as approved by the Human Protection Committee was obtained in all patients.

RESULTS

A total of 41 eligible were treated. For purposes of data analysis, the patients were seperated into 2 groups as follows (Table 1).

TABLE 1. CLINICAL FEATURES OF 41 PATIENTS

	Superior Sulcus Chest wall (11)	Other Cases (30)	Total (41)
M:F	6.5	20:10	26:15
Age median	53 yr	55 yr	56
range	43-73	29-64	29-73
Stage	$T_3N_0 - 7$ $T_3N_1 - 2$ $T_3N_2 - 2$	$T_1N_2 - 3$ $T_2N_2 - 20$ $T_3N_2 - 7$ $T_1N_2 - 3$ $T_2N_2 -20$ $T_3N_2 - 9$	$T_3N_1 - 2$ $T_3N_0 - 7$
Adenocarcinoma	6	17	23
Squamous cell	2	9	11
Large cell	2	3	5
Mixed	1	1	2

The objective response after 2 cycles of CAP chemotherapy was as follows: (Table 2)

TABLE 2. RESPONSE AFTER 2 CYCLES OF CAP

	Superior Sulcus chest wall (11)	Other Cases (30)	Total (41)
Response			
PR	4 - 44% } 78%	12 - 43% } 75%	16 - 43% } 76%
MR	3	9	12
SD	2	4	6
PD	0	3	3

Only 3 patients had progressive disease, occurring in extra thoracic sites, and were removed from the study. Radiotherapy was started in the remaining patients, but subsequent surgery could not be carried out in 2 patients due to a fatal stroke (1) or CNS metastases (1). Thus, thoracotomy was performed in 36 patients with the following results. (Table 3).

TABLE 3. SURGICAL EXPLORATION OF 36 PATIENTS

Unresectable (severe fibrosis)	-	1
Radical pneumonectomy	-	18
Lobectomy c̄ chest wall resection	-	10
Lobectomy c̄ mediastinal node dissection	-	6
Bilobectomy	-	1

One patient who could not be resected because of fibrosis had received 5000 rad pre-op (considered a protocol viola- tion). The remaining 35 patients had radical resection of the primary lung cancer and draining lymph nodes without any residual gross disease. Histopathologic findings were varia- ble and will be the subject of a subsequent report. Major complications included subsequent benign pericardial effu- sions in 3 cases, and one case each of lung abscess, broncho- pleural fistula, radiation esophagitis, and fatal lung fail- ure. Post-operative radiotherapy was accomplished without difficulty. Adjuvant CAP would not be completed in all patients because of compliance and subjective toxicity (chronic fatigue, weight loss and anorrhexia).

Patterns of failure can be summarized as follows:

TABLE 4. PATTERNS OF FAILURE IN ALL 41 PATIENTS

Progressive disease	-	3
Relapse	-	16
? relapse (no autopsy)	-	2
Fatal stroke	-	1
Fatal post-op lung failure	-	1
Death from myeloma	-	1
No relapse	-	17(41%)

Disease relapse to date in 16 patients (44% of 36 sur- gical cases) was distributed as follows: CNS only - 3; chest only - 2; extra thoracic - 5; multiple sites - 6. Since prophylactic cranial radiotherapy was added to the protocol, no CNS relapses have occurred. The median follow-up of living patients is 2 years with 11 patients followed for 30+ months. Of 11 patients presenting with superior sulcus or chest wall lesions (T_3), 6 (55%) are disease-free with a median follow-up time of 31+ months, while of the remaining 30 patients, 12 (40% are disease-free with a median follow- up time of 29+ months.

COMMENT

While considerable progress has occurred in the man- agement of patients with advanced NSCLC, including improved chemotherapy programs (Hoffman, et al 1983) and demonstra- tion of a dose-response effect with radiotherapy including the need for careful technique (Choi, et al 1981; Perez, et al 1982), long term survival has not dramatically improved. Treatment failure is mainly due to distant metastases, although local control can be a significant problem with inadequate radiotherapy (Mountain, et al 1980; Perez, et al 1982). In our study, we have attempted to define patients with marginally resectable Stage III disease, who can then be treated aggressively with curative intent. The CAP chemotherapy resulted in a high initial regression rate of 76% (PR = 43%, MR = 33%) and after radiotherapy surgical resection without gross residual disease was possible in all but 1 patient. The rationale for so-called neoadjuvant chemotherapy has been discussed in detail (Frei 1982) and relates to control of micro-metastases as well as increasing the local control of the primary cancer by surgery and/or radiotherapy. The median survival of our patients of 31+ months is encouraging and may translate into a significant improvement in long-term survival for patients with Stage III M_0 marginally resectable disease. An earlier study at our Center in patients with marginally resectable NSCLC employing pre-op radiotherapy followed by surgery showed a median survival of 24 mo. (Sherman, et al 1978). While the survival curve for Pancoast/chest wall lesions (T_3) in the present study appears to be similar to other sites (N_2) longer follow-up will be required before firm conclusions can be made. Patients with Pancoast (superior sulcus) tumors have a better prognosis than other categories of NSCLC with a reported 5-yr. survival rate of 35% after pre-op radiotherapy and aggressive surgery (Paulson 1975).

Patients with more advanced limited Stage III disease (including bilateral mediastinal metastases and unilateral supraclavicular nodes) which are "categorically" unresectable, treated by us with CAP and radiotherapy (Fram, Skarin et al 1985) have a poor prognosis with a median survival of only 9 mo. More effective chemotherapy regimens are required before the overall prognosis for all patients with Stage III limited disease can be improved.

REFERENCES

Caldwell WL, Bashaw MA (1968). Indication for and Results of Irradiation of Carcinoma of the LUng. Cancer 22:999.
Choi NCH, Doucette JA (1981). Improved Survival of Patients with Unresectable Non-Small-Cell Bronchogenic Carcinoma by an Innovated High-Dose En-Bloc Radiotherapeutic Approach. Cancer 48:101.

Eagan RT, Ingle JN, Frytak S (1977). Platinum-based poly-chemotherapy versus dianhydrogalactitol in advanced non-small cell lung cancer. Cancer Treat Rep 61:1339.

Eagan RT, Lee RE, Frytak S, Scott M, Ingle JN, Creagan ET, Nichols WC (1981). Thoracic radiation therapy and Adriamycin/cisplatin-containing chemotherapy for locally advanced non-small-cell lung cancer. Cancer Clin Trials 2:381.

Fram R, Skarin A, Balikian J, Amato D, Leslie N, Malcolm A, Frei E III (1985). Combination Chemotherapy Followed by Radiation Therapy in Patients with Regional Stage III Un-resectable Non-Small Cell Lung Cancer. Cancer Treatment Reports (In Press).

Frei E III (1982). Clinical Cancer Research: An Embattled Species. Cancer 50:1979.

Hellman S, Kligerman MD, Von Essen DF (1964). Sequelae of Radical Radiotherapy of Carcinoma of the Lung. Radiol 82: 1055.

Hoffman PC, Bitran JD, Golomb HM (1983). Chemotherapy of Metastatic Non-Small Cell Bronchogenic Carcinoma. Seminars in Onc 10:111.

Martini N, Flehinger BJ, Zaman MB, Beattie EJ (1980). Pro-spective study of 445 lung carcinomas with mediastinal lymph node metastases. J Thorac Cardiovasc Surg 80:390.

Mountain CF, McMurtrey MJ, Frazier OH (1980). Regional Extension of Lung Cancer. Int J Radiation Oncol Biol Phys 6:1013.

Overholt RH, Neptune W, Ashraf M (1975). Cancer of the Lung - A 42 year Experience. Am Thor Surg 20:5.

Paulson DL (1975). Carcinomas in the superior pulmonary sulcus. J Thorac Cardiovasc Surg 70:1095.

Perez CA, Stanley K, Grundy G, Hanson W, Rubin P, Kramer S, Brady LW, Marks JE, Perez-Tamayo R, Brown S, Concannon JP, Rotman M (1982). Impact of Irradiation Technique and Tumor Extent in Tumor Control and Survival of Patients with Unresectable Non-Oat Cell Carcinoma of the Lung. Cancer 50:1091.

Petrovich A, Stanley K, Cox JD, Paig C (1981). Radiotherapy in the Management of Locally Advanced Lung Cancer of All Cell Types: Final Report of a Randomized Trial. Cancer 48:1335.

Sherman DM, Neptune W, Weichselbaum R, Order SE, Piro AJ (1978). An Aggressive Approach to Marginally Resectable Lung Cancer. Cancer 41:2040.

Takita H, Hollinshead AC, Rizzo DJ, Kramer CM, Chen TY, Bhayana JN, Edgerton F (1979). Treatment of Inoperable Lung Carcinoma: A Combined Modality Approach. Ann Tho-racic Surg 28:363.

Primary Chemotherapy in Cancer Medicine, pages 133-139
© 1985 Alan R. Liss, Inc.

CHEMOTHERAPY PRECEDING RADIOTHERAPY IN STAGE III
NON-SMALL CELL LUNG CANCER

Jacques A. Wils[*], Irwan Utama[+], Andre Naus[++] and
Tom A. Verschueren[$]

*Departments of Internal Medicine, [+]Pulmonary
Diseases and [++]Biochemistry, St. Laurentius
Hospital, 6043 CV Roermond, The Netherlands and
[$]Radiotherapeutisch Instituut Limburg,
6419 PC Heerlen, The Netherlands

ABSTRACT

Thirty-seven patients with stage III non-small cell lung
cancer were treated with the sequential administration of
chemotherapy, consisting of Cisplatinum, VP-16 and Adriamycin, and radiotherapy. The response rate in 33 evaluable
patients was 82 percent. The median survival for all evaluable patients was 11 months; 5 patients actually survived
more than 24 months but all ultimately relapsed. It is concluded that treatment of advanced non-small cell lung cancer with the currently available tools is still unsatisfactory. Despite a high response rate our treatment protocol
had only a modest impact on survival. Obviously, a concert-
ed effort will be required to improve these results and
will probably involve the development of new and better
drugs.

INTRODUCTION

Non-small cell lung cancer (NSLC) is generally considered
relatively refractory to chemotherapy. In stage III NSLC
(TNM classification, UICC, Genova, 1978) radiotherapy is
considered by many physicians as the treatment of choice.
However, in recent years high response rates have been reported in NSLC using combination chemotherapy with Cisplat-

inum and Vindesine or VP-16 [1,2]. Regimens containing Adriamycin without Vindesine or VP-16 have also produced a significant percentage of response[3]. In an earlier study we
demonstrated that the sequential use of chemotherapy and
radiotherapy is better than radiotherapy alone[4]. After a-
nalysis of that study, all further patients with stage III
NSLC were treated with the combined modality. We now report
our final results after a median follow-up period of 32
months.

PATIENTS AND METHODS

Between July 1979 and July 1984, 51 eligible patients were
diagnosed as having stage III NSLC which, according to the
TNM classification, includes all $T_{1-3}N_2M_0$ tumors. In table
1 the patient eligibility criteria are shown. The first 33
patients were treated with a randomized phase II trial comparing the sequential use of chemotherapy and radiotherapy
with radiotherapy alone. Analysis of this study demonstrated significantly superior survival with the combined modality treatment (11 vs 5 months); therefore the following
18 patients were also treated with chemotherapy preceding
irradiation, resulting in a total of 37 patients who received the combined modality treatment. Irradiation was
given by linear accelerator (photons of 5Mv) with an initial target volume encompassing both the tumour and areas
of lymphnode drainage, including the supraclavicular re-
gions. In 2.5 Gy daily fractions given 4 times a week with
AP and PA portals, a total target dose was given of 45.0 Gy.
The second part of the treatment consisted of an additional
15.0 Gy using the same scheme on a smaller target volume,
encompassing the primary and the adjacent part of the
mediastinum but not the spinal cord. The total dose was
therefore 60.0 Gy. The patients who were subsequently
treated with cytostatic drugs received the same treatment
policy, but the total target dose in the initial plan was
reduced to 40.0 Gy and the additional dose in the second
part of the treatment to 10.0 Gy. Each treatment plan was
designed with the aid of a computer assisted planning
system.
Chemotherapy consisted of Cisplatinum, 60 mg/m^2 , day 1,
i.v.; Adriamycin, 40 mg/m^2, day 1, i.v.; and VP-16, 200 mg,
i.v., day 1 and 200 mg orally on days 3 and 5. Cycles were
repeated every 4 weeks. In patients who received the combi-

nation of chemotherapy and radiotherapy, 2 cycles of chemotherapy were given before radiotherapy and 4 cycles thereafter. The time interval between chemotherapy and radiotherapy was 4 weeks.

TABLE 1 Eligibility Criteria

Histologically proven stage III non-small cell lung cancer

Age $\leq$ 70 years

Karnofsky index $\geq$ 70%

No previous treatment with chemotherapy or radiotherapy

Complete response was defined as total disappearance of all evidence of tumour. Because of the difficulty in measuring lesions demonstrated on chest X-rays, especially after radiotherapy, a partial remission was defined as a clear decrease in size of the lesions seen on X-rays, agreed upon by two investigators. It has been shown that the clinical outcome in patients with measurable or evaluable disease is the same [2,5]. Progression was defined as an increase in tumour volume of 25% or more, or the appearance of new lesions.

RESULTS

In table 2 the patient characteristics are shown. Of the 37 eligible patients 4 were considered to be not evaluable because of early death, within 4 weeks of starting the treatment. In table 3 a summary of the results is given. Twenty-seven patients showed an objective response while in 5 patients a complete response was observed. The median duration of response was 10 months and the median overall survival 11 months. The median follow-up for all patients is now 32 months. Five patients actually survived for more than 2 years but all of them ultimately relapsed.

Table 2. Patient characteristics

Entered	37
Not evaluable	4
Number of evaluable patients	33
Median age (range)	63 (41-70)
Median Karnofsky index (range)	80 (70-100)
Median weight loss (range)	5% (0-10%)
Histology	
Squamous	27
Adenocarcinoma	3
Large cell anaplastic	3

Table 3. Results

CR	5/33
PR	22/33
CR + PR	27/33
Median duration of response	10 months
Median survival (all patients)	11 months

Figure 1 shows the survival curve for all patients.

The toxicity of the chemotherapy schedule was considerable, with gastro-intestinal disturbances and alopecia seen in

almost all cases. Hematological problems which were generally manageable, manifested themselves primarily as anaemia;
packed cells were given if hemoglobin concentration fell to
less than 6.0 mmol/l. Dose reductions according to the
nadir of the leucocytes were not made. Only very few patients had leucocyte nadirs of less than $1.0 \times 10^9/1$ and
all had full recovery upon the next scheduled course. There
was no clinical renal toxicity and there were no toxic
deaths.
The radiotherapy was well tolerated and no major complications of the myelum, heart and lungs were observed.

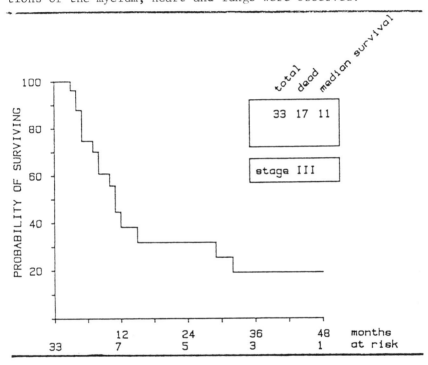

Figure 1. Survival curve (Kaplan-Meier) for all evaluable
         patients.

DISCUSSION

For patients with NSLC, chemotherapy with Cisplatinum and
VP-16 or Vindesine had been reported to give a relatively
high incidence of remission. It has been suggested that the
addition of a third drug, such as Adriamycin, which was used

in this study, does not enhance therapeutic results[6]. However, the data on the activity of Adriamycin used in combination regimens in NSLC are conflicting[3,7,8].
It is the general practice in oncology to compare responders with non-responders. The survival benefit which is found for responders is then easily interpreted as a result of the treatment. However, the finding of a longer survival in responders must be cautiously interpreted. It may well be that patients respond and have a longer survival because of unknown biological factors and thereby have an inherently better prognosis. The only way to show that treatment itself prolongs survival is to compare the overall survival of a treated group of patients with a matched control group, ideally executed in a randomized trial. Therefore, the response rate in NSLC must not be overemphasized, as overall survival is the most important treatment parameter.

There have been a number of published non-randomized trials focusing on the combined use of chemotherapy and radiotherapy; most of these studies employed chemotherapy following radiotherapy. We have performed a randomized trial comparing chemotherapy preceding irradiation with radiotherapy alone and have found significantly better survival for the combined modality. However, the median survival of 11 months for all patients who were treated with chemotherapy preceding irradiation remains rather low. About 30 percent may survive 2 years, but at this point, all our surviving patients (survival time > 2 yrs) have relapsed.
In conclusion, we feel that for stage III NSLC patients with a relatively good performance status, the sequential use of chemotherapy and radiotherapy is better than radiotherapy alone. It is obvious that further studies are needed to improve therapeutic results in patients with advanced NSLC.

REFERENCES

1. Gralla RJ, Casper ES, Kelsen DP et al.
   Cisplatinum and vindesine combination chemotherapy for advanced carcinoma of the lung: a randomized trial investigating two dosage schedules.
   Ann Intern Med 1981, 95, 414-420.

2. Longeval E, Klastersky J.
   Combination chemotherapy with cisplatinum and eteposide

in bronchogenic squamous cell carcinoma and adenocarcinoma.
Cancer 1982, 50, 2751 - 2756.

3. Britell JC, Eagan RT, Ingle IN et al.
Cis-dichlorodiammineplatinum alone followed by Adriamycin plus cyclophosphamide at progression versus cis-dichlorodiammineplatinum, Adriamycin and cyclophosphamide in combination for adenocarcinoma of the lung.
Canc Treat Rep 1978, 62, 1207 - 1210.

4. Wils JA, Utama I, Naus A, Verschueren TA.
Phase II randomized trial of radiotherapy alone versus the sequential use of chemotherapy and radiotherapy in stage III non-small cell lung cancer. Phase II trial of chemotherapy alone in stage IV non-small cell lung cancer.
Eur J Cancer Clin Oncol 1984, 20, 911 - 914.

5. Eagan RT, Fleming TR, Schoonover V.
Evaluation of response criteria in advanced lung cancer.
Cancer 1979, 44, 1125 - 1128.

6. Klastersky J.
Therapy of non-small cell bronchogenic carcinoma; the experience of the EORTC lung cancer working party (Belgium).
Proc of 13th Int Congress of Chemotherapy, Vienna, 1983, 205, 53 - 57.

7. Luedke DW, Luedke SL, Petruska P et al.
A randomized prospective study of vindesine versus doxorubicin and cyclophosphamide in the treatment of epidermoid lung cancer.
Cancer 1983, 51, 778 - 782.

8. Wils JAMJ, Ribot JG.
Sequential combination of vincristine, adriamycin and cyclophosphamide (VAC) and radiotherapy in advanced non-small cell lung cancer.
Neth J of Med 1982, 25, 43 - 46.

Primary Chemotherapy in Cancer Medicine, pages 141–152
© 1985 Alan R. Liss, Inc.

RADIOTHERAPY OF SMALL CELL LUNG CANCER. AN ANALYSIS WITH
SPECIAL REFERENCE TO AUTOPSY FINDINGS

Heine H. Hansen, M.D., Kell Østerlind, M.D.
A. Gersel Pedersen, M.D., John Elliott, M.D.
Department of Oncology II
Finsen Institute, 49, Strandboulevarden 49
DK-2100 Copenhagen, Denmark

Treatment with chemotherapy either alone or combined
with radiotherapy has become standard management for patients
with small cell lung cancer (SCLC). This mode of treatment
yields an overall tumor response of approximately 80-90%
with 25-40% achieving a complete remission of their disease.
Most studies demonstrate an overall median survival around
14-16 months for patients initially having limited disease
and 9-11 months for patients with extensive disease. Only
5-10% of all patients achieve prolonged disease-free
survival (1). Substantial improvement has thus occurred in
the overall management, however, the majority of patients
relapse and die of their disease. In view of these disappointing results a variety of treatment strategies have been
suggested as possible ways of improving the therapeutic efficacy of the currently available treatment modalities. These focus in particularly on an improvement of the systemic
treatment with combination chemotherapy with application of
more intensive induction treatments, "late intensification",
kinetic scheduling of drugs, high-dose chemotherapy with
autologous bone-marrow rescue and cyclic alternating non-
cross-resistant chemotherapy. All these concepts are at
present under active investigation in small cell carcinoma
together with the development of new active cytostatic agents.

The role of purely localized therapeutic modalities such
as radiotherapy and surgery has been an issue of increasing
interest during the last years, in connection with the development of better systemic treatment. It is the purpose of
this paper to analyse the role of radiotherapy to the primary treatment of SCLC both with respect to chest irradiation

and CNS-irradiation and particularly the influence of radiotherapy on the patterns of failure and thereby also its implication for future therapy.

In general, the major object of most therapeutic trials
of SCLC has been to concentrate on the improvement of tumor
response rates and the survival. It is recognized that both
of these are important factors but a careful analysis of the
reasons for treatment failure in SCLC is just as important
as a means of guiding planned modifications to existing
therapy in order to bring about improved disease control.
The progressive evolution of treatment strategy in Hodgkin's
disease is a good example of the value of such an approach.

Reliability of Patterns of Failure

Attempts to assess patterns of treatment failure are
immediately met with certain difficulties. Both clinical
and autopsy studies can provide useful information, but
each approach has its limitations. Analysed clinically,
treatment failure is usually expressed in terms of the first
site or sites of disease progression. Detection of relapse
is thus biased by the procedures, which are available or
which are more or less arbitrarily chosen by the investigator in the evaluation of disease. Inevitably such an approach
will underestimate the true extent of treatment failure, as
metastatic disease at many sites will escape detection and
the true extent of treatment failure as metastatic disease
will not be disclosed. Thus the clinical relapse pattern
will be determined at least in part by the methods and the
thoroughness of clinical evaluation. Relapse at sites which
readily give rise to symptoms or at sites which are readily
assessed by a routine restaging investigations will undoubt-
ly be overrepresented, whilst relapse at sites which tend
to remain clinically silent will be underrepresented in such
a study. Furthermore, the evidence for clinical relapse is
usually indirect and may be unreliable. The reliability of
clinical data will be influenced by the varying and often
modest sensitivity and specificity of the various procedures that are used for the evaluation. Of interest is a study of 30 patients with SCLC where pathological findings at
autopsy were correlated with the results of clinical evaluation just before death (2). Chest radiographic findings
were accurate in diagnosing the presence or absence of par-
enchymal, mediastinal and pleural disease in 87%, 70% and

63% of cases, respectively. Physical examination was accurate in the evaluation of hepatic metastases in only 52% of patients, although accuracy was improved by the addition of isotopic liver scanning and serum liver function tests. The diagnosis of local recurrence is especially problematic after thoracic irradiation when radiographic changes secondary to radiation-induced fibrosis may lead to misinterpretation. Nevertheless, by pointing to the first site of treatment failure, meticulous clinical studies can indicate particular locations where disease control is especially poor and at which more effective therapy should be specifically directed.

Autopsy evaluation permits a more thorough assessment of the true extent of treatment failure but often weeks or months after the first treatment failure has occurred. The routine sampling undertaken at post-mortem examinations may furthermore lead to insufficient screening of specific sites, especially the skeleton and the central nervous system. This insufficiency is reflected by a wide range of values for metastases to specific sites due to different sampling procedures employed in individual institutions.

How the pattern of disease spread is influenced by the effect of a variable duration of time without specific antineoplastic treatment prior to death has never been evaluated. The extent of spread of disease may become relatively independing of, and therefore fail to reflect the influence of prior therapy.

Post-mortem evaluation gives however, histological proof of residual disease and provides a necessary complement to clinically derived data. With these qualifications and shortcomings in mind both clinical and autopsy studies are considered in relation to use of radiotherapy in the treatment of SCLC.

Thoracic Irradiation

Small cell lung cancer is the most radiosensitive histologic subtype of bronchial carcinoma. Regression of the intrathoracic tumor greater than 50% has been documented in 80-90% of prior treated patients with SCLC receiving a variety of radiotherapy schedules (3, 4). Despite its apparent sensitivity, thoracic irradiation alone has no significant impact upon the median survival of patients with SCLC although occasional long-term survivors are seen.

In analysing early data focusing on radiotherapy alone, it is quite evident that SCLC failure after radiotherapy alone relates both to distant sites and to local recurrence as pointed out in several articles from the late 1970ties (5, 6, 7).

With the introduction of effective chemotherapy the possibility to control even disseminated disease emerged and new studies were necessary to define the role of radiotherapy to the primary chest tumor in patients with no clinical evidence of extrathoracic dissemination.

The high frequency of primary site relapse in small cell lung cancer treated by chemotherapy alone inevitably led to the concept of integrating local irradiation with systemic treatment. The objective was to obtain more effective long-term local tumor control and with this, improved survival. The results of several major combined modality studies have now been reported as shown in table 1 even some of the results are preliminary and not published in extent. Comparing median survival no difference is observed and no distinct tendency is observed either in the data available at 2 or 5 years survival respectively.

Table 1. Selected randomized trials of chemotherapy versus chemotherapy plus radiotherapy

No. pts	MST Months		% alive at 2-years		% alive at 5-years		Study period	Comments	Reference
	CT	CT+RT	CT	CT+RT	CT	CT+RT			
32	12	11.5	N.A.*		N.A.			limit.dis.	Stevens et al. (8)
154	11.5	10.5	11	8	4	3	1976-1979	abstract + unpubl. data	Finsen group (9)
84	14.5	14.5	N.A.		N.A.		1977-1979	-	Fox et al. (10)
63	12	17	15	32	N.A.		1977 -	ongoing trial	NCI-VA Group (11)
25	11	9	8	0			1975-1976	all pts had extensive disease	Williams et al. (12)
371	7.5	81	8	8	N.A.		1979-1982	all stages	Souhami et al. (13)
304	11	14	N.A.		N.A.		1978-1982	preliminary report. All pts had limited disease.	Perez et al. (14)

x not available.

In all studies the clinical relapse pattern indicates that combined modality of treatment using chest irradiation plus chemotherapy significantly decreases the local relapse rate. On the other hand autopsy data from 6 studies of patients with irradiated SCLC indicate that regional tumor persists in a substantial proportion of patients following radiotherapy (table 2). In these studies dose and schedule of radiotherapy vary considerable. Unfortunately, there are no major clinical studies, in wich a systemic analysis of the reasons for radiotherapeutic failure has been assessed in relation to irradiation dose, fractionation, adequacy of treatment fields and tumor bulk, even though it is often stressed that these characteristics of radiation therapy have an important influence on response, site of relapse and survival in SCLC (20).

Table 2. Autopsy incidence of residual tumor after thoracic irradiation

No. of patients	XRT dose schedule	No. with residual tumor at primary site (%)	Reference
27	30-40 gray, 20 fractions in 4 wks	21 (78%)	Deeley (1966) (15)
17	45-70 gray in 5-10 wks	11 (65%)	Rissanen et al. (1968) (16)
7	Not given	2 (29%)	Abadir and Muggia (1975) (17)
13[a]	30 gray in 2 wks or 50-60 gray in 7-9 wks	10 (77%)	Ajaikumar and (18) Barkley
18	30 gray, 15 fractions in 3 wks	14 (78%)	MRC Lung Cancer (7) Working Party (1981)
99[b]	40 gray - split-course	81 (82%)	Finsen Group (1985) (19)

a) patients also received single agent chemotherapy
b) all patients also received combination chemotherapy with 3-4 drugs

Autopsy data from randomized trials are scarce, but of interest are the data from the randomized Finsen study as presented in table 3. It is noteworthy that significantly fewer patients had invasion of the pericardium following radiotherapy than did patients, who received no radiotherapy. On the other hand patients, who received combined chemo- and radiotherapy had significantly higher degree of non-malig-

nant pericarditis indicating a detrimental effect of the combined modality of treatment. Overall the results of post-
mortem examinations confirm the relatively ineffectiveness
of local irradiation in sterilizing the intrathoracic disease, when it is given as a part of a combined modality
schedule. The explanation of this is unclear. Tumor dose is
certainly an important factor. In a combined modality study
reported by Choi and Carey, local control rate assessed clinically increased with increasing tumor dose from 60% with
tumor dose of 30 Gy to 80% control with a tumor dose of 48
Gy (21). Holoye et al. reported local recurrence in only 1
of 16 patients (6%) receiving 60 Gy (22). However, the correlation between the total dose of irradiation and local
control is not close and other factors undoubtfully contribute to local control. It has been suggested that many radiation failures may be a result of reseeding of tumor cells
from metastatic sites or may represent marginal recurrence.

Table 3.   Results of post-mortem examinations in 44 patients who received
chemotherapy and 46 patients who received combined chemo-
and radiotherapy ₓ

	Chemotherapy	Chemo- and radiotherapy	
Patterns in patients with residual tumor: (fractions and per cent)			
Primary site	31/41 (76)	30/38 (79)	NS
Mediastinal glands	30/40 (75)	24/36 (67)	NS
Pleura	12/43 (28)	10/39 (26)	NS
Pericardium	12/43 (28)	3/45 (7)	p = 0.02
Non-malignant pericarditis	6/44 (14)	14/16 (30)	p = 0.05
Abdominal glands	9/33 (27)	5/21 (24)	NS
Liver	30/43 (70)	23/39 (59)	NS
Adrenals	12/43 (28)	13/39 (33)	NS
Bone-marrow	8/27 (30)	6/22 (27)	NS
Brain	14/33 (42)	12/28 (43)	NS

(NS: No significant difference - 95% confidence limits)
ₓ Data modified from Elliott et al. (19)

If reseeding was the cause one would expect a slightly different distribution of metastases to the lung with a higher
percentage of peripheral pulmonary lesions. It is possible
that the schedule of radiotherapy in combined modality treat-

ment programs might influence upon both local control and toxicity. Further controlled clinical studies are necessary in order to identify the optimal approach achieving the maximum local control without compromising the ability to administer sufficient chemotherapy to eliminate distant metastases. A careful registration of autopsy findings in these clinical studies are also needed in order to shed some additional light on this important issue.

It should also be emphasized that the contribution of local radiotherapy in combined modality schedule might be increased by the use of CT-scanner in the planning, although its contribution to the efficiency of local radiotherapy of SCLC has not yet been assessed. Improved local disease control may also be obtained by the use of other types of irradiation such as neutrons, negative pi-mesons, and other types of high linear energy transfer radiation although these means will be outside the scope of most institutions. The use of radiosensitisers has turned out to be less efficient than first believed while hyperthermia is still in an investigative phase.

CNS-metastases

The management of CNS-metastases from SCLC poses an increasingly important problem. The inability of most chemotherapeutic agents to penetrate the blood brain barrier, together with therapeutic advances resulting in prolonged survival, has led to an increase in the frequency of CNS-metastases.

CNS-relapse usually accompanies progression of systemic disease but may also be the primary site of failure. Primary CNS-relapse is however, often soon followed by progression of systemic disease and reports of CNS-metastases as the only autopsy evidence of disease in patients dying in complete systemic remissions are uncommon (8-10%). Thus, the majority of CNS-metastases is diagnosed either at presentation, at autopsy or in association with progression of systemic disease, and only the minority of CNS-metastases presents as the only site of relapse.

Nevertheless the occurrence of CNS-relapse is associated with considerable morbidity and should be prevented if possible. The prediction that some form of CNS-prophylaxis would be necessary together with systemic therapy as patient survival improved appears to have been accurate (23), but the exact place of such therapy in the overall management of SCLC remains uncertain. There is good evidence from both nonrandomized and randomized studies that prophylactic cranial irradiation (PCI) will effectively delay or prevent CNS-recurrence. The combined results of 11 non-randomized studies including 355 patients yielded a CNS-relapse rate of only 8% after PCI (24).

In some randomized studies, PCI produced a statistically significant decrease in the rate of CNS-relapses (25,26, 27,28). In non-randomized trials autopsy findings have confirmed the protective effect of PCI. Matthews reported a 29% incidence of CNS-metastases after PCI, compared with a 63% incidence of CNS-disease without PCI (29). However, in a randomized controlled trial the Finsen group was not able to demonstrate significant difference of brain metastases in the group of patients, who received PCI compared to the patients who did not receive PCI. However, when compared to larger cumulated groups of patients PCI seemed to reduce the risk of brain metastases (19).

None of the trials have demonstrated any prolongation of median survival in PCI treated patients. This is of course hardly surprising as a survival benefit will only be expected in the few patients in whom CNS-relapse is presented. Our present inability to control systemic disease in the majority of patients effectively limits the application of PCI. It would therefore seem reasonable to restrict its use to patients achieving a complete remission. More recently, however, an increasing number of reports have been reported on late CNS-complications secondary to prophylactic PCI, including a psycho-neurologic syndrom characterized by personality changes and confusion (30, 37, 32). Advantages and adverse effects of PCI in patients having achieved a complete remission thus have to be defined and it is awaiting a prospective randomized trial which should include a careful evaluation not only of survival and clinical and post-mortem relapse pattern, but also an evaluation of neuro-psychiatric status of the patients.

In summary very few conclusions concerning the use of elective thoracic and cranial irradiation can be drawn, but the use of thoracic irradiation might improve local disease control when given in adequate dosis in patients with limited disease as evidenced by decreasing local recurrence rate and it might also improve the prospects for long-term survival when applied with intensive combination chemotherapy. Improvement in radiotherapy techniques may also contribute in the future to increase local control. CNS-prophylaxis in the form of cranial irradiation may be worthwile as an elective procedure in patients with complete response, although considerable toxicity may turn out to restrict the benefit.

Distant metastatic spread is however still the dominant factor in the failure to cure patients with apparent localized disease of SCLC and the patterns of failure and the autopsy data clearly points to the need for the development of more effective systemic treatment with new chemotherapeutic regimens.

1. Hansen HH (1982). Management of small-cell anaplastic carcinoma, 1980-1982. In Ishikawa S. Hayata Y, Suemasu K (eds): "Lung Cancer 1982", Amsterdam, Excerpta Medica, pp 31-54.
2. Chak LY, Daniels JR, Sikic BI, Torti FM, Lockbaum P, Carter SK (1982). Patterns of failure in small cell carcinoma of the lung. Cancer 50: 1857.
3. Carr DT, Childs DS Jr, Lee RE (1972). Radiotherapy plus 5-FU compared to radiotherapy alone for inoperable and unresectable bronchogenic carcinoma. Cancer 29: 375.
4. Salazar OM, Rubin P, Brown JC, Feldstein ML, Keller BE (1976). Predictors of radiation response in lung cancer: a clinicopathological analysis. Cancer 37: 2636.
5. Cox JD, Byhardt RW, Wilson FJ, Komaki R, Eisert DR, Green berg M (1978). Dose-time relationships and the local control of small-cell carcinoma of the lung. Radiology 128: 205.
6. Stanley K, Cox JD, Petrovich Z, Paig C (1981). Patterns of failure in patients with inoperable carcinoma of the lung. Cancer 47: 2725.
7. Medical Research Council Lung Cancer Working Party (1981). Radiotherapy alone or with chemotherapy in the treatment of small-cell carcinoma of the lung: the results at 36 months. Br J Cancer 44: 611.
8. Stevens E, Einhorn L, Rohn R (1979). Treatment of limited small cell lung cancer. Proc. Am Ass Cancer Res/Am Soc Clin Oncol 20: 435.
9. Hansen HH, Dombernowsky P, Hansen HS, Rørth M (1979). Chemotherapy versus chemotherapy plus radiotherapy in regional small-cell carcinoma of the lung. Proc Am Ass Cancer Res/Am Soc Clin Oncol 20: 277.
10. Fox RM, Woods RL, Brodie GN, Tattersall MH (1980). A ran-

domized study: small cell anaplastic lung cancer treated by combination chemotherapy and adjuvant radiotherapy. Int J Radiat Oncol Biol Phys 6: 1087.

11. Cohen MH, Lichter AS, Bunn PA, Jr., Glatstein EJ, Ihde DC, Fossieck BE, Jr., Matthews MJ, Minna JD (1980). Chemotherapy-radiation therapy (CT-RT) versus chemotherapy (CT) in limited small cell lung cancer (SCLC). Proc Am Ass Cancer Res/Am Soc Clin Oncol 21: 448.

12. Williams C, Alexander M, Glatstein EJ, Daniels JR (1977). Role of radiation therapy in combination with chemotherapy in extensive oat cell cancer of the lung: a randomized study. Cancer Treat Rep 61: 1427.

13. Souhami RL, Geddes DM, Spiro SG, Harper PG, Tobias JS, Mantell BS, Fearon F, Bradbury I (1984). Radiotherapy in small cell cancer of the lung treated with combination chemotherapy: a controlled trial. Brit Med J 288: 1643.

14. Perez CA, Einhorn LE, Oldham RK, Greco FA, Cohen HJ, Silberman H, Krauss S, Hornback N, Comas F, Omura G, Salter M, Keller JW, McLaren J, Kellermeyer R, Storaasli J, Birch R, Dandy M (1984). Randomized trial of radiotherapy to the thorax in limited small-cell carcinoma of the lung treated with multiagent chemotherapy and elective brain irradiation: A-preliminary report. J.Clin Oncol 2: 1200.

15. Deeley TJ (1966). A clinical trial to compare two different tumour dose levels in the treatment of advanced carcinoma of the bronchus. Clin Radiol 17: 299.

16. Rissanen PM, Tikka V, Holsti LR (1968). Autopsy findings in lung cancer treated with megavoltage radiotherapy. Acta Radiol Oncol Radiat Phys Biol 7: 433.

17. Abadir R, Muggia FM (1975). Irradiated lung cancer. Radiology 114: 427.

18. Ajaikumar BS, Barkley HT, Jr. (1979). The role of radiation therapy in the treatment of small cell undifferentiated bronchogenic carcinoma. Int.J Radiat Oncol Biol Phys 5: 977.

19. Elliott JA, Østerlind K, Hirsch FR, Hansen HH (1985). Metastatic patterns in small cell lung cancer. Correlation of autopsy findings with clinical parameters in 537 patients. J Clin Oncol. In press.

20. White JE, Chen T, McCracken J, Kennedy P, Seydel HG, Hartman G, Mira J, Khan M, Durrance FY, Skinner O (1982). The influence of radiation therapy quality control on survival, response and sites of relapse in oat cell carcinoma of the lung. Cancer 50: 1084.

21. Choi CH, Carey RW (1976). Small cell anaplastic carcino-

ma of the lung: reappraisal of current management. Cancer 37: 2651.

22. Holoye PY, Samuels ML, Lanzotti VJ, Smith T, Barkley HT Jr. (1977). Combination chemotherapy and radiation therapy for small cell carcinoma. JAMA 237: 1221.

23. Hansen HH (1973). Should initial treatment of small cell carcinoma include systemic chemotherapy and brain irradiation? Cancer Chemother Rep 4: 239.

24. Bunn PA, Jr., Nugens JL, Matthews MJ (1978). Central nervous system metastases in small cell bronchogenic carcinoma. Semin Oncol 5: 314.

25. Jackson DV, Jr., Richards F II, Cooper MR et al. (1977). Prophylactic cranial irradiation in small cell carcinoma of the lung. A randomized study. JAMA 237: 2730-2733.

26. Maurer LH, Tulloh M, Weiss RB et al. (1980). A randomized combined modality trial in small cell carcinoma of the lung: comparison of combination chemotherapy-radiation therapy versus cyclophosphamide-radiation therapy effects of maintenance chemotherapy and prophylactic whole brain irradiation. Cancer 45: 30.

27. Beiler DD, Kane RC, Bernath AM, Cashdollar MR (1979). Low dose elective brain irradiation in small cell carcinoma of the lung. Int.J.Radiat Oncol Biol Phys 5: 941.

28. Aroney RS, Aisner J, Wesley MN, Whitacre MY, Van Echo DA, Slawson RG, Wiernik PH (1983). Value of prophylactic cranial irradiation given at complete remission in small cell lung carcinoma. Cancer Treat Rep 67: 675.

29. Matthews MJ (1979). Effects of therapy on the morphology and behaviour of small cell carcinoma of the lung: a clinico-pathologic study. In: Muggia F, Rozencweig M (eds) Lung Cancer: Progress in therapeutic research. New York, Raven, pp. 155-165.

30. Johnson BE, Ihde DC, Lichter AS, Johnston-Early A, Cohen MH, Walsh T, Weinstein Z, Becker B, Whang-Peng J, Glatstein E, Carney DN, Minna JD, Bunn PA (1984). Five to 10 year follow-up of small cell lung cancer (SCLC) patients disease free at 30 months: Chronic toxicities and late relapses. Proc Am Ass Cancer Res/Am Soc Clin Oncol 3: 218.

31. Lee JS, Lee YY, Umsawasdi T, Welch S, Kalter S, Farha P, Murphy WK, Valdivieso M (1984). Neurotoxicity (NT) in long-term survivors (LTS) of small cell lung cancer (SCLC). Proc Am Ass Cancer Res/Am Soc Clin Oncol 3: 220.

32. Sculier JP, Feld R, Evans WK, Shepherd FA, Payne DG, Pringle J, Yeoh JL, Quirt IC, Curtis JE, Myers R, Herman JG, De Boer G (1984).Neurological complications in pa-

tients (PTS) with small cell lung cancer (SCLC). Proc Am
Ass Cancer Res/Am Soc Clin Oncol 3: 222.

SECTION V
HEAD AND NECK CANCER

Primary Chemotherapy in Cancer Medicine, pages 155–157
© 1985 Alan R. Liss, Inc.

NEOADJUVANT CHEMOTHERAPY FOR HEAD AND NECK CANCER
INTRODUCTION

Paul van den Broek, M.D.

Chairman Dept. of Otorhinolaryngology

Nijmegen, The Netherlands

Head and neck cancer comprises about 4% of all malignant tumors. For a country such as Holland, with 14 million
inhabitants, this represents about 1600 new cases per year.
The most frequently occurring tumors are those of the upper
respiratory and digestive passages and these therefore have
an important inpact on vital primary functions like breathing,
speaking and eating and also of course on cosmetic concerns.
Anatomically they form a very diverse group; the most common
sites are the larynx and the oral cavity. Other less frequently involved sites are the naso-, oro- and hypopharynx,
nose and sinuses, salivary glands and the ear. However, the
distribution of the various anatomical sites can differ
widely with geographical location.

More than 75% of the tumors are squamous cell carcinomas, while the other 25% consist of such carcinoma as anaplastic and adenocarcinoma. The non-Hodgkin lymphomas comprise around 6% of head and neck tumors. The carcinomas
appear to be related to life style, as evidenced by the pre-
ponderence of heavy smokers and/or alcohol consumers, among
these patients. The role of industrial carcinogens (asbestos,
sawdust, leather processing products, nickel) in head and
neck cancers have also been confirmed.

Head and neck cancer is primarily a loco-regional
problem; metastases are rarely present when patients begin
treatment. More than 50% of recurrences are at the primary
site.

Surgery and radiotherapy are the classical modalities of treatment and over the past 20 years great advances have been made in this field, resulting in an improvement of the loco-regional control rate. However the limits of these treatments seem now to have come within sight. The results of treatment expressed in crude survival rates appear to vary considerably for the different sites and are related to factors such as stage, histology, age and treatment. The average crude survival figures for different sites are listed in table I.

Table I. AVERAGE FIVE-YEAR SURVIVAL

RATES FOR CANCER OF THE HEAD AND NECK

Site	%
Lip	85
Larynx	60
Floor of mouth/tongue	40
Oropharynx	30
Nasopharynx	30
Hypopharynx	15
Nasal cavity/sinuses	30

A further improvement in the control rate at the primary site and the treatment of local recurrences and metastases can probably only be achieved with systemic therapy. While different chemotherapeutic agents have been shown to be effective on squamous cell carcinoma of the head and neck, the measured effects on these tumors have been very variable and as yet unpredictable. The drugs which have been the most intensively studied are Methotrexate, Bleomycine, 5-Fluorouracil and most recently, Cisplatinum. Single agent regimens have been widely replaced because of inferior initial responses. Trials with multidrug schemes are now being widely conducted in a joint effort to improve the treatment results, especially for advanced stages of head and neck cancer. However, in spite of a sometimes dramatic initial response, the effect of chemotherapy has never been longlasting and it remains to be proven that chemotherapeutic agents can improve survival in head and neck cancer. Therefore the quality of life as influenced by the often serious side effects should be taken into account when weighing the advantages in terms of survival time.

In this section the results of different treatment regimens are presented from various authoritative centres in the world. Together they are a partial reflection of the state of the art in chemotherapeutic treatment of head and neck cancer. However, they also underline the great need for well-planned randomised clinical trials to further explore the potential benefits of this treatment modality.

Primary Chemotherapy in Cancer Medicine, pages 159–167
© 1985 Alan R. Liss, Inc.

INCREASED SURVIVAL IN STAGE III AND IV SQUAMOUS CELL
CARCINOMAS OF THE HEAD AND NECK USING AN INITIAL 24-HOUR
COMBINATION CHEMOTHERAPY PROTOCOL WITHOUT CISPLATIN:
6 YEAR FOLLOW-UP

L.A. Price M.D., Bridget T. Hill Ph.D., K.
Macrae Ph.D.
Imperial Cancer Research Fund Laboratories
and Department of Medical Statistics,
Charing Cross Hospital, London

Since 1973 we have carried out a series of studies to
determine whether the prognosis in advanced squamous cell
carcinoma of the head and neck can be improved by the use
of initial combination chemotherapy followed by local
treatment. We first showed, using standard agents, that intensive chemotherapy could be given safely to patients
with advanced disease and that a response rate of at least
70% could be achieved (1). We then demonstrated that this
combination of vincristine, methotrexate, bleomycin and
5-fluorouracil +/- adriamycin, given according to certain
theoretical stem cell kinetic concepts could be integrated
safely with radiation therapy and/or surgery. We also
showed that the chemotherapy response rate was significantly higher in previously unirradiated patients (2,3).
Subsequently, we have established the value of this drug
combination as initial treatment. From January 1975 -
December 1983 one hundred and seventy eight patients have
been treated in this study and we now report a detailed
analysis of the results together with long term survival
figures with a median follow-up of 6 years on the first
158 patients treated.

PATIENTS AND METHODS

One hundred and seventy-eight patients were entered into
this study. 175 patients were considered eligible with
histologically proven squamous cell carcinomas of the head
and neck, who had not received prior therapy of any kind
and were judged free of metastases beyond the regional
lymph nodes. No patients were considered resectable for

cure prior to chemotherapy. There were 71 patients with Stage IV tumours and 104 with Stage III disease. The drug protocol used is shown in Figure 1.

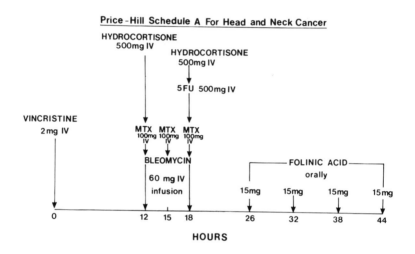

Fig. 1. Schedule A Chemotherapy Protocol

Standard medical precautions detailed earlier (4) were observed in all patients. The therapeutic strategy was to give the first course of Schedule A chemotherapy on day 1, the second on day 14 and to assess response to chemotherapy on day 28. Local "curative" therapy with radiotherapy and/or salvage surgery was started on day 28 and overall response was assessed within one month of its completion. A response (partial) was defined as a reduction of at least 50% in the product of two perpendicular diameters of all measurable lesions. A complete remission (CR) was defined as the absence of clinically detectable disease. The response rates were compared using the chi-squared test with the Yates' correction. P-values were determined by the two-tailed test. Survival was calculated by a life table method and compared using a log rank test.

RESULTS

Response to Chemotherapy

One hundred and sixty-seven patients were assessed for response to initial Schedule A chemotherapy. One hundred and thirty patients were male and 37 female, with an age range of 13 - 80 years (median 57 years). One hundred and eight patients (65%) had an objective response to chemotherapy and 59 (35%) were classed as non-responders although 16 had a minimal 20-30% response. The response rate to initial chemotherapy was higher in the 96 patients with Stage III disease being 70%, than in the 71 patients with Stage IV disease where the figure was only 58%. Chemotherapy response was not significantly influenced by sex or histologic tumour grade. However, as shown in Table 1, site and age are important predictive factors.

TABLE 1
Factors Influencing Chemotherapy Response

	Chemotherapy Responders/Non-Responders			
	Overall	(%)	Stage III	Stage IV
Site:				
Oral Cavity	29/8	(78)	22/6	7/2
Oropharynx	19/15	(56)	10/2	6/13
Nasopharynx	18/3	(86)	6/1	12/2
Hypopharynx	12/11	(52)	7/6	5/5
Larynx	29/21	(58)	20/13	9/8
Others	4/2		2/1	2/1
Age:				
49 years	37/8	(82)	21/3	16/5
49 years	69/53	(57)	43/27	26/26

Oral cavity and nasopharyngeal lesions do significantly better compared with all other sites: $p < 0.05$ and $p < 0.01$ respectively, whilst hypopharyngeal tumours respond poorly, $p < 0.1$. Patients aged 49 or younger are more likely to respond to chemotherapy than older patients $p < 0.01$.

Response to Local Therapies

Response to local therapy after chemotherapy was assessed in 167 patients: 63% had radiation only, 32% had radiation plus surgery and 5% surgery only. An overall CR rate of

63% was achieved with results by stage being 74% and 49% for Stage III and IV disease respectively. For all patients as a group this CR rate was significantly greater in chemotherapy responders (76%) than in chemotherapy non-responders (39%), p > 0.001. Analyses by stage showed improved figures for chemotherapy responders (80%) versus non-responders (60%) in Stage III disease and highly significant benefit in Stage IV disease with figures of 69% for chemotherapy responders versus 23% for non-responders, p < 0.001.

Toxicity

Toxicity associated with Schedule A chemotherapy was minimal and there was 100% patient compliance. Significant side effects observed in this study are summarised in Table 2.

TABLE 2
Incidence of Side Effects in 175 Eligible Patients

Side Effect:	No. of Patients (%)	
Myelosuppression	5	(3%)
Mucositis (mild)	18	(10%)
Nephrotoxicity	0	
Peripheral neuropathy	8	(5%)
Pulmonary (chest pains)	1	
Skin rash	14	(8%)
Alopecia	10	(6%)
Nausea & vomiting	14	(8%)
Malaise & lethargy	9	(5%)
Deaths from treatment (protocol violations)	2	(1%)

No. of patients WITHOUT any side effects 107 (61%)
No. of patients WITH some side effects   68

They necessitated no change of chemotherapy dosage or timing except for one patient who developed a severe skin reaction and bleomycin was omitted from the second chemotherapy course. Myelosuppression was negligible with only one patient having a WBC nadir below 2000 per mm^3. This patient, with known impaired renal function (creatinine clearance of 70 ml per min) in whom the stated medical precautions were not observed, since a prolonged folinic acid "rescue" was not administered, died from the treatment. The second death also resulted from a protocol violation since the second course of chemotherapy was administered when the patient's white cell count was 3000 per mm^3 but their normal level was 10,000 per mm^3.

Survival

Overall survival data for the first 158 eligible patients treated are available with a median follow-up of 69 months. These, summarized in Table 3, show that all patients with Stage III disease had a median survival of 30.4 months, whilst the figure for patients with Stage IV disease was only 18.2 months.

TABLE 3
Median Durations of Survival in Months

	Stage III	Stage IV
All eligible patients	30.4	18.2
Chemotherapy responders	32.3	20.4*
Chemotherapy non-responders	17.1	8.5*
Patients in CR after local therapy	66+**	52.4**
Patients with RD at assessment	8.0**	7.8**

* p = 0.01   ** p = 0.0001

Chemotherapy responders lived longer than non-responders. Response to Schedule A chemotherapy is therefore a good prognostic sign. By stage these differences were significant only in Stage IV disease being 20.4 versus 8.5 months, $p < 0.01$. The importance of achieving a final complete remission is emphasized by these data. All patients achieving a CR after local therapy lived significantly longer than those with residual disease (RD) at assessment ($p < 0.00001$). This difference was significant irrespective of stage. This point is also illustrated in Figure 2, which also demonstrates that improved survival figures are noted in those patients achieving a complete remission who are aged < 49 years, compared with the older patient group. Finally, it should be noted that all patients alive at five years are disease free and 75% of these patients responded to initial chemotherapy.

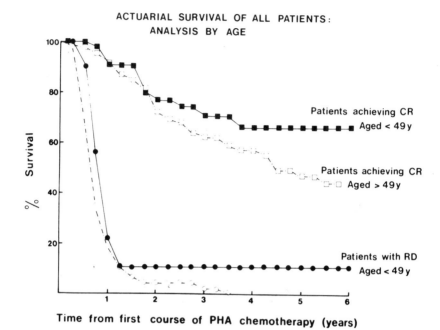

Fig. 2. Actuarial Survival Data

CONCLUSIONS

1. In this large series of 167 patients a high response rate (65%) can be achieved safely using our non cis-platinum containing chemotherapy protocol.
2. Age, site and stage appear significant predictive factors for response to Schedule A chemotherapy.
3. Schedule A chemotherapy does not compromise subsequent radiation therapy: 80% of all patients were given full dose uninterrupted radiotherapy.
4. Chemotherapy responders lived longer than non-responding patients: in Stage IV disease this increase in survival of chemotherapy responders is statistically significant (p < 0.01).
5. Significantly more chemotherapy responders achieve a complete remission than non-responders, p < 0.001 for all patients: by stage this difference reached statistical significance only for Stage IV disease (p < 0.001).
6. Achievement of complete remission increases survival very significantly, irrespective of disease stage.

TABLE 4
Summary of Toxicities from Some Recent Studies Using Cis-
Platinum-Containing Drug Combinations Compared with Price-
Hill Schedule A Chemotherapy

Drugs Used	Days on Treatment per Course	Nausea and Vomiting	Significant Myelo-Toxicity	Renal Toxicity	Ref.
CDDP* +VCR +BLM	5	71%	27%	10%	(5)
CDDP +BLM	9	moderate	2%	9%	(6)
CDDP +BLM	9	100%	5%	20%	(7)
CDDP +VCR +BLM	7	100%	2%	19%	(8)
CDDP +5FU	4	66%	37%	22%	(9)
CDDP +BLM +MTC	5	100%	2%	0%	(10)
VCR +BLM +MTX +5FU	2	8%	3%	0%	Our data

*CDDP - cis-platinum: VCR - vincristine:
 BLM - bleomycin: 5FU - 5-fluorouracil:
 MTC - mitomycin C: MTX - methotrexate.

(reproduced in part from 11)

This study was closed in January 1984. These patients will now be followed up so as to provide 10-year survival data, including detailed site by site analysis. Unfortunately it has not been possible at the Royal Marsden Hospital to carry out a randomised prospective controlled clinical trial so as to establish beyond doubt the role of initial chemotherapy in head and neck cancer. This type of study is clearly indicated. The major advantage of this Schedule A chemotherapy protocol is its lack of toxicity compared with a number of currently used cis-platinum containing schedules (see Table 4) <u>without</u> loss of therapeutic effect. Using the same theoretical principles outlined earlier (2) we have recently shown in a small feasibility study that it is also possible to combine cis-platinum safely with Schedule A. In view of data from several centres there may now be a case for a randomised study in advanced squamous cell carcinomas of the head and neck comparing, as initial therapy, Schedule A chemotherapy with or without cis-platinum.

REFERENCES

1. Price LA, Hill BT, Calvert AH, et al: Kinetically-based multiple drug treatment for advanced head and neck cancer. Br Med J 3: 10-11, 1975
2. Price LA, Hill BT: A kinetically-based logical approach to the chemotherapy of head and neck cancer. Clin Otolaryngol 2: 339-345, 1977
3. Price LA, Hill BT, Calvert AH, et al: Improved results in combination chemotherapy of head and neck cancer using a kinetically-based approach: a randomised study with and without adriamycin. Oncology 35: 26-28, 1978
4. Price LA, Hill BT: Safe and effective induction chemotherapy without cisplatin for squamous cell carcinoma of the head and neck: impact on complete response rate and survival at five years following local therapy. Med Ped Oncol 10: 535-548, 1982
5. Al-Sarraf M, Drelichman A, Jacobs J, et al: Adjuvant chemotherapy with cis-platinum, oncovin, and bleomycin followed by surgery and/or radiotherapy in patients with advanced previously untreated head and neck cancer: final report, in Salmon SE, Jones SE (eds): Adjuvant Therapy of Cancer III. New York, Grune and Stratton, 1981, pp 145-152

6. Hong WK, Pennachio J, Shapsay St, et al: Adjuvant chemotherapy with cis-platinum and bleomycin infusion prior to definitive treatment for advanced Stage III and IV squamous cell head and neck carcinoma, in Salmon SE, Jones SE, (eds): Adjuvant Therapy of Cancer III. New York, Grune and Stratton, 1981, pp 153-160
7. Pennachio JL, Hong W, Shapsay S, et al: Combination of cis-platinum and bleomycin prior to surgery and/or radiotherapy alone for the treatment of advanced squamous cell carcinoma of the head and neck. Cancer 50: 2795-2801, 1982
8. Spaulding MB, Kahn A, De Los Santos R, et al: Adjuvant Chemotherapy in advanced head and neck cancer: an update. Am J Surg 144: 432-436, 1982
9. Decker DA, Drelichman A, Jacobs J, et al: Adjuvant chemotherapy with cis-diamminodichloroplatinum II and 120-hour infusion with 5-fluorouracil in Stage III and IV squamous cell carcinoma of the head and neck. Cancer 51: 1353-1355, 1983
10. Israel L, Aguilera J, Soudant J, et al: Bleomycin and cis-platinum with or without mitomycin C in 110 previously untreated patients with head and neck cancer. Am J Clin Oncol 5: 305-311, 1983
11. Hill BT, Price LA, Busby E, et al: Positive impact of initial 24-hour combination chemotherapy without cis-platinum on 6-year survival figures in advanced squamous cell carcinomas of the head and neck. Adjuvant Therapy of Cancer IV (SE Jones and SE Salmon, eds) Grune and Stratton, New York, 1985, in press.

Primary Chemotherapy in Cancer Medicine, pages 169–175
© 1985 Alan R. Liss, Inc.

INDUCTION CHEMOTHERAPY WITH METHOTREXATE, BLEOMYCIN AND
HYDROXYUREA WITH OR WITHOUT CISPLATIN IN ADVANCED SQUAMOUS
CELL CARCINOMA OF THE HEAD AND NECK : A STUDY OF THE SWISS
GROUP FOR CLINICAL CANCER RESEARCH (SAKK)

R. Abele, H.P. Honegger, M. Wolfensberger,
R. Grossenbacher, B. Mermillod, F. Cavalli.
Division of Oncology
University Hospital
CH-1211 Geneva 4 (Switzerland)

The value of chemotherapy in squamous cell carcinoma
of the head and neck had been tested since 1972 in Swiss
pilot studies. Combination chemotherapy had been used, initially with methotrexate and bleomycin (Broquet 1974; Medenica 1976). Later hydroxyurea - administered orally - had
been added to this 2-drug program (Medenica 1981, Medenica
1981). The addition of cisplatin, at various dosages, had
also been tested and an effective and safe out-patient program, with a short hydration and a relatively low cisplatin
dose, had been defined.

As it appeared that chemotherapy may be very effective
as induction treatment in advanced disease (Medenica 1981),
this program was used in this setting, as a tentative to
improve the rate of local control and the poor prognosis of
advanced disease.

In 1982, the Swiss Group for Clinical Cancer Research
(SAKK) decided to initiate a randomized phase II trial,
using the "standard" regimen of methotrexate, bleomycin and
hydroxyurea as well as the same regimen plus cisplatin. The
randomization was chosen to have homogeneous and comparable
patient population. Since the potential for patient accrual
was limited, we did not embark on a randomized phase III
trial. Untreated patients as well as patients with reccurent
disease were eligible. The trial was closed to patient entry
in December 1983, after having observed a superior response
rate to the cisplatin-containing regimen (Abele 1984, Abele

1985). Since the vast majority of patients were previously untreated, a separate analysis had been done for this particular subgroup, and is the subject of this report.

MATERIALS AND METHODS

Patients with advanced squamous cell carcinoma of the head and neck were included in this study, after classification in the T.N.M. system and general examination. Only advanced disease patients were eligible. Normal serum biochemical and hematological values were required at entry. Patients were stratified in 2 groups : oral cavity and oropharyngeal primary tumors and hypopharynx + larynx primaries. A randomization in the 2 treatment regimens was performed, differing only by the addition of cisplatin. Regimen A consisted in a combination of methotrexate (30 mg/m2), bleomycin (15 mg) both intravenously weekly and hydroxyurea (1000 mg/m2) administered orally 3 times per week. Regimen B was similar to A but cisplatin (60 mg/m2) was given intravenously prior to all other drugs with 2 liters of fluids on day 1. Cycles were repeated on day 29. In case of myelosuppression, methotrexate and cisplatin were reduced by 33% and temporarily omitted for leukocyte values below 3.0 and/or platelet values below 80 x 10^9/liter. Cisplatin was not given in case of serum creatinine elevation above 120 micromol/liter. A minimum of 1 month of treatment should be given to patients in order to be evaluable for response. The duration of this inductive chemotherapy was not defined initially, but left to the investigator's decision. Subsequent local treatment was not standardized in this study. It was decided by investigators in each participating center, according to their personal practice.

Standard criteria of response were used for response evaluation by the first 4 authors, who reviewed the flow sheets. Survival was determined from day 1 to death or lost to follow up, and plotted with the Kaplan-Meier method.

RESULTS

Sixty-two patients were entered in this study. Six were considered as ineligible, based on inadequate laboratory values at entry (4 patients) and presence of a previous tu-

mor of other origin (2 patients). Twelve were considered as
inevaluable, mainly because of lack of adequate documentation. Therefore, only 44 patients were fully evaluable, 25 in
regimen A and 19 in regimen B. Table 1 shows patient demographic data. Stage III-IV disease was present in 41 patients.
Only 3 patients with T2 N0 disease were included in the study, a conservative approach being preferred to mutilating
surgery.

	Regimen A	Regimen B	Total (%)
Number	25	19	44
Mean age in years	57.3	59.6	58.3
(range)	(40.9-73.5)	(46.7-71.3)	(40.9-73.5)
Performance index :			
0 - 1	21	18	39 (87%)
2 - 3	4	1	5 (11%)
Male : female	23 : 2	16 : 3	39 : 5

Table 1 : Evaluable patient demographic data

One cycle of induction chemotherapy was given to 7 patients, 20 patients received 2 cycles, and 17 received 3 or
more cycles. In regimen A, seven partial remissions were observed (response rate 28%). Regimen B yielded 4 complete and
10 partial responses (overall response rate 74%). The difference in the response rates was statistically highly significant, with a P value of 0.0027 in favor of the cisplatin-
containing regimen. Table 2 shows the details of the responses in both regimens, according to primary tumor location.
Allthough the numbers are too small to draw valid conclusions,
responses have been seen in all locations. Among the 4 complete responses in regimen B, 2 patients were subsequently
operated and residual tumor was histologically found in both
cases. On the other hand, a partial remitter patient with
primary originating in the floor of mouth had no residual tumor found in the pelvimandibular resection piece. Dense fi-
brotic tissue with discrete inflamation was only observed.

After induction chemotherapy, local treatment consisted
in exclusive radiation therapy in 18 patients and surgical or
combined treatment in 17 patients. A total of 9 patients did
not receive local treatment, because of absence of response
to chemotherapy and/or too poor condition.

	Regimen A					Regimen B				
	CR	PR	NC	P	Tot	CR	PR	NC	P	Tot
Oral cavity										
- buccal mucosa		1			1		2*			2
- lower alveolus					0	1		1		2
- tongue			1	1	2		1	1		2
- floor of mouth		1	6		7		4			4
Oropharynx										
- anterior wall		2			2	1**	1	1		3
- lateral wall		2	4		6	1	1			2
- superior wall					0	1				1
Hypopharynx										
- junction		1	2	1	4					0
- piriform sinus		2	1		3			1	1	2
Larynx										
- supraglottic					0		1			1
	0	7	15	3	25	4	10	4	1	19

* 2 patients with stage II (T2 N0) disease
** stage II (T2 N0) disease

Table 2 . Evaluation of the response according to primary tumor location and regimen.

Median survival for the evaluable patients was 16.2 months (95% confidence interval 11.2 to 21.4 months) (figure 1). Survival did not differ according to treatment regimens, nor to primary tumor locations. Responders to chemotherapy had a median survival of 17.3 months, whereas patients with no change or progressive disease had a survival of 13.9 and 3.8 months, respectively.

A significant more severe hematologic toxicity was observed in regimen B in the first cycle of treatment (table 3) No patient had World Health Organization grade 3 and 4 toxicity in regimen A. In regimen B, grade 3 and 4 toxicity was seen in 1 patient for hemoglobin, 4 patients for leukocytes, and 4 patients for platelets. One of these patients died of a septicemia, with acute renal failure in regimen B.

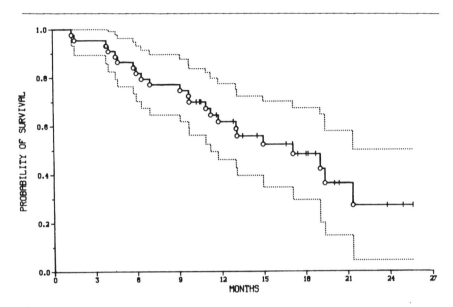

Fig. 1. Probability of survival in all evaluable patients.

	Hemoglobin (g/liter)	Leukocytes (x 10^9/l)	Platelets (x 10^9/l)
Regimen A	12.8	4.6	191
range	9.9 - 16.0	2.3 - 7.4	70 - 420
Regimen B	11.7	3.3	140
range	6.7 - 14.1	0.7 - 5.3	22 - 284
P value	0.02	0.002	0.02

Table 3. Hematologic toxicities : median lowest values in 51 evaluable patients (first cycle only).

In the first cycle, non hematologic toxicities consisted in grade 1 and 2 nausea and vomiting in 38% of the patients in regimen A and in 48% in regimen B. Stomatitis was more frequently seen in regimen B (39% of the patients) than in A (17% of the patients). Grade 1 and 2 serum creatinine elevation was observed in 1 patient in each regimen. Other toxicities consisted in mild alopecia (10% in A, 9% in B), and in skin toxicity (7% in A, 13% in B). probably related to bleomycin and hydroxyurea administration. No other toxicities were observed. in particular no clinically detectable lung toxicity.

Unusual surgical or radiation therapy complications were not reported by local investigators.

CONCLUSIONS

The results of this study show a significant higher response rate to a cisplatin-containing regimen in patients previously untreated for squamous cell carcinoma of the head and neck. A 74 % response rate, including 4 complete and 10 partial remissions, is reported in 19 patients.

This higher response rate is obtained at the cost of an increased hematologic and non hematologic toxicity rate. However, the toxicities seem to be acceptable by patients and had been reversible,except in 1 patient. In our opinion, this increased toxicity to chemotherapy in untreated patients is justified, since the remission rate is quite elevated.

Nevertheless, the survival of this group of patients remains low and does not differ according to induction chemotherapy regimens. The survival is merely the reflection of the patient selection, and we had shown that the vast majority had very advanced disease.

In conclusion, a cisplatin-containing regimen, used in untreated patients, is very effective and statistically superior to a "standard" non cisplatin-containing regimen. Since no benefit in survival had been observed, the definite value of this induction chemotherapy remains unsettled. Larger groups of patients and prolonged observation may be necessary to establish proven benefit in survival. Anatomical subgroups of head and neck squamous cell carcinomas should probably be separately studied in order to draw more precise conclusions. It seems that the main objective to reach is a high complete remission rate. This condition may then lead to an increase in survival of patients previously untreated for advanced head and neck cancer.

REFERENCES

Abele R, Honegger HP, Grossenbacher R, Kaplan E, Mermillod B, Cavalli F (1984). Randomized trial of methotrexate (M), bleomycin (B), hydroxyurea (HU) with versus without cisplatin in advanced squamous cell carcinoma of the head and neck. Proc Am Soc Clin Oncol 3 : 186.

Abele R, Honegger HP, Wolfensberger M, Grossenbacher R, Mermillod B, Cavalli F (1985). Methotrexate (M), bleomycin (B), hydroxyurea (HU) versus M+B+HU and cisplatin (C) in stage III-IV squamous cell carcinoma of the head and neck : A randomized study. Cancer Chemother Pharmacol 14 (suppl.) : 1.

Broquet MA, Jacot-Descombe E, Montandon A, Alberto P (1974). Traitement des carcinomes épidermoïdes oro-pharyngo-laryngés par combinaison de méthotrexate et de bléomycine. Schweiz med Wschr 104 : 18-22.

Medenica R, Alberto P, Lehmann W (1976). Traitement des carcinomes épidermoïdes oro-pharyngo-laryngés disséminés par combinaison de méthotrexate et de bléomycine à petites doses. Schweiz med Wschr 106 : 799-802.

Medenica R, Alberto P, Lehmann W (1981). Combined chemotherapy of head and neck squamous cell carcinomas with methotrexate, bleomycin and hydroxyurea. Cancer Chemother Pharmacol 5 : 145-149.

Medenica R, Lehmann W, Pipard G (1981). Adjuvant chemotherapy of advanced head and neck squamous cell carcinoma, prior to surgery and radiotherapy. Proc Am Assoc Cancer Res and ASCO 22 : 430.

Primary Chemotherapy in Cancer Medicine, pages 177-189
© 1985 Alan R. Liss, Inc.

THE ROLE OF INDUCTION CHEMOTHERAPY IN ADVANCED HEAD AND
NECK CANCER: THE WAYNE STATE UNIVERSITY EXPERIENCE

J. A. Kish, M.D.
Assistant Professor of Medicine

J. Ensley, M.D.
Assistant Professor of Medicine

J. Crissman, M.D.
Professor of Pathology

A. Weaver, M.D.
Professor of Surgery

J. Jacobs, M.D.
Assistant Professor of Otolaryngology

J. Kinzie, M.D.
Associate Professor of Radiation Oncology

M. Al-Sarraf, M.D.
Professor of Medicine
Wayne State University
Detroit, Michigan 48201 U.S.A.

INTRODUCTION

The chemotherapy of head and neck cancer is in its evolu-
tionary stage. The initial goal was palliative therapy for
local failures and those with systemic disease. Single agents
predominated, particularly methotrexate with response rates of
8-63%, bleomycin with response rates of 6-45%, and cis-platinum with response rates of 14-41% (Al-Sarraf, 1984). The introduction of cis-platinum in the mid 1970's and the success
achieved in other malignancies with combination chemotherapy
stimulated the use of combination chemotherapy for head and
neck cancer. Many cis-platinum containing combinations from
single institutions have been evaluated in patients with

recurrent and advanced disease. Responses range from 48-100% (Weaver, Fleming, et al., 1984). Responses are higher in previously untreated patients. As noted, bleomycin was most commonly aligned with cis-platinum. This presents a major problem in a head and neck cancer population which has marginal pulmonary function to begin with.

Alternative chemotherapy combinations required exploration. Thus, the trials of cis-platinum (CACP) and 5-fluorouracil (5-FU) infusion developed at Wayne State University. Retrospectively, in vitro synergism had been reported with these drugs in L1210 leukemic bearing mice (Gale, Atkins 1976; Gale, Atkins 1977; Kline 1974; Schabel, Trader 1979; Speer, Lapis 1971; Woodman, Sirica 1973). The data from three sequential pilot studies with cis-platinum combination chemotherapy as initial treatment in 191 patients with emphasis on response and survival will be presented. It is to be noted that the initial goals of induction or preoperative chemotherapy were to objectively test and measure the antitumor effects of the drug combinations, evaluate side effects, and carefully scrutinize the feasibility of combining chemotherapy with surgery and/or radiation.

MATERIALS AND METHODS

A total of 191 patients were entered into the three trials at two Wayne State University affiliated hospitals, Harper-Grace Hospitals in Detroit and Veterans Administration Medical Center in Allen Park; 77 in Trial I, 26 in Trial II and 88 in Trial III. All patients had advanced stage III and IV head and neck cancer. Patients with distant metastases and multiple primary malignancies were ineligible. All patients had a performance status of 1-3; adequate renal function as demonstrated by a serum creatinine of $\geq$ 60 ml/min; and adequate bone marrow reserve with a WBC of $\geq$ 4 x 10^3/mm^3 and a platelet count of $\geq$ 100 x 10^3/mm^3. Patients receiving bleomycin were required to have a vital capacity of $\geq$ 60% predicted, CO diffusion capacity $\geq$ 75% predicted and/or a PO$_2$ on room air of 70 mm Hg.

All patients were initially evaluated by a surgeon, radiation therapist and medical oncologist. Surgical planning was done prior to chemotherapy. The extent of eventual resection was not altered by subsequent responses to chemotherapy or radiation.

Patients were reevaluated by all three modalities after induction chemotherapy. Those considered surgically resectable advanced to the previously determined operative procedure. Patients who were not resectable after induction chemotherapy or refused surgery received 5000 rads over three to five and one-half weeks to the primary lesion and local lymph nodes three weeks after completion of chemotherapy. Patients who became resectable following chemotherapy and radiation moved on to resection while patients still inoperable or who continued to refuse surgery received an additional 1600 rads to the gross residual disease.

Trial I patients received cis-platinum, vincristine and bleomycin. Trial II patients received cis-platinum and 96 hour 5-FU infusion. Trial III patients received cis-platinum and 120 hour 5-FU infusion. All doses of cis-platinum were preceded by 24 hours of hydration with 2 liters of D_5 0.45 N.S. with 40 meq KCl and an immediate I.V. bolus of 12.5 gms mannitol in one liter D_5 0.45 N.S. with 20 meq KCl was administered over 4 hours. The 5-FU infusion was 1000 mg/m^2/d in two liters D_5 0.45 N.S. over 24 hours x 4 days in Trial II and x 5 days in Trial III. Utilization of an 8-inch peripheral line, subclavian or Hickman catheter assured continuous large vein access for 5-FU infusion. Chemotherapy regimens are demonstrated in Table 1.

TABLE 1
Chemotherapy Regimens for Induction Chemotherapy Trials

	Trial I COB* x 2	Trial II CACP+5FU x 2	Trial III CACP+5FU x 3
Cis-platinum	100 mg/m^2 I.V. day 1	100 mg/m^2 I.V. day 1	100 mg/m^2 I.V. day 1
Oncovin	1 mg I.V. days 2 and 5	-	-
Bleomycin	30 U/day 24 hr infusion days 2-5		
5-Fluorouracil	-	1000 mg/m^2/d 24 hr infusion days 1-4	1000 mg/m^2/d 24 hr infusion days 1-5

*C = cis-platinum; O = oncovin; B = bleomycin

The patient population consisted of 156 males and 35 females. Ages ranged from 15 years to 84 years with a median of 56. Twenty-three percent of the patients presented with a second primary cancer in the upper aerodigestive tract. The majority of patients are stage IV, representing a variety of T and N stages (Table 2).

TABLE 2
T and N Stage of Patients for Induction
Chemotherapy Trials

	T_0	T_1	T_2	T_3	T_4	Total	%
N_0			3	13	37	53	27.7
N_1			1	16	7	24	12/6
N_2		1	1	30	16	48	25.1
N_3	4	4	7	27	24	66	34.6
Total	4	5	12	86	84		
	(2.1%)	(2.6%)	(6.3%)	(45%)	(44%)		

All patients are being followed until death. Any patients who received one course of chemotherapy, even if she/he refused further treatment has been included for evaluation for response, toxicity and survival in this report. All deaths occurring after enrollment into these studies are considered cancer deaths. Any patient lost to followup even if they had no evidence of disease (NED) was considered a cancer death at that point.

Responses to initial induction chemotherapy are defined as: Complete Response (CR) - complete resolution of primary and nodal lesions as determined by physical exam, endoscopic and radiologic examinations; Partial Response (PR) - if a 50% or greater reduction in perpendicular dimensions of measurable primary lesion and/or local lymph node is noted; No Response (NR) response less than PR, stable disease or progression of the cancer while on chemotherapy.

RESULTS

Overall response to induction chemotherapy was high for

all groups. In Trial I, 61/77 (80%) responded (CR + PR). In Trial II, 23/26 (88%) responded, and in Trial III, 83/88 (94%) responded. These overall response rates are not statistically significant by the chi square test. However differences in the complete response rates--Trial I 29%, Trial II 19% and Trial III 54% are statistically significant at p = 0.04 (Table 3).

TABLE 3
Response to Chemotherapy by Treatment Regimen

	Trial I COB x 2	Trial II CACP+5-FU x 2 96 hr	Trial III CACP+5-FU x 3 120 hr	
CR	22 (29%)	5 (19%)	48 (54%)	p = 0.04
PR	39 (51%)	18 (69%)	35 (39%)	
NR	16 (20%)	3 (12%)	5 (7%)	
CR+PR/Total	61/77 (80%)	23/26 (88%)	79/88 (94%)	

No significant difference is response was noted between clinical stages III or IV. Response according to T and N status was evaluated. The highest CR rate of 79% was seen in T_4N_0 patients who received 3 courses of 5-FU and cisplatinum. The lowest complete response was in T_4N_3 (20%) (Table 4). No statistically significant difference in response could be elicited on basis of sex, race, or tumor morphology.

TABLE 4
Response to Three Courses of 5-FU and CACP by T and N Stage

	T_4N_0	T_4N_1	T_4N_2	T_4N_3
CR	11	2	2	3
PR	1	2	1	11
NR	2	-	-	-
CR/Total	11/14 (79%)	2/4 (50%)	2/3 (67%)	3/14 (21%)

With minimum followup of 24 months and median followup of 42 months, median survival for the entire patient population is 14.5 months. Median survival in Trial I is 53 weeks, in

Trial II, 50 weeks, and in Trial III the median survival has
not been reached at 66+ weeks (Fig. 1).

Overall Survival For Treatment Groups

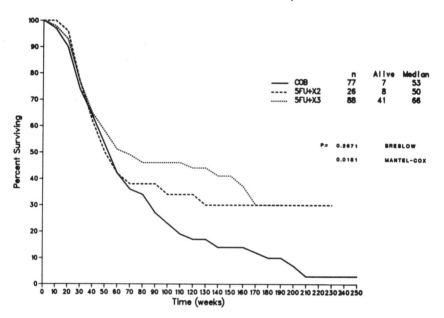

Figure 1. Overall survival by treatment group for induction
chemotherapy.

Comparing actual survival curves at 18 months, patients in
Trial III showed survival advantage, with 38/61 (62%) (24
patients had not yet reached 18 months survival) alive vs.
11/26 (42%) in Trial II and 31/77 (40%) in Trial I. This
difference is statistically significant at p = 0.001. In
comparing treatment sequence, chemotherapy + surgery + radiation therapy vs. chemotherapy + radiation therapy + surgery
vs. chemotherapy + radiation therapy, no significant difference was noted. Responders to initial chemotherapy had
statistically better survival as compared to non-responders to
chemotherapy (p = 0.05) regardless of the subsequent definitive therapy of surgery and/or radiation (Fig. 2).

Overall Survival By Response

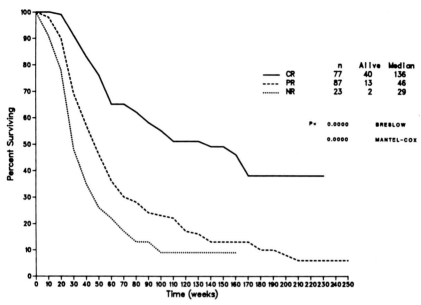

Figure 2. Overall survival by response for 187 patients in three chemotherapy induction trials. NOTE: Patients with unknown primaries were excluded.

Patients with T_4N_0 enjoyed a better survival overall compared to T_4N_3 (Fig. 3).

Toxicities encountered during induction chemotherapy are summarized in Table 5. Pulmonary toxicity, rash, fever and alopecia were encountered primarily in Trial I patients who received bleomycin. Mild to moderate reversible renal impairment, defined as a rise in the serum creatinine of 1.6 mg% to 4 mg% was encountered in some patients within all groups and was associated with the cis-platinum component of each regimen. Nausea and vomiting related to platinum was common in all three groups. Myelosuppression was encountered more frequently in Trial III which received a total higher dose of cis-platinum, an extra day of 5-FU and the three total courses of chemotherapy.

Survival T4N0 vs. T4N3

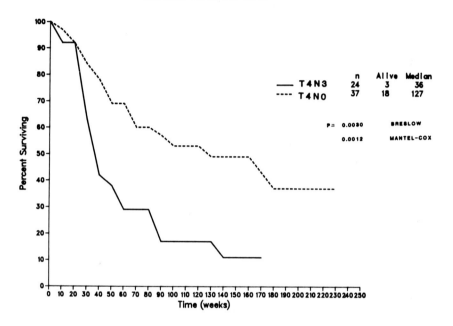

Figure 3. Overall survival for patients in induction chemotherapy comparing T_4N_0 vs. T_4N_3.

TABLE 5
Incidence of Drug Toxicity for Induction Chemotherapy Trials

	Trial I COB x 2	Trial II CACP+5-FU	Trial III CACP+5-FU
Leukopenia	27	27	39
Thrombocytopenia	4	4	9
Nausea/vomiting	71	70	64
Diarrhea	–	–	16
Stomatitis	7	8	15
Renal	10	27	33
Skin	13	–	4
Fever	30	–	–
Alopecia	52	4	6
Pulmonary	5	–	–
Phlebitis	–	8	9

DISCUSSION

The concept of a multimodality approach utilizing induction chemotherapy prior to definitive local therapy is gaining increased acceptance in the management of advanced squamous carcinoma of the head and neck. Most effective combinations are based on earlier studies which utilized cisplatinum with bleomycin and a variety of other drugs producing response rates of 48-100% (Weaver, 1984). In our first pilot study (1977-1979)ₐ patients were given two courses of cisplatinum, Oncovin^R (Lilly) and bleomycin infusion (COB). The complete response rate was 29% with 51% partial response (Al-Sarraf, Drelichman 1981). Since the majority of patients with squamous carcinoma of the head and neck are heavy cigarette smokers with marginal pulmonary function, many potential candidates for the COB trial were rejected. The second pilot with cis-platinum and 96 hour infusion 5-FU was an attempt to circumvent the pulmonary function requirements of bleomycin and identify a new effective combination (Al-Sarraf, Drelichman 1981; Kish, Drelichman 1982). 5-Fluorouracil alone has a 31% response rate in squamous carcinoma of the head and neck (Amer, 1979). In vitro synergism between 5-FU and cis-platinum has been demonstrated (Gale, Atkins 1976; Gale, Atkins 1977; Kline 1974; Schabel, Trader 1979; Speer, Lapis 1971; Woodman, Sirica 1973). Two courses of a 96 hour 5-FU infusion with cis-platinum produced response rates very similar to the COB regimen without the additional toxicity of bleomycin (Kish, Drelichman 1982). Patients tolerated this combination well and it was effectively followed by surgery and/or radiation.

The third pilot study started in 1980 involved 120 hour infusion of 5-FU and cis-platinum for 3 courses. Although the overall response rates did not differ significantly from the first two trials, the complete response rate of 54% was superior (p = 0.04) (Rooney, Kish 1985).

The explanation for this increase in complete response may be related to several factors: patient selection, staging, number of courses of chemotherapy and actual drug related effects. This was not a randomized trial and patient selection for study may have been biased by the surgeon's decision regarding surgery. The stages may not be evenly distributed and several subgroups existed within clinical staging groups. In addition, a higher response was seen in patients with large primaries and no neck nodes. By increasing the time of the

5-FU infusion to 120 hours and the number of courses to three, the CR rate reached statistical significance. In 1979, Schabel et al. reported therapeutic synergism was seen between 5-FU + cis-platinum in mice bearing L1210 leukemia treated with cis-platinum alone, 5-FU alone or both. Sixty percent of the animals treated with drug combinations were cured and median life span (MLS) of combination drug treated animals (although dying of leukemia) exceeded MLS of other mice treated with either agent alone (Schabel, Trader 1979).

With a minimal followup of 24 months on every patient and a median followup of more than 42 months, the survival of patients who received the 3 courses of the 5-FU and cis-platinum combination was statistically superior to the survival of the other patients. This difference in survival is particularly emphasized in patients with a histological CR. Of 32 patients with clinical CR in whom a surgical specimen was available, 13 with negative histology are still alive. Only two of the 19 patients with positive histology are still alive. The median survival for the patients with positive histology is 104 weeks which is better than anticipated in advanced head and neck cancer (Al-Kourainy, Crissman 1985). This increase in survival reflects the CR obtained with chemotherapy.

Many patients who experience a good response to chemotherapy may subsequently refuse definitive local treatment and jeopardize their potential chance for increased quality longevity. In the group of patients with the highest CR rate, that is cis-platinum + 5-FU 120 hours x 3, 21/48 (44%) who were CR refused surgery. There were 11 patients who refused any other therapy after chemotherapy and radiation (see Table 6). In addition, despite vigorous attempts at objectivity, it is difficult for the surgeon to perform the pre-chemotherapy planned surgery when no tumor may be grossly visible. Thus, the exact sequence of multimodality therapy needs to be defined.

It must be noted that single arm, single institution pilot studies, regardless of the number of patients, have the limited objective of establishing feasibility, toxicity and effectiveness of induction chemotherapy. Only well designed randomized prospective levels can establish the role of combined modality therapy by comparing disease free survival and overall survival.

TABLE 6
Compliance to Local Therapy by Response
to Induction Chemotherapy

	COB (2 courses)			5-FU + CACP (2 courses)			5-FU + CACP (3 courses)		
	CR	PR	NR	CR	PR	NR	CR	PR	NR

Response to Chemotherapy and Surgery Compliance

	CR	PR	NR	CR	PR	NR	CR	PR	NR
Yes	10	20	7	2	10	1	17	20	2
No	10	16	9	1	5	2	10	11	1
Refused	2	3	0	2	3	-	21	4	2

Response to Chemotherapy and Radiotherapy Compliance

	CR	PR	NR	CR	PR	NR	CR	PR	NR
Yes	18	34	13	3	15	3	42	28	3
No	1	2	2	-	3	-	-	3	1
Refused	3	3	1	2	-	-	7	4	1

Patients Refused Further Chemotherapy

	CR	PR	NR	CR	PR	NR	CR	PR	NR
Chemotherapy Only	1	2	2	1	2		7	4	1

Several conclusions can be derived from this work. Induction chemotherapy can be safely and effectively administered to patients with advanced head and neck cancer prior to definitive local therapy. Cis-platinum containing combinations, particularly cis-platinum and 5-FU infusion, produce high response rates with marked increase in CR rates. Patients who are clinically CR to chemotherapy and those with pathologic CRs have a prolonged survival. There is a high attrition rate from local therapy in patients who achieve a CR to chemotherapy.

Several questions are raised by this work. Is there any other chemotherapy which can produce a higher CR rate? Does achievement of a CR reflect actual therapy effect or select out a favorable prognosis group? What is the appropriate number of courses of chemotherapy and the most appropriate sequence of therapies? The Head and Neck Contracts Program evaluated one course of chemotherapy prior to definitive therapy. A response rate of 48% was seen (Wolf, Makuch 1984). It was highly optimistic to expect significant anti-tumor response with one course of therapy. With the introduction of the 5-FU + cis-platinum regimen which shows increases in CR with increasing number of courses, one cannot justify less than three courses. Studies utilizing chemotherapy post-operatively, followed by radiation therapy, have been performed. The chemotherapy is well tolerates in this group and the definitive surgical procedure is per- formed. These studies have not been randomized and prolonged survival data is not available yet (Al-Sarraf, Kinzie, 1984; Weaver, Jacobs, 1984). When to use the chemotherapy is as crucial a question as which drugs and how many cures.

Currently, several cooperative groups in the United States are randomizing patients to local therapy alone vs. local and systemic therapy with chemotherapy between surgery and radiation. This should help define the role of chemotherapy in operable disease and the most appropriate sequence of multimodality therapy.

REFERENCES

Amer MH, Al-Sarraf M, Vaitkevicius VK (1979). Factors that affect response to chemotherapy and survival of patients with advanced head and neck cancer. Cancer 43:2202.

Al-Kourainy K, Crissman J, Ensley J et al. (1985). Achievement of superior survival of histologically negative vs. histologically positive clinically complete responders to cis-platinum (CACP) combination in patients with locally advanced head and neck cancer. Abstr submitted to AACR.

Al-Sarraf M (1984). Chemotherapy strategies in squamous cell carcinoma of the head and neck. Critical Reviews in Oncology/Hematology, Vol 1, Issue 4, p. 323.

Al-Sarraf M, Drelichman A, Jacobs J et al (1981). Adjuvant chemotherapy with cis-platinum, Oncovin and bleomycin followed by surgery and/or radiotherapy in patients with advanced previously untreated head and neck cancer. Final report. In Jones SE and Salmon SE (eds): "Adjuvant Therapy of Cancer III", New York: Grune & Stratton, p. 145.

Al-Sarraf M, Drelichman A, Peppard S et al. (1981). Adjuvant cis-platinum and 5-fluorouracil 96 hour infusion in previously untreated epidermoid cancers of the head and neck. (Abstr) Proc ASCO 22:428.

Al-Sarraf M, Kinzie J, Marcial V et al. (1984). Combination of cis-platinum and radiotherapy in patients with advanced head and neck cancer: Radiation Therapy Oncology Group Progress Report. (Abstr) Proc ASCO 3:180.

Gale GR, Atkins LM, Meischen SJ et al. (1976). Combination chemotherapy for L1210 leukemia with platinum compounds and cyclophosphamide plus other selected anti-neoplastic agents. J Natl Cancer Inst 57:1363.

Gale GR, Atkins LM, Meischen SJ et al. (1977). Chemotherapy of advanced L1210 leukemia with platinum compounds in combination with other anti-tumor agents. Cancer Treat Rep 61:445.

Kish J, Drelichman A, Jacobs J et al. (1982). Clinical trial of cis-platinum and 5-FU infusion as initial treatment for advanced squamous carcinoma of the head and neck. Cancer Treat Rep 66:471.

Kline I (1974). Potentially useful combinations of chemotherapy detected in mouse tumor systems. Cancer Chemo Rep (Pt 2) 4:33.

Rooney M, Kish J, Jacobs J, Kinzie J, Weaver A, Crissman J, Al-Sarraf M (1985). Improved complete response rate and survival in advanced head and neck cancer after three-course induction therapy with 120-hour 5-FU infusion and cisplatin. Cancer 55:1123.

Schabel FM Jr, Trader MW, Laster WR Jr et al. (1979). Cis-dichlorodiammine platinum (II): Combination chemotherapy and cross resistance studies with tumors of mice. Cancer Treat Rep 63:1459.

Speer RJ, Lapis S, Ridgway H et al. (1971). Cis-platinum diamminodichloride (PDD) in combination therapy of leukemia L1210. Weekly Med Bull 1:103.

Weaver A, Fleming S, Ensley J et al. (1984). Superior clinical response and survival rates with initial bolus and cisplatin and 120 hour infusion of 5-FU before definitive local therapy for locally advanced head and neck cancer. Amer J Surg 148:525.

Weaver A, Jacobs JR, Al-Sarraf M et al. (1984). Combined modality therapy with surgery, chemotherapy and radiotherapy in patients with head and neck cancer: Radiation Therapy Oncology Group Study. Proc ASCO 3:180.

Wolf G, Makuch R, Baker S (1984). Predictive factors for tumor response to preoperative chemotherapy in patients with head and neck squamous carcinoma. Cancer 54:2869.

Woodman RJ, Sirica AE, Gang M et al. (1973). The enhanced therapeutic effects of cis-platinum (II) diamminodichloride against L1210 leukemia when combined with cyclophosphamide or 1,2 bis(3,5-dioxopiperazine-1Yl) propane of several other anti-tumor agents. Chemotherapy 18:179.

Primary Chemotherapy in Cancer Medicine, pages 191-197
© 1985 Alan R. Liss, Inc.

SEQUENTIAL RESPONSE PATTERNS TO CHEMOTHERAPY AND
RADIOTHERAPY IN HEAD AND NECK CANCER: POTENTIAL IMPACT OF
TREATMENT IN ADVANCED LARYNGEAL CANCER.

*WK Hong, GM O'Donoghue, S Sheetz, S Fofonoff, EB Dorman,
J Welch, CW Vaughan, DD Karp, B Willett, and S Strong.

Departments of Otolaryngology, Radiation Therapy, and
Medical Oncology. Boston Veterans Administrative Medical
Center, Boston University School of Medicine, Boston, MA.

*Section of Medical Head and Neck Oncology, The
University of Texas System Cancer Center M. D. Anderson
Hospital and Tumor Institute, Houston, Texas.

Surgery and/or radiotherapy have been the standard
therapies for locally advanced squamous cell carcinoma of
the head and neck region. Despite major improvement in
these therapeutic techniques, the control rate in cases of
advanced cancer remains poor. More recently, induction
chemotherapy as initial treatment has been used in
previously untreated squamous cell carcinoma of the head and
neck. For the last 6 years at the Boston Veterans
Administration (V.A.) Medical Center, initial induction
chemotherapy followed by surgery and/or radiotherapy has
been employed in the treatment of advanced head and neck
cancer. The use of chemotherapy and radiotherapy has
allowed us to moniter and correlate sequential response
patterns produced by each modality of treatment. We have
observed that responders to chemotherapy can be predicted to
have further response to subsequent radiotherapy.
Conversely, patients who initially fail to respond to
chemotherapy subsequently fail to respond to radiotherapy.
Similar reports from other investigators (1,2,3,4) and
therapeutic strategies in the treatment of advanced
laryngeal cancer (e.g. better preservation of voice function
even if overall survival rates remain unchanged) will be
discussed.

Patients and Methods
    From January 1977 to July 1984, 110 patients with
advanced squamous cell carcinoma of the head and neck were
treated at Boston V.A. Medical Center. These patients were
placed on one of three nonrandomized protocols. During the
first trial, patients were treated with one of the following
three regimens of induction chemotherapy: 1) Cisplatin at
120 mg/m^2 on days 1 and 22 plus bleomycin at 15 u/m^2 by
intravenous push on day 3, followed by a continuous infusion
of bleomycin at 15 u/m^2 per day for 7 days (64 patients); 2)
single-agent bleomycin infusion at 15 u/m^2 per day for 7
days (23 patients); 3) (the most recent protocol) Cisplatin
at 100 mg/m^2 by intravenous push plus 5-fluorouracil 1,000
mg/m^2 per day by a continuous infusion for 5 days for 3
courses (22 patients). Following the initial induction
chemotherapy, evaluation of the response to chemotherapy
with either indirect or direct endoscopy was performed
within 2 weeks of completion of chemotherapy. Complete
response (CR) and partial response (PR) were defined as
complete regression and greater than 50 percent regression
of clinically measurable disease. Anything less than a
partial response or stable disease was classified as a
nonresponse (NR). After surgery and/or radiotherapy were
completed, another evaluation was undertaken to assess
complete response or presence of residual persistent disease
(RD). Forty-six patients (Table 1) who had sequential
chemotherapy and radiotherapy with no surgery were
evaluated.

    Among these 46 patients, 20 patients (larynx: 10;
hypopharynx: 10) who had sequential chemotherapy and
radiotherapy without laryngectomy (patient refusal: 7;
medical contraindication for surgery: 3; surgeon's refusal
because of dramatic response: 6; other: 4) were separately
also evaluated and analyzed. All patients were then
followed closely at monthly intervals for recurrence and
survival.

Table 1.

Patient Characteristics

Total No.	46		Sites of Primary	
Median age 58.9	(45 - 76)		Oral Cavity	11
			Oropharynx	10
Sex	All Male		Hypopharynx	11
			Larynx	10
P.S.	> 80	28	Nasopharynx	2
	< 80	18	Sinus	2
Stage	II	1	Chemotherapy Regimens	
	III	7		
	IV	38	Cisplatin + Bleomycin 25	
Tumor Differentiation			Bleomycin	13
WD and MD		25		
P.D.		21	Cisplatin + 5-FU	8

Results

Tumor response was significantly higher with cisplatin-containing regimens than with bleomycin alone. Table 2 shows the association between the initial response to chemotherapy and the response following radiotherapy.

Of the 28 patients who had a PR to initial chemotherapy, 22 (79%) attained a CR after radiotherapy. Of the 11 patients who failed to achieve a PR to chemotherapy, only 2 (18%) subsequently attained a CR after radiotherapy (P = 0.0002). Table 3 shows sequential response patterns of patients with operable advanced laryngeal and hypopharyngeal cancer.

Table 2.

Response to Chemotherapy and Subsequent
Response to Radiotherapy

Response to Chemotherapy	Response to Radiotherapy		P value
	Final CR	R.D.	
CR (7)	7 (100%)	0	
PR (28)	22 (79%)	6	.0002
NR (11)	2 (18%)	9	

Table 3.

Sequential CT and RT in Patients With
Operable Laryngeal and Hypopharyngeal Cancer

```
                CT            RT
                      CR (1)
      Larynx   ------ PR (7) ----- CR (8)
       (10)           NR (2)       RD (2)

                CT            RT
   Hypopharynx ---- CR (2) ------ CR (8)
       (10)         PR (6)        RD (2)
                    NR (2)
```

Overall median survival of patients who received sequential
chemotherapy and radiotherapy was 17 months. Median
survival in the final CR group was 35 months compared to
only 9.9 months in patients with persistent residual
disease. The patterns of relapse in 31 patients who

attained final CR were local regional metastasis in 9 and local regional plus distant metastasis in 6 patients. Median survival of patients with advanced laryngeal cancer was 25 months; median survival of those with hypopharyngeal cancer was 31 months.

Discussion

The greatest therapeutic challenge for patients with advanced squamous cell cancer of the head and neck is achievement of CR and long-term disease-free survival. Many studies have shown the feasibility of induction chemotherapy prior to surgery and/or radiotherapy without a subsequent increase in morbidity. These data clearly show that initial response to chemotherapy in patients with head and neck cancer predicts further response to subsequent radiotherapy. Glick et al. (3) described 29 patients treated with cisplatin and bleomycin followed by radiotherapy. The patients who achieved a PR with chemotherapy had a 67 percent CR rate following radiotherapy. Conversely, in the group of patients with less than a PR to chemotherapy, only 20 percent achieved a CR to subsequent radiotherapy. Ensley et al. (1) reported their experience with 48 patients who received a cisplatin-containing regimen prior to full-dose radiotherapy. Only one of the 14 nonresponders (7%) to chemotherapy achieved a CR, while 20 of 34 PRs (58%) to chemotherapy were converted to CRs after radiotherapy. Ervin et al. (2) recently reported their experience with 93 patients who received neoadjuvant chemotherapy before standard local treatment. For patients achieving notable tumor reduction to 2 cm or less, radical radiotherapy alone appeared to be as effective as surgery plus radiotherapy, which would indicate that surgery does not improve local control and survival rates.

In patients with laryngeal or hypopharyngeal cancer who had received sequential chemotherapy and radiotherapy without laryngectomy, it would appear that a reasonable median overall survival was achieved (25 and 31 months, respectively, with 3-year actuarial survival rate in 34 percent).

Conclusions
    1.   Sequential chemotherapy and radiotherapy to head
and neck cancer is a more logical approach to treatment than
either radiotherapy alone or simultaneous chemotherapy and
radiotherapy, because no increased adverse reactions has
been noted in patients who are receiving sequential
chemotherapy and radiotherapy.

    2.   Response to chemotherapy may predict conversion to
CR by radiotherapy, while failure to respond to chemotherapy
may predict poor response to radiotherapy.

    3.   Sequential chemotherapy and radiotherapy trials are
very attractive in head and neck cancer because they enable
the physician to monitor tumor regression carefully and to
determine an absence of response and the need for surgical
salvage.

    At present, this approach to laryngeal cancer is being
tested nationally by randomized trials in the V.A.
Cooperative Study Group according to the following schema:

    Treatment of Operable Laryngeal Squamous Cancer

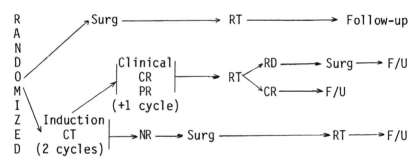

    Any progress from this approach would be a great
contribution to the treatment of advanced laryngeal cancer,
because the larynx would be preserved and quality of life
would be improved.

REFERENCES

1. Ensley JF, Jacobs JR, et al (1984). The Correlation Between Response to Cisplatinum Combination Chemotherapy and Subsequent Radiotherapy in Previously Untreated Patients with Advanced Squamous Cell Cancers of the Head and Neck. Cancer 54: 811-814.

2. Ervin TJ, Weichselbaum RR, et al (1984). Advanced Squamous Carcinoma of the Head and Neck. Arch Otolarygol 110: 241-245.

3. Glick JH, Marcial V, et al (1980). The Adjuvant Treatment of Inoperable Stage III and IV Epidermoid Carcinoma of the Head and Neck With Platinum and Bleomycin Infusions Prior to Definitive Radiotherapy: An RTOG Pilot Study. Cancer 46: 1919-1924.

4. Nervi C, Arcangeli G, et al (1978). The Relevance of Tumor Size and Cell Kinetics As Predictors of Radiation Response in Head and Neck Cancer. Cancer 41: 900-906.

Primary Chemotherapy in Cancer Medicine, pages 199-203
© 1985 Alan R. Liss, Inc.

PRELIMINARY RESULTS OF A RANDOMIZED STUDY ON PREOPERATIVE
INTRA-ARTERIAL CHEMOTHERAPY COMBINED WITH SURGERY AND
IRRADIATION FOR CARCINOMAS OF THE FLOOR OF THE MOUTH.

B. LUBOINSKI*

INSTITUT GUSTAVE ROUSSY

VILLEJUIF - FRANCE

Since 1960, several centers have used intra-arterial
chemotherapy for the treatment of head- and neck carcinomas.
Used as induction chemotherapy, it produces better results
than those obtained by intravenous therapy, despite its use
during long periods of monochemotherapy.
Studying 189 cases treated at the Gustave Roussy Institute
it was possible to demonstrate a statistically significant
relationship between the intensity of the response to chemotherapy and survival (1). However, one cannot conclude from
these results that there is an equally close relationship
between the chemotherapy itself and survival. The positive
responses could simply be a function of the patient's inherent prognostic state. In fact, we now have evidence that
the better responses are obtained for patients with small
lesions and specifically clinical node involvement.
In order to demonstrate the contribution of chemotherapy to
response, a randomized trial was necessary. This trial was
realised by the Head and Neck group of the E.O.R.T.C.

MATERIAL AND METHODS

Carcinomas of the floor of the mouth with extension to the
mandible or with a borderline of more than 2 cms with the

*EORTC - HEAD AND NECK COOPERATIVE GROUP
I.G.R. - J. RICHARD, H. SANCHO-GARNIER
N.C.I. Milan - R. MOLINARI
C.A.C. Lille - J.L. LEFEBVRE
C.A.C. Caen - F. BLANCHET
I. JULES BORDET - P. DOR

mandible were chosen for this trial.
The two arms of the trial were:
- Surgery alone or with post-operative radiotherapy, determined by the quality of the margin and extension to the
cervical nodes .
- Intra-arterial chemotherapy preceding surgery with or
without post-operative radiotherapy determined by the same
factors.

Were excluded:
Patients with prior treatment, advanced tumors with need
for major reconstructive surgery, patients with bilateral
neck node involvement or nodes with fixation to the deep
muscles.

SURGERY

The primary was treated by composite resection with or
without interruption of the mandible. The margins were as
large as possible and always included a safety margin beyond the limits of the tumor prior to the chemotherapy.
Frozen sections were performed to study the margin. Patients
classified as N_0 (UICC) were treated by bilateral supra-
hyoid neck dissection. A radical neck dissection was performed only when frozen section indicated node metastasis.
For patients with clinical homolateral node involvement, a
radical neck dissection was performed with ispilateral
modified neck dissection.

RADIOTHERAPY

Post-operative radiotherapy was performed only in cases of
positive margins or of histological involvement of the
nodes. The dose given was 50 Gy on both sides of the neck,
with an additional 15 Gy at the location of nodes with
capsular rupture. In instances of positive margins, the
dose given was 65 Gy to the floor of the mouth and sub-
mandibular area; 50 to 65 Gy was also given to the neck in
case of node involvement. In instances of bone involvement,
a wide resection was performed on the mandible.

CHEMOTHERAPY

Chemotherapy was given intra-arterially, on one or both
sides, depending on the extension of the tumor. Every 12
days the following regimen was administered: 15 mg of Bleomycin each day by continuous infusion and 1 mg of Vincristin on days 1, 5 and 9 in a one-hour infusion. In

instances of technical failure, involving insertion of the
catheter, or in case of problems arising during the treatment, the same regimen was administered intravenously.
Surgery was performed 10 to 21 days after the completion of
chemotherapy, and post-operative radiotherapy 3 to 6 weeks
after surgery.
The clinical response to chemotherapy was evaluated 10 days
after its end. A 6-step scale was used by the pathologist
to define the histological response of the tumor to chemotherapy (from 1: no pathological regression to 6: no trace
of tumor in the specimen) (2).
Follow-up consisted of re-examination every 3 months.
In evaluating the results of chemotherapy, survival was the
primary criterium, although rates of local, nodal and metastatic recurrence were also valuable indicators.

RESULTS:

The results of randomization were:
  Surgery: 62 cases
  Chemotherapy + surgery: 64 cases

There were no statistically significant differences in the
two treatment groups, including the state of the main
prognostic factors; i.c. extension of the primary (T) and
nodal involvement (N):

	SURG.	CHEMO.		SURG.	CHEMO		SURG.	CHEMO.
T2	29	26	NO	42	37	N-	28	27
T3	29	27	N1,2	16	23	N+R-	14	10
T4	4	11	N3	4	4	N+R+	18	23
						N+R?	0	1

Intra-arterial chemotherapy was performed as scheduled in
74% of the cases. In 17% of the cases, catheterization was
not possible and chemotherapy was given intravenously.
In 9%, intra-arterial administration was stopped due to
technical failure (displacement, obstruction of the catheter). Toxicity was low. One patient succumbed due to an
error in the regimen, and in 4 cases (2 intra-arterial,
2 intravenous), the chemotherapy was suspended due to
allergic reaction.

CLINICAL RESPONSE TO THE CHEMOTHERAPY

	PRIMARY	NODES
CR:	4 (6%)	2
PR:	27 (42%)	1

(PR defined as a 50% or greater decrease in tumor load)

HISTOLOGICAL RESPONSE:

of 57 cases studied; the histological response was:
poor (grades 1, 2) in 35 cases (61%)
good or very good (3 to 6) in 22 cases (39%)

Survival data have not yet been compiled as all the patients
have not completed the necessary follow-up.
It is notable that the preliminary results indicate a better
survival rate for those patients treated with chemotherapy
(fig. 1). The difference between the two groups is of
borderline significance (p = 0,07).

Fig. 1, Survival:carcinoma of the floor of the mouth

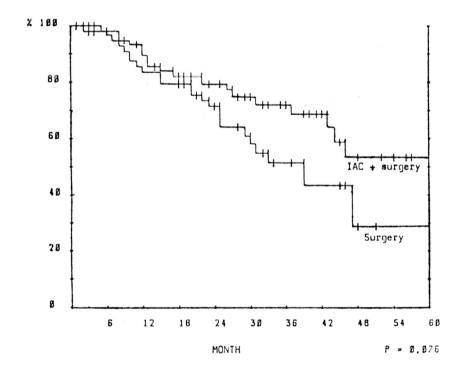

However, the group receiving chemotherapy did seem to have a lower rate of local recurrences (5 cases) than the group treated with surgery alone (15 cases).

DISCUSSION

These preliminary results must be interpreted with care. Nevertheless, they do represent the first time that a randomized trial has pointed in the direction of improved survival with induction chemotherapy. Furthermore, the results of recent years with polychemotherapies promise even greater responsiveness than was seen in this 8-year old trial.
This study is to be expanded to include different primary localizations. In fact, precisily the same study was con-comitantly executed, by several other centers, on carcinoma of the tonsillar area, treated by the commando procedure. This second randomised study shows absolutely no difference between the two arms. It should be quite obvious that the results of such studies must be separately reported and analyzed; mixing the results from separate localizations could mask the positive results of one with the negative results of another.
The Head and Neck Group of the EORTC has recently begun a new randomized trial. On induction chemotherapy for carci-noma of the tonsillar area treated by the commando proce-dure. The chemotherapy is administered intravenously and consists of 5-FU and Cis-platin.

BIBLIOGRAPHY

1. - RICHARD J.M., SNOW G.B. - Present role of chemotherapy in head and neck cancer. Reprinted from Excerpta Medica International Congress, Series N° 365 Cancer of the Head and Neck. Proceedings of an International Symposium. Montreux, Swizerland, 1975.
Excerpta Medica, Amsterdam-Oxford

2. - MICHEAU C., RICHARD J.M. - Actions tissulaires de la chimiothérapie intra-artérielle (CIA) dans les cancers pelvi-linguaux et leurs métastases ganglionnaires (à propos de 47 cas).
Ann. Oto-laryng. Paris 1975, t. 92, n° 9, p 499-508.

SECTION VI
GYNAECOLOGICAL CANCER

Primary Chemotherapy in Cancer Medicine, pages 207–211
© 1985 Alan R. Liss, Inc.

CHEMOTHERAPY PRECEDING SURGERY OR IRRADIATION IN CARCINOMA OF THE OVARIES

Nina Einhorn, M.D., Bo Nilsson, B. Sc., Kerstin Sjövall, M.D.
Dpt of Gynaecological Oncology, Epidemiological Unit, Dpt of Obstetrics and Gynaecology, Karolinska Hospital, S-104 01 STOCKHOLM/Sweden

Chemotherapy preceding surgery or irradiation in carcinoma of the ovary with loco-regional confined disease has until now been used in small numbers of patients and experience with neo-adjuvant therapy in ovarian cancer is still limited. Although the percentage of patients with regional confined disease is small radical surgery in these patients has had great impact on survival. However, as many as 63% of the patients have at the time of diagnosis disease spread beyond the pelvis (Einhorn et al. 1984).

In discussing neo-adjuvant therapy in ovarian carcinoma it is necessary to point out the need for non-invasive diagnostic methods. Once the patient is undergoing laparatomy for a diagnosis of an ovarian mass and the tumour is easily resectable it is doubtful that neo-adjuvant therapy can be justified. In order to find out if neo-adjuvant therapy is of value in carcinoma of the ovary we have to:

1. develop methods for non-invasive diagnosis

2. review the historical series for information

At the Gynaecological Department of Radiumhemmet a non-invasive procedure in the diagnosis of ovarian masses has been developed during the 1950´s. A fine-needle aspiration biopsy instrument developed by Franzen and evaluated by Ångström has been extensively utilized during the last 20 years for the diagnosis of ovarian masses (Franzen et al. 1969; Ångström et al. 1972) (Fig. 1, 2).

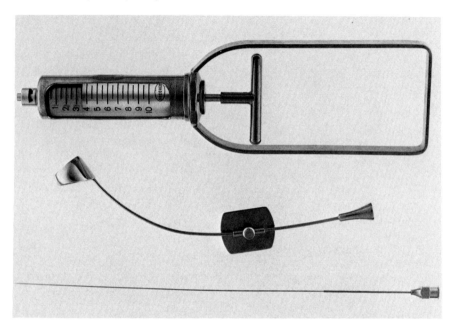

Fig. 1. Franzen instrumentary

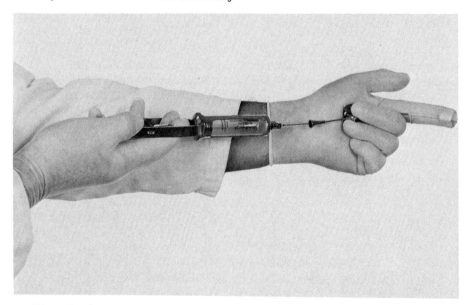

Fig. 2. Arrangements for pelvis puncture

Fine-needle aspiration biopsy gave us the opportunity to apply the philosophy of Hans-Ludvig Kottmeier who already declared in 1961 that aggressive and extensive surgery is valid for mucinous cancer but not for serous and endometrioid neoplasms fixed to surrounding tissues (Kottmeier 1961). This was the rational behind the Radiumhemmet policy where preoperative fine-needle aspiration biopsy diagnosis made it possible to use pre-operative chemotherapy and radiotherapy in patients with loco-regional disease.

Material and Methods

During the years 1974-1979 770 patients with carcinoma of the ovaries have been treated at Radiumhemmet; 186 patients in stage IA-IIA underwent primary radical surgery (Table 1).

Table 1.
Carcinoma of the ovary, distribution by stage of disease

Stage	No	%
IA	130	17.0
IB	25	3.2
IC	10	1.3
IIA	21	2.7
IIB	103	13.4
IIC	28	4.6
III	288	37.0
IV	165	21.0

Total   770

In the remaining 584 patients 416 were diagnosed by thin-needle aspiration biopsy or surgical biopsy without undergoing any debulking procedure. In 58 patients only limited debulking was performed and 110 had radical initial surgery leaving less than 2 cm of tumour mass.

Results

Among the 474 cases with large tumour masses left in the abdomen 92 patients died before any meaningful treatment. In 280 cases despite preoperative measures no debulking surgery was possible, while 102 patients were surgically debulked after preoperative treatment. In 67 of these cases debulking surgery was possible following preoperative chemotherapy and irradiation and in 33% after chemotherapy alone.

Thirty-seven patients treated by preoperative chemotherapy and irradiation were debulked leaving less than 2 cm of tumour. Likewise 18 patients were successfully debulked after chemotherapy alone. The 5-year survival rate for these two groups was similar, 41% and 44% respectively. (Table 2)

Table 2.

Percentage of patients treated with preoperative therapy (102 patients)

Therapy	% pat	Survival
Chemotherapy + irr	67%	41%
Chemotherapy	33%	44%

In stage IIB and IIC with regional confined disease only 76 of 131 patients had primary surgical resectable tumour. These patients had 52% 5-year survival.Nineteen patients treated preoperatively with chemotherapy and irradiation were carried through to debulking surgery and the survival rate was 45% (Table 3).

Table 3.

Regional confined disease with and without preoperative measures

Treatment	No pat	Survival
Primary operation < 2 cm	76	52%
Preoperative treatment	19	45%

Discussion

In 76% of patients at diagnosis the disease is spread outside the gynaecological organs. Within this group there is a sub-group of patients where the disease is still confined to the true pelvis, yet still difficult to surgically debulk. These patients are in stage IIB and IIC and in present material the ones where preoperative therapy was used. In the group of patients with early disease where the surgery can be easily performed it is difficult to study the value of neo-adjuvant therapy as most of the patients undergo primary operation. For the future one must ask if it is justified to diagnose the early disease patient by non-

invasive measures to open the way for the use of adjuvant
therapy before surgery. Until now there has been very little
data available to answer this question. This is where fine-
needle aspiration biopsy may make a large contribution
allowing one to study by non-invasive means the value of
preoperative neo-adjuvant therapy. Today the group of patients
in stage IIB and IIC diagnosed by biopsy and operated after
preoperative measures is the best one to study. The conclusion drawn from such data can be interpreted in different
ways but there is no doubt that preoperative measures either
by chemotherapy or chemotherapy combined with irradiation
can give the same survival rate as for the patients treated
primarily with successful surgery. The modern trends to debulk primary ovarian carcinoma patients as radically as
possible may have to be re-evaluated. There is probably a
group of patients where neo-adjuvant therapy would be highly
useful. There is at the present moment one established method
to diagnose an ovarian mass before surgery. Fine-needle
aspiration biopsy is an excellent tool in the hands of an
experienced clinician and cytologist.

Monoclonal antibody technique has opened another
possibility for primary diagnostic measures. Still there has
to be more investigation to confirm the sensitivity and
specificity of these tests.

Einhorn N, Nilsson B, Sjövall K (1984). Factors influencing
  survival in carcinoma of the ovary. Study from a well defined Swedish population. Cancer in press.
Franzén S, Giertz G, Zajicek J (1960). Cytological diagnosis
  of prostatic tumours by transrectal aspiration biopsy: A
  preliminary report. Br J Urol 32:193.
Ångström T, Kjellgren O, Bergman F (1972). The cytologic
  diagnosis of ovarian tumors by means of aspiration biopsy.
  Acta Cytol 16:336.
Kottmeier HL (1961). Radiotherapy in the treatment of
  ovarian carcinoma. Clin Obst Gynec 4:865.

Primary Chemotherapy in Cancer Medicine, pages 213-215
© 1985 Alan R. Liss, Inc.

ROLE OF INTERVENTION SURGERY IN STAGE III-IV
EPITHELIAL OVARIAN CARCINOMA.

H.Hoogland, G.Blijham, H.Bron, A.Eekhout,
H.van Geuns, J.Haest, H.Huiskes, J.Kornman,
H.de Koning Gans, F.Lalisang, J.v.d.Meulen,
P.Moorman,J.Stoot,P.Tushuizen,J.Vreeswijk,J.Wils.
Gynecologic Oncology Group, Comprehensive Cancer
Center Limburg, The Netherlands.

Initial debulking surgery is generally considered to be
one of the mainstays in the treatment of advanced stage
(III and IV) ovarian cancer. The amount of residual tumor
after debulking surgery has been described as one of the
major prognostic indicators (Griffiths et al, 1979); in a
multivariate analysis (Neijt, 1983) only initial stage,
type of chemotherapy and residual tumor were found to predict for histological complete remission and prolonged
survival. These findings, however, do not necessarily
imply the surgical debulking procedure to be an important
therapeutic manoeuvre (Richardson et al, 1985).
The degree of success of surgery may at least in part be
a reflection of the degree of invasiness and bulkiness of
the initial tumor load; these latter factors may carry
the important prognostic information which then is not
altered by performing surgery or not. Moreover, initial
surgery may be associated with considerable morbidity
(Blyth et al, 1980; Bereck et al, 1980; Castaldo et al,
1980) and may cause a delay in the start of chemotherapy.
We investigated the prognosis of patients with non-
debulkable ovarian cancer treated with primary chemotherapy; the results suggest that primary debulking surgery
is not a prerequisite to obtain durable histological
complete remissions.

PATIENTS AND TREATMENT.
    Thirty-three patients with stage III-IV epithelial
ovarian cancer were treated with primary chemotherapy.
In all these patients primary debulking to lesions less
then 1.5 cm was judged to be impossible. Chemotherapy

consisted of Cyclophosphamide (C) 500 mg/m², Adriamycin
(A) 50 mg/m², and CDDP (P) 50 mg/m², all administered i.v.
on day 1 every 4 weeks. All patients were treated with 9
courses of CAP or till progression; in some patients with
a favourable response after 3 courses, intervention surgery with,if needed and possible, debulking to lesions
< 1.5 cm was performed. In case of clinical complete res-
ponse after 9 courses second look surgery was performed
and treatment stopped.

RESULTS.

Table 1. Results of Primary Treatment with CAP in Non-
Debulkable Patients with Stages III-IV Ovarian
Cancer.

Number of patients	33
Histological CR after 9 courses	8 (24%)
Relapses at 26 months median follow-up	0

As can be seen in table 1, eight patients (24%) obtained
a histological complete remission (HCR) after 9 courses;
none of these patients have relapsed sofar. In 6 of these
patients a clinical CR was already apparent after 3 courses; in some cases additional cytoreductive surgery was
performed at that point. These results can be compared to
those obtained in simultaneously treated patients with
bulky (lesions > 5 cm) stage III-IV ovarian cancer in
which initial debulking to lesions < 1.5 cm was possible.
Of 12 such patients 7 obtained HCR at second look surgery
after 6 courses of CAP; 2 patients have relapsed sofar.

DISCUSSION.
    In a number of randomized trials CDDP-containing chemo-
therapy has been shown to induce HCR in around 30% of unselected stages III-IV ovarian cancer patients; the majority of these complete responders will have the prospect
of prolonged survival or even cure (Decker et al, 1982;
Edwards et al, 1983; Neijt, 1983). We were surprised
to find a 24% HCR-rate in a population of patients with
such bulky or invasive disease that effective cytoreductive
surgery was precluded. In the majority of these patients
virtually all cytoreduction was eventually reached with
9 courses of CAP without any appreciable contribution of
surgical removal. This favorable result in patients with
very bulky or invasive cancers suggests to us that up-front
chemotherapeutic cytoreduction may be even more effective

in patients with less bulky disease; the 58% HCR-rate obtained with initial debulking followed by CAP may well be equalled by chemotherapy alone. With the advent of efficacious chemotherapy the role of locoregional debulking will diminish;this has been the case in malignant lymphoma and testicular cancer, in which diseases the role of surgery and/or radiotherapy has in some instances been changed from cytoreductive before to adjuvant therapy after powerfull chemotherapy. We suggest that time may have come for such a transition to make in ovarian cancer; a randomized trial comparing initial surgery with initial chemotherapy is highly warranted.

REFERENCES.
Griffiths CT, Parker LM, Fuller AF (1979). Role of cytoreductive surgical treatment in the management of advanced ovarian cancer. Cancer Treat Rep 63: 235-240.
Neijt JP. Combination chemotherapy in the treatment of advanced ovarian cancer (1983). Thesis, Utrecht, Holland.
Richardson GS, Scully RE, Nikzui N, Nelson JH (1985). Common epithelial cancer of the ovary. N Engl J Med 312: 415-424.
Bereck JS, Hacker NF, Lagasse LD, Leuchter RS (1982). Lower uterine tract resection as part of cytoreductive surgery for ovarian cancer. Gynecol Oncol 13: 87.
Blyth JG, Wahl TP (1982). Debulking surgery: does it increase the quality of survival. Gynecol Oncol 14: 396.
Castaldo TW, Petrilli ES, Ballon SC, Lagasse LD (1980). Intestinal operations in patients with ovarian carcinoma. Am J Obstet Gynecol 139: 801.
Decker DG, Fleming TR, Malhasian GD, Webb MJ, Jefferies JA, Edmonson JH (1982). Cyclophosphamide plus cis-platinum: a combination treatment program for stage III and IV ovarian carcinoma. Obstet Gynecol 60: 481-487.
Edwards CL, Herson J, Gershenson DM,Copeland LJ, Wharton JT (1983). A prospective randomized trial of Melphalan and cis-platinum versus Hexamethylmelamine, Adriamycin and Cyclophosphamide in advanced ovarian cancer. Gynecol Oncol 15: 261-277.

Primary Chemotherapy in Cancer Medicine, pages 217-223
© 1985 Alan R. Liss, Inc.

CYTOREDUCTIVE SURGERY WITH OR WITHOUT PRECEDING CHEMOTHERAPY
IN OVARIAN CANCER

J.P. Neijt, E.J. Aartsen, J. Bouma, A.P.M. Heintz,
M. van Lent, A.C.M. van Lindert
Netherlands Joint Study Group for Ovarian Cancer,
Department of Internal Medicine,
Utrecht, University Hospital.

Cytoreductive surgery (debulking surgery) is of major
importance in the treatment of ovarian cancer. The purpose
of this procedure is to minimize the tumor burden before
treatment is instituted. Cytoreductive surgery seems only
valuable if all gross tumour is excised. In a retrospective
study, Griffiths showed that despite 'debulking', there were
no long-term survivors if a mass greater than 1.5 cm in diameter was left behind. In his report including 102 patients
with stage II or III ovarian carcinoma, the diameter of the
largest residual tumor mass below 1.5 cm was correlated
with survival as an independent prognostic factor, but this
correlation disappeared with mass size above 1.5 cm
(Griffiths 1975). Similar conclusions could be drawn from a
review on ovarian cancer from the M.D. Anderson Hospital and
Tumour Institute (Houston); even patients with multiple
small metastases throughout the abdomen had a far better
prognosis than those with one single mass larger than 1 cm
(Smith 1979). Several other studies confirmed that patients
in whom cytoreductive surgery resulted in small tumor ag-
gregates will have a good chance of achieving a negative
second-look (Schwartz 1983). It is not yet clear from these
data whether the optimum point for providing a significant
survival benefit is 1, 1.5, or even 2 cm. The optimum size
is probably different for monochemotherapy and combination
chemotherapy as postoperative treatment.

Unfortunately, cytoreductive surgery is not always feasible in all patients at the initial laparotomy. This is the
case when the patient has a low performance status, when
tumor masses are located around the pancreas and splenic

pedicle, and when there   are large numbers of implants on
the peritoneal surfaces. In these patients debulking surgery sometimes may be easier when it is performed after a
few cycles of successful chemotherapy (intervention cytoreductive surgery). The decrease in the tumor mass facilitates
removal and makes the ablative procedure less extensive.

The selection factors that predict the outcome of surgery and subsequent cytotoxic treatment are not well under-
stood. These factors, i.e. the questions concerning the
timing of the debulking procedure and the relationship between surgical intervention and treatment outcome, will be
discussed and documented from material of the Netherlands
Joint Study Group for ovarian cancer. This group initiated
a study to compare the efficacy of two combination regimens
in ovarian cancer. Patients with FIGO stage III and IV previously untreated epithelial cancer were randomized to receive either combination chemotherapy consisting of hexamethylmelamine, cyclophosphamide, amethopterin (methotrexate), and 5-fluorouracil (Hexa-CAF), or combination chemotherapy that included cyclophosphamide, hexamethylmelamine,
adriamycin, and cisplatin (CHAP-5). Nine institutions par-
ticipated in this study. Numbers of eligible patients allocated to the Hexa-CAF and CHAP-5 regimen were 94 and 92,
respectively. The distribution of the different prognostic
factors was the same for both regimens.

It was concluded that results produced with CHAP-5
were significantly superior to those achieved with Hexa-CAF
with regard to response, progression-free survival and survival. In the study, maximum debulking(the removal of as
much tumor as possible) was recommended for all patients
before chemotherapy was initiated. As shown in Table 1, debulking surgery resulting in tumor remnants of less than 1
cm succeeded in only 18% of the patients and most patients
had tumor masses of more than 2 cm prior to the start of
chemotherapy.

The effect of the remaining tumor mass on survival was
most obvious when curves were computed separately for patients with tumor remnants of less than 1 cm, 1-2 cm, and
more than 2 cm (see Figure 1).

Patients who had residual tumor with a diameter of
less than 1 cm prior to chemotherapy survived longer than
patients with larger tumors. However, the survival curve

TABLE 1

Tumor Mass at Diagnosis and Residual Tumor after Debulking
Surgery in 186 Patients

Largest cross-sectional diameter	Tumor mass at diagnosis No. of pat. (%)		Residual tumor after debulking No. of pat. (%)	
microscopic	0		8	(4)
1 cm	0		26	(14)
1 - 2 cm	1	(1)	23	(12)
2 - 5 cm	22	(12)	41	(22)
5 cm	159	(86)	88	(47)
unknown	4	(2)	0	

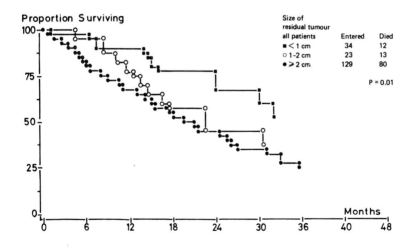

Figure 1. Survival of patients according to the largest
cross-sectional tumor diameter prior to the initiation of chemotherapy.

for patients who had residual tumor with diameters between 1 and 2 cm was similar to that for patients who had larger tumor remnants (p = 0.335). The effect of cytoreductive surgery on survival was more pronounced in the patient group treated with CHAP-5 (see Figure 2) than in the patients on Hexa-CAF, who did not receive significant benefit from cytoreductive surgery (p = 0.09).

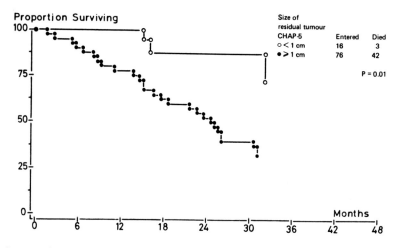

Figure 2. Survival following treatment with CHAP-5 in relation to the largest cross-sectional tumor diameter prior to the initiation of chemotherapy.

To identify whether the tumor residuum prior to chemotherapy was an independent prognostic predictor, a multivariate analysis was performed. The analysis revealed that the residual tumor prior to chemotherapy was a significant predictor for a complete remission documented at laparotomy (CRL) and long term survival. Other significant predictors were the cytotoxic treatment and FIGO stage (Neijt 1984). Every tumor reduction by surgery prior to the initiation of therapy lead to enhancement of the probability that a patient will reach a complete remission at second-look. Patients with FIGO stage III and a residuum of less than 1 cm had an almost 80% chance of obtaining a CRL after treatment with

CHAP-5. However, 4 patients with stage IV disease and small
residuals did not reach a complete remission. Only two factors predicted successful cytoreduction: a good performance
status and normal pretreatment body weight. However, age,
FIGO stage, histological type, histological grade and leucocyte count did not influence the outcome of the procedure.

In 18% of the patients, intervention cytoreductive
surgery was performed. This debulking procedure was performed prior to the third cycle of chemotherapy (early
intervention) or thereafter (late intervention). When intervention surgery was successful and debulking resulted in
tumor residuals of less than 1 cm, survival was prolonged
irrespective of the time when the procedure was performed.
There were no differences in the survival of the patients
who underwent successful cytoreductive surgery before the
third cycle of chemotherapy versus those operated thereafter (p = 0.38). There was a tendency for patients with
residual tumor of less than 1 cm in diameter after intervention debulking to have inferior survival compared with
those who had successful debulking prior to chemotherapy
(see Figure 3), but the difference was not significant.

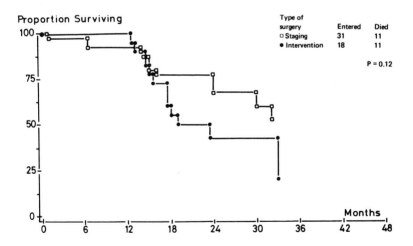

Fig. 3: Survival following cytoreductive surgery resulting
in tumor residuals of less than 1 cm, either at the
staging laparotomy (staging) or during chemotherapy
(intervention cytoreductive surgery).

As shown above, the outlook for the patient with advanced ovarian cancer can be improved by means of strategies other than new, powerful drug combinations. Surgical
resection of the tumor mass prior to institution of chemotherapy is also an important factor in the achievement of
higher complete response rates and significant prolongation
of survival. As shown here, the probability that a patient
will achieve a long-lasting response increases with decreasing size of the residual tumor prior to chemotherapy.
A significant effect on survival will be obtained when all
tumor masses are reduced to a size of 1 cm or less. There
has been much discussion about whether cyto-reductive surgery should be performed prior to chemotherapy or thereafter. If cytoreductive surgery is performed after chemotherapy has been initiated and the tumor has begun to respond (intervention-cytoreductive surgery), the tumor load
is therefore decreased and the surgical procedure less extensive. On the other hand, there is always a slight chance
that the patient will not respond to chemotherapy due to the
presence of resistant tumor cells which were not removed
surgically prior to the onset of cytotoxic treatment. In our
study both surgical strategies were performed. A retrospective analysis raises a number of problems concerning patient
selection requiring that the results be considered with
care. Conclusions concerning the timing of the procedure
can scarcely be drawn. However, it can be deduced from our
data that successful cytoreductive surgery reducing the
tumor to a size of 1 cm or less always improves survival,
irrespective of whether the procedure is performed before
or during the administration of chemotherapy and that the
most suitable candidates for extensive initial surgery are
the patients in a good general condition and with a high or
normal body weight.

REFERENCES

Griffiths CT (1975). Surgical resection of tumor bulk in the primary treatment of ovarian carcinoma. Natl Cancer Inst Monogr 42:101.

Neijt JP, Ten Bokkel Huinink WW (1984). Randomised trial comparing two combination chemotherapy regimens (Hexa-CAF vs CHAP-5) in advanced ovarian carcinoma. The Lancet II:594.

Schwartz PE (1983). Current status of the second-look operation in ovarian cancer. In: "Clinics in Obstetrics and Gynaecology", Philadelphia: Saunders, p 245.

Smith JP, Day GT (1979). Review of ovarian cancer of the University of Texas Systems Cancer Center MD Anderson Hospital and Tumor Institute. Am J Obstet Gynecol 135: 984.

Primary Chemotherapy in Cancer Medicine, pages 225-237
© 1985 Alan R. Liss, Inc.

VINCRISTINE, BLEOMYCIN, MITOMYCIN C, CISPLATIN COMBINATION
CHEMOTHERAPY AS ADDITIVE TREATMENT TO RADIOTHERAPY IN POOR
RISK PATIENTS WITH SQUAMOUS CELL CARCINOMA OF THE UTERINE
CERVIX

J.B. Vermorken*, M.E.L. v.d. Burg, A.J. Subandono,
C. Mangioni, C.F. De Oliveira, P. Zola, A.T. van
Oosterom, S. Pecorelli, A.C.M. van Lindert.

*Free Univ. Hosp., Amsterdam, The Netherlands

INTRODUCTION

    Traditionally, chemotherapy has been limited to a pal-
liative role in those patients with cervical cancer who present with distant metastases or who have recurrent disease
following primary local therapies and for whom salvage procedures, such as irradiation or pelvic exenteration, are in-
appropriate or have failed. The development of even this role
has been hampered by a number of factors, including:1) limited numbers of patients at individual institutions; 2) decreased pelvic vascular perfusion; 3) renal compromise; 4)
inevaluable pelvic disease; 5) limited bone marrow reserve;
and 6) histology. Nevertheless, currently available information indicates that cervical cancer is responsive to cytotoxic therapy. With former single agent chemotherapy responses were observed in 10-25% of cases which seldom were
complete, mostly of short duration and generally not having
any impact on survival (Wasserman, Carter 1977; Muscato et
al 1982). It should be realized that response criteria used
in the past have occasionally varied from those used nowa-
days (WHO 1979). At present, cisplatin is considered the most
active single drug in this disease, showing a 27% response
rate when used in first-line (Baker 1980; Thigpen et al 1979;
Bonomi et al 1982). About 10% complete remissions can be expected and responding patients do live longer. Combination
chemotherapy improves the response rate up to 50%, including
a larger number of complete remissions (Muscato et al 1982;
Green, Young 1983). Although overall remission duration is
still of the order of 4-6 months, some patients who achieve
complete remission have a long-term disease free survival
(Alberts et al 1981; Vermorken et al 1984).

Improved information about the natural history of cervical cancer that has been provided by more sensitive roentgen-
ologic techniques and the practice of staging laparotomy have
helped to identify those patients who are at particular high
risk for failure with conventional therapy. These include
patients with advanced disease (Stages III and IVA) and those
with pelvic or para-aortic nodal involvement found at initial
surgery. In the latter group of patients (FIGO Stages IB and
IIA) the 5-year survival rate decreases to 50% or less when
pelvic nodes contain metastatic cancer (Piver, Chung 1975;
Hsu et al 1972; Fuller et al 1982; Bleker et al 1983). In
patients with nodal disease various factors are of additional
importance for predicting recurrence, including the number
of positive nodes, the extension of the tumor beyond the cervix, the size and stage of the primary cervical tumor and also its biological properties (Fuller et al 1982; Noguchi et
al 1983). In this respect it is of importance to realize that
patients with three or more node groups involved or those
with para-aortic lymph node involvement have a very poor prognosis.

Only a few data are available on the use of primary
chemotherapy (preceding radiotherapy) in these poor-risk categories of cervical cancer patients (Table 1). So far, in a
limited number of patients, such a procedure seemed feasible
with cisplatin-containing regimens.

Table 1. Chemotherapy(CT) preceding radiotherapy(RT) in poor-
risk patients with carcinoma of the uterine cervix

FIGO Stage	# pts	CT	# cycl	Resp rate %	Compl.[+] CT+RT	Reference	
IIIB	22	BMP	1	50	N.I.	Merwe et al	(1983)
IIIB	7	BOMP	2	71	-	Surwit et al	(1983)
IIIB/IV	10	PVB	3	60	-	Friedlander et al	(1983)
IIIB/IVA	25	BOMP*	3	48	0/19	Kavanagh et al	(1984)
IIB- IVB	9	BMP	2-4	78	2/9°	Bauer et al	(1984)
IIB- IVA	11	P	6	78	1/10°°	Jobson et al	(1984)
IB /IIA	30	BP	2	N.I.	-	Hakes et al	(1984)

B=bleomycin; O=vincristine; V=vinblastine; P=cisplatin;
M=methotrexate (in BMP) or mitomycin C (in BOMP); N.I.= not
indicated; °= prolonged treatment breaks due to thrombocytopenia; °°= one patient refused RT and one developed chronic
leucopenia; *= intra-arterial CT; [+] = complications.

During the past five years the EORTC Gynecological Cancer Cooperative Group (G.C.C.G.) performed several studies
in patients with disseminated squamous cell carcinoma of the
uterine cervix (SCCUC) (Vermorken et al 1984). The first
trial (protocol 55802) studied the efficacy and toxicity of
a bleomycin-mitomycin C based regimen to which vincristine
and cisplatin were added (VBMP). The overall response rate
in 50 evaluable patients was 40% and median time to progression was 48 weeks and 32 weeks for patients with complete response (16%) and partial response respectively. Of interest
was that the complete remission rate in patients with only
distant metastases was 30% (for patients with only lung and/
or lymph node metastases 40%) and some of these patients had
long term disease-free survival. The toxicity of the VBMP
regimen was acceptable to the patients. Bone marrow toxicity
was cumulative, but in general no severe myelosuppression was
observed during the first four cycles. These results prompted
some members of the EORTC G.C.C.G. to start a feasibility
study, investigating the use of VBMP as additive treatment to
radiotherapy in the primary treatment of poor-risk patients
with SCCUC. The main objectives of this study were to explore
the interaction of VBMP and radiotherapy with regard to toxicity and to investigate whether the use of VBMP would interfere with giving radiotherapy at full doses. This report will
summarize the current results of this ongoing feasibility
study (study coordinator: M.E.L. v.d. Burg, RRTI, Rotterdam).

PATIENTS AND METHODS

Patients eligible for the study are those with histologically confirmed SCCUC FIGO stages IIB distal, III and IVA
(advanced local disease) and those with high common iliac or
para-aortic nodal metastases found at initial surgery for
stages IB and IIA, who give informed consent. Ineligibility
criteria include age > 70 years, a life expectancy < three
months, performance status < 60%,prior chemotherapy or radiotherapy, other histology than squamous cell carcinoma, uncontrolled active infection, creatinine clearance < 60 ml/min,
WBC < 4.0 x 10^9/l, platelets < 100 x 10^9/l, bilirubin $\geq$ 25
μmol/l, severe pulmonary dysfunction, additional malignances
except for skin cancer, overt psychosis and marked senility.

The chemotherapy regimen used in this feasibility study
is identical to that used in protocol 55802 (mentioned above).
Each course consists of 1.4 mg/m² (maximum 2 mg) vincristine
i.v. on day 1 followed six hours later by a continuous infu-

sion of bleomycin for 48 hours, 15 mg/day on days 1 and 2.
At the end of the bleomycin infusion 6 mg/m² mitomycin C is
given i.v. (day 3). After a therapy-free interval of 22-24
hours, cisplatin is given over three hours with adequate hydration. Patients are prehydrated with 1 liter of normal saline and receive 4 liters after the end of cisplatin administration over 24 hours. Mannitol and furosemide are not giv-
en on a routine basis. When diuresis is less than 600 ml per
six hours, 100 cc 20% mannitol is given. If this is not effective within two hours, mannitol is given again in combination with 5-10 mg furosemide. The chemotherapy regimen is
repeated at four-week intervals. Unless there is evidence of
disease progression after the first VBMP cycle patients are
supposed to receive two cycles of VBMP before the start of
radiotherapy (interval between chemotherapy and radiotherapy
± four weeks). The radiotherapy schedule is variable and radiotherapy is given according to standard procedures in each
participating center (see also under RESULTS). After termination of the radiotherapy another two cycles of VBMP should
be given to those patients, who have shown a response during
the first two VBMP cycles before the radiotherapy. In case of
no change of disease after the first two cycles further VBMP
therapy after radiotherapy is at the discretion of individual
investigators. Chemotherapy dose modifications have been described earlier in relation to protocol 55802.(Vermorken et al
1982). However, contrary to the previous study, patients will
not receive further chemotherapy in case the second cycle of
VBMP has to be postponed for more than two weeks.

Initial work-up includes complete medical history and
physical examination (clinical staging if possible under anesthesia), urinalysis, creatinine clearance, complete blood
counts (CBC) with differential, platelet counts, blood chem-
istry (liver function tests, creatinine, electrolytes), radiological survey (chest, abdomen, IVP), ultrasound examination of the pelvic lesions, CT-scanning of the whole abdomen,
electrocardiogram, audiogram and pulmonary function tests;
lymphangiography is optional. During VBMP cycles CBC, platelet
counts and serum creatinine are performed on days 13 and 20.
Physical examination, evaluation of tumor status, renal and
liver function tests, CBC, platelet counts and radiological
survey of the chest are repeated prior to each treatment
course and before radiotherapy. During radiotherapy, CBC and
platelet counts are performed at least weekly next to urinalysis and renal function tests at regular intervals. Toxicity
is recorded during treatment period and monthly therafter up

to one year after the initiation of therapy; after the first
year every three months up to three years. Response to treatment is determined after each chemotherapy course and after
the radiotherapy and during follow-up at intervals as indicated above for the registration of toxicity. Complete remission is defined as a disappearance of all clinically detectable disease. A partial remission is defined as an estimated
decrease in tumor mass of 50% or more, whithout the appearance of new lesions. Stable disease is defined as an estimated decrease of less than 50% in tumor size, or an increase
of less than 25%. Progressive disease is defined as an estimated increase in tumor size of more than 25%, or the appearance of new lesions. Survival is dated from the commencement
of treatment.

Patients

Since 1982 a total of 64 eligible patients entered in
the study, of whom 60 are currently evaluable for toxicity
and survival and 54 are evaluable for response. It is too
early to evaluate three patients and one patient is considered inevaluable, because for unknown reasons cisplatin was de-
leted from the schedule. The median age of the 60 evaluable
patients at start of treatment was 57 years (range 23-70 yrs)
and their median performance status 100%(range 70-100%).FIGO
stages at initial diagnosis were as follows: IB (4 patients),
IIA (3), IIB (12), IIIA (1), IIIB (33), IVA (6) and IVB (1).
The patient with Stage IVB disease had involved inguinal
nodes and tumor depositions in the vulva. Eight patients had
initial surgery:for Stage IB disease (4 patients), Stage IIA
(2 patients), Stage IIB (1 patient) and Stage IVA (1 patient)
respectively. Five patients had no evidence of disease (NED)
clinically afterwards, two patients still had evaluable residual disease and in one patient (initially with Stage IB
disease) inguinal nodes were found involved as well at time
of admission to the referral center.

RESULTS

Treatment Evaluation

Three of the 60 evaluable patients did not receive radiotherapy at all. In one case because of patient's refusal

after reaching a partial remission on two cycles of VBMP
(duration 5.5 months), in two cases because of progressive
disease. Of these latter two patients one showed a very rapid
progression of the disease leading to death after three months;
the second patient developed bone metastases within two months
from the start of chemotherapy, but is still alive with disease after eight months. Three patients received only one
cycle of VBMP. In all cases this was followed immediately by
radiotherapy because of either documented progression after
the first cycle of VBMP, or patient's refusal of the second
VBMP course and in one case this was due to protocol violation. All the other patients received two cycles of VBMP followed by radiotherapy, while 33 patients received VBMP cycles
after the radiotherapy as well. In total, 178 cycles of VBMP
were administered. Radiotherapy was given either by external
teletherapy without shielding, followed by intracavitary
brachytherapy given as a booster or with shielding of the
effective area of intracavitary brachytherapy during external teletherapy or by external teletherapy alone. External
teletherapy was applied either with a Cobalt 60 teletherapy
unit or megavoltage equipment to a total dose of about 40-60
Gy delivered in 20-30 fractions in about 5-6 weeks. Para-
aortic lymph nodes irradiation was given as a routine or on
indication. Intracavitary brachytherapy was mostly applied
by means of an afterloading applicator using Radium 226, Cobalt 60 or Cesium 137 sources which delivered the dose either
with a low-dose rate or with a high-dose rate. For comparison of the different radiotherapy schedules the TDF (time-
dose fractionation) value was used as a quantitative measure of the biological effect (Orton 1974; Ellis 1971). In
table 2 the TDF values of the radiotherapy regimens used on
several reference points (point A, pelvic wall, para-aortic
region) are summarized. A distinction is made between patients,
who underwent surgery and those who did not. Data of seven
patients are not included for the following reasons: no radiotherapy given (3 patients), early tumor death (radiotherapy given only for 4 days: 1 patient), no data (1 patient),
discontinuation of radiotherapy because of toxicity (see section toxicity below: 2 patients). In relation to the data giv-
en in table 2 it is of importance to realize that minimal
requirements for optimal radiotherapy dose/TDF value, as was
defined by the Subcommittee for Radiotherapy of the G.C.C.G.
in 1984, are for advanced local disease: at point A= 120, at
"poire" isodose=120, pelvic wall=70, para-aortic region=66.
For patients after radical surgery these requirements are the
following: at point A (in case positive resection margins

of the vagina and paracervical areas are present)=95, pelvic wall=66, at the para-aortic region=66. The latter group of patients are considered to have positive nodes (common iliac and/or para-aortic).

Table 2. Evaluation of radiotherapy schedules in 53 evaluable patients: TDF values at different reference points

Treatment Group	# pts	Time-dose fractionation value		
		point A	pelvic field	PAO region
Stage IB/IIA/IIB (surgery)	8	77 (60-105)	74 (60-90)	72 (60-99)/N=4
Stage II/III/IV (no surgery)	45	115 (66-128)	92 (66-115)	76 (60-84)/N=18

Toxicity

Hematological and non-hematological toxicities are summarized in tables 3 and 4. Hematological toxicity in general was acceptable throughout the three phases of therapy (see table 3).However,an increasingpercentage of WHO grade III toxicities (WBC 1.0-1.9 x 10^9/l; platelets 25-49 x 10^9/l) was encountered in each successive phase; in 5 out of 56 evaluable patients during the first two VBMP cycles (9%), in 6 out of 44 evaluable cases during radiotherapy (14%) and in 6 out of 32 evaluable cases during VBMP after radiotherapy (18%), while an additional patient during this last mentioned phase showed grade IV toxicity (for platelets).

Table 3. Hematological toxicity observed during VBMP + radiotherapy related to different treatment phases.

Treatment Phase	Hb(mmol/l) median range	WBC($x10^9$/l) median range	Plts($x10^9$/l) median range
VBMP before RT	6.9 5.1-9.4	3.7 1.2-8.6	138 46-290
Radiotherapy	6.6 4.5-9.2	2.9 1.8-7.4	140 28-300
VBMP after RT	6.0 4.7-8.7	2.6 1.4-4.5	110 20-300

Sixteen patients had interruptions of the radiotherapy treatment. In 14 patients this was only for a short period,

two weeks or less. The reasons for this interruption were:
myelosuppression (in 3 cases), gastrointestinal (4), fever
without evidence of infection (3), severe skin reaction (2),
the development of a tumor fistula (1) and infection (1).
In two patients treatment was discontinued permanently because of myelosuppression. One of these two patients developed an isolated thrombocytopenia during radiotherapy. At the
time that the platelet counts were still in the normal range
(154×10^9/l) there was a severe drop in hemoglobin (4.5 mmol/l),
without clear evidence of bleeding, for which red cell trans-
fusion was needed. Thereafter both a coagulation disorder and
an important rise in transaminases were found next to low
platelet counts (28×10^9/l). Radiotherapy was stopped at that
time (TDF value at point A and pelvic wall: 32). Very slowly
the platelets recovered in eight weeks time, however radiotherapy never was restarted. The tumor progressed and the
patient died 5.7 months after the start of therapy. The second patient stopped radiotherapy after a total dose of 34 Gy
(TDF value at point A and pelvic wall: 56). The reason for
this was chronic leucopenia. However, the lowest WBC value
during radiotherapy was 1.8×10^9/l (for platelets 120×10^9/
l) and the decision to discontinue radiotherapy is debatable.
The patient received only one cycle of VBMP before radiotherapy (protocol violation) without bone marrow toxicity (lowest
values for WBC and platelets 4.1 and 150×10^9/l, respectively). The patient is alive with still evidence of disease
(tumor reduction < 50%). Both patients described above had
FIGO Stage IIIB disease.

Table 4. Non-hematological side effects observed during VBMP+
radiotherapy treatment and during follow-up.

Type of Toxicity	Incidence and grade of tox* VBMP				Radiotherapy				Late toxicity		
	1	2	3	4	1	2	3	4	mild	moderate	severe
Nausea/vomiting	10	30	4	1	18	10	–	–	–	–	–
Diarrhea	8	3	1	–	12	11	5	–	–	–	–
Fever	9	10	–	–	–	3	–	–	–	–	–
Infection	1	2	–	–	–	–	1	–		–	1
Skin	2	–	–	–	4	3	2	2	2	3	1
Neurotoxicity	6	2	2	–	–	–	–	–	–	–	–
Lung fibrosis	–	–	–	–	–	–	–	–	–	1	–
Ileus	–	–	–	–	–	–	–	–	1	–	2
Perforation	–	–	–	–	–	–	–	–	–	–	2
Proctitis	–	–	–	–	–	–	–	–	4	1	2

*WHO criteria

The non-hematological side effects observed during VBMP
treatment were not different from those observed during our
previous study in patients with disseminated SCCUC. In addition to what is listed in table 4, about one third of the
patients had alopecia (grade 1-3), two patients had phlebitis,
one patients had stomatitis and one complainted of bowel
cramps. The main toxicities observed during radiotherapy were
nausea/vomiting and diarrhea. But, additionally 15 patients
complained of bowel cramps. According to some collegues, the
skin reactions observed during radiotherapy may have been
somewhat more severe than with radiotherapy alone in some instances. During follow-up after treatment some severe side
effects have been encountered (see table 4), including skin
fibrosis, ileus, perforation and proctitis. Two patients died
without evidence of disease. The first patient had Stage IIB
disease. She received two cycles of VBMP followed by a modified radiotherapy program because of the position of the
ileum near the intracavitary source (Cathetron/high dose rate).
At 9 months she complained of severe diarrhea and lost weight
excessively. At 11 months she was admitted because of urinary
retention and hydronephrosis was found at ultrasound examination. Clinical features of peritonitis developed and she died
shortly therafter (survival 11.5 months). At autopsy no tumor
was found, but peritonitis was evident (and empyema in the
lower abdomen) with bowel adhesions, a large recto-vaginal
fistula and a small recto-vescical fistula. The second patient
had a Stage IIIB disease. She received two cycles of VBMP, and
the same difficulties during intracavitary brachytherapy (Se-
lectron/high dose rate) were encountered as in the first
patient. The total TDF value at the lower pelvic area and at
point A was 126, and at the higher pelvic area and the para-
aortic region 76. The patient received two further cycles of
VBMP after radiotherapy. Six months after the end of radiotherapy the patient had surgery for a small bowel perforation.
This patient had severe proctitis as well (with diarrhea and
bloody stools) and she ultimately developed a recto-vaginal
fistula. The patient died 14 months after the start of therapy while being in complete remission clinically. Autopsy was
not allowed. Both lethal complications were seen in the same
institute and were not felt to be clearly related to the addition of VBMP to the radiotherapy by the local radiotherapist. Two patients needed surgical intervention because of
ileus. Both patients underwent radical surgery one year and
two and a half year previously for stages IB and IIB disease
respectively. The first patient received only two cycles of
VBMP followed by adequate radiotherapy (including irradiation

to the para-aortic region); the second patient did not receive radiotherapy to the para-aortic region, but did receive
four cycles of VBMP in total.

Response and Survival

Data on response and survival are summarized in tables
5 and 6. The response rate to VBMP before radiotherapy, according to WHO criteria, was somewhat disappointing when compared with the data obtained with the same regimen in patients
with disseminated SCCUC. Excluding the patients who refused
a second cycle (1) or who did not receive this because of
protocol violation (1) only 17 out of 53 evaluable patients
responded (32%), and no complete remissions were observed.
No clear explanation can be given for this, although tumor
volume and necrosis next to a difficult tumor evaluation at
this site might play a role.

Table 5. Response to VBMP + radiotherapy

Treatment Phase	# Eval. pts	Complete response	Partial response	No change	Progressive disease
2 x VBMP	53+	–	17	29	7
2 x VBMP + RT	49	13	24	7	5
Overall*	54°	25	13	4	12

*Ultimate result after the end of whole treatment period
°In one patient not available, + one patient only one cycle

During the observation period of the study 28 patients showed progression during treatment or relapsed. The site of progression was at distance (metastases) in 13 patients, only
loco-regional in six, both in seven and unknown in two.

Table 6. VBMP+radiotherapy feasibility study: Survival Status

FIGO Stage	#Eval pts	Alive rec–	rec+	follow-up*	Dead tumor+	tumor–	survival
IB	4	3	–	54,87,101	1	–	43
IIA	3	2	–	38,72	1	–	92
IIB	12	8	1	42(25–117)	2	1(51)	33,98
IIIA	1	1	–	52	–	–	–
IIIB	33	15	5	51(18–104)	12	1(63)	57(11–102)
IVA	6	1	2	35,45,80	3	–	21,22,25
IVB	1	–	1	92	–	–	–
Total	60	30	9	52(18–117)	19	2	52(11–102)

*Weeks: median (range); rec= recurrence

CONCLUSIONS

This feasibility study indicates that the addition of VBMP to radiotherapy in the primary treatment of poor-risk patients with squamous cell carcinoma of the uterine cervix is a feasible procedure. Radiotherapy could be given to full extent in 55 out of the 57 patients, who received this combined modality program. Moreover, the reasons to discontinue radiotherapy in one of the two patients, in whom this occurred, were debatable. Severe late side effects, such as skin fibrosis (1), proctitis (2), ileus (2) and bowel perforation (2) have been observed. Although there is a suggestion of an enhancement of the radiotherapy effects to the skin, it is not clear whether the other side effects are related to the addition of VBMP to radiotherapy. In order to establish the value and the risks of this combined treatment a randomized trial, comparing VBMP + radiotherapy with radiotherapy alone, is required.

REFERENCES

Alberts DS, Martimbeau PW, Surwitt EA, Oishi N (1981). Mitomycin C, bleomycin, vincristine and cisplatin in the treatment of advanced, recurrent squamous cell carcinoma of the cervix. Cancer Clin Trials 4:313.
Baker LH (1980). Cis-platin in treatment of cervical and endo-endometrial cancer patients. In Prestayko JW, Crooke ST, Carter SK (eds):"Cis-Platin: Current Status and New Developments", New York: Academic Press, pp 403-409.
Bauer K, Knapp R, Bloomer W, Bast Jr R, Canellos G (1984). Cis-DDP, bleomycin, MTX-LCV (PBM) chemotherapy in advanced, previously untreated carcinoma of the cervix (CaC). Proc Am Soc Clin Oncol 3:169.
Bleker OP, Ketting BW, van Wayjen-Eecen B, Kloosterman GJ (1983). The significance of microscopic involvement of the parametrium and/or pelvic lymph nodes in cervical cancer stages IB and IIA. Gynecol Oncol 16:56.
Bonomi P, Bruckner HW, Cohen C, Marshall R, Blessing J, Slayton R (1982). A randomized trial of three cis-platin regimens in squamous cell carcinoma of the cervix. Proc Am Soc Clin Oncol 1:110.
Ellis F (1971). Nominal standard dose and the RET. Br J Radiol 44:101.
Friedlander M, Kaye SB, Sullivan A, Atkinson K, Elliot P, Coppleson M, Houghton R, Solomon J, Green D, Russel P,

Hudson CN, Lanflands AO, Tatterdall MHN (1983). Cervical carcinoma: A drug-responsive tumor - Experience with combined cisplatin, vinblastine and bleomycin therapy. Gynecol Oncol 16:275.

Fuller AF, Elliot N, Kosloff C, Lewis JL (1982). Lymph node metastases from carcinoma of the cervix, stages IB and IIA: Implications for prognosis and treatment.Gynecol Oncol13:165.

Green JA, Young RC (1983). Gynecological tumors. In Pinedo HM, Chabner BA (eds):"Cancer Chemotherapy 1983", Amsterdam, Elsevier, pp 369-397.

Hakes T, Wertheim M, Daghestani A, Nori D, Clark D, Lewis Jr J (1984). Adjuvant chemotherapy for poor-risk stage IB/IIA cervix carcinoma patients- A pilot study with cisplatin/bleomycin. Proc Am Soc Clin Oncol 3:171.

Hsu C, Cheng Y, Su S (1972). Prognosis of uterine cervical cancer with extensive lymph node metastases. Am J Obstet Gynecol 114:954

Jobson V, Homesley H, Muss H, Welander C, Ferree C, Wells B (1984). Cisplatin chemotherapy (CT) followed by radiotherapy (RT) in patients with advanced cervical carcinoma. Proc Am Soc Clin Oncol 3:170.

Kavanagh J, Wallace S, Delclos L, Rutledge F (1984). Update of the results of intra-arterial (IA) chemotherapy for advanced squamous cell carcinoma of the cervix. Proc Am Soc Clin Oncol 3:172.

Merwe A v.d., du Toit J, Smit B (1983). Combination chemotherapy in stage IIIB cervical cancer; comparative five year survival results of cis-diammine dichloroplatinum, methotrexate, bleomycin & radiotherapy versus radiotherapy. Proc Am Soc Clin Oncol 2:146.

Muscato MS, Perry MC, Yarbro JW (1982). Chemotherapy of cervical carcinoma. Semin Oncol 9:373.

Nogushi H, Shiozawa K, Tsukamoto T, Tsukahara Y, Iwai S, Fukuto T (1983). The postoperative classification for uterine cervical cancer and its clinical evaluation. Gynecol Oncol 16:219.

Orton CG (1974). Time dose factors (TDFs) in brachytherapy. Br J Radiol 17:603.

Piver MS, Chung WS (1975). Prognostic significance of cervical lesion size and pelvic node metastases in cervical carcinoma.Obstet Gynecol 46:507.

Surwit EA,Alberts DS, Aristizabal S, Deatherage KJ, Heusinkveld R (1983). Treatment of primary and recurrent, advanced squamous cell cancer of the cervix with mitomycin-C + vincristine + bleomycin (MOB) plus cisplatin (PLAT). Proc Am Soc Clin Oncol 2:153.

Thigpen T, Shingleton H, Homesley H (1979). Phase II trial of cis-platin as first or second line treatment for advanced squamous cell carcinoma of the cervix. Proc Am Soc Clin Oncol 20:288.

Vermorken JB, v.d.Burg MEL, Rotmensz N, Dalesio O.(1984). EORTC Gynecological Cancer Cooperative Group (G.C.C.G.) 1977-1984. In "Decimo Corso di Aggiornamento in Oncologia Medici", Rome, pp 615-626.

Wasserman TH, Carter SK (1977). The integration of chemotherapy into combined modality treatment of solid tumors VIII. Cervical Cancer. Cancer Treat Rev 4:25.

WHO handbook for reporting results of cancer treatment (1979). Geneva: World Health Organization.

SECTION VII
GASTROINTESTINAL CANCER

Primary Chemotherapy in Cancer Medicine, pages 241–252
© 1985 Alan R. Liss, Inc.

CHEMOTHERAPY-BASED MULTI-MODALITY THERAPY OF
ESOPHAGEAL CANCER

David Kelsen, M.D.
Associate Attending Physician
Solid Tumor Service
Memorial Sloan-Kettering Cancer Center
Associate Professor of Clinical Medicine
Cornell University Medical College
New York, New York

The prognosis for patients with epidermoid cancer of the esophagus
treated with surgery or radiation therapy alone or in combination is
dismal,even when the tumor is clinically limited to the local-
regional area. The reason for such poor survival in patients with
potentially curable disease can be at least partly explained by the
results of several recent autopsy series (Table I).[1,2] In these
studies, most patients were found to have distant metastases, with
or without local recurrence or residual tumor. The major sites of
metastatic disease were lymph nodes, lung, liver, adrenal glands, and
trachea-bronchus. The extent of tumor found at autopsy did not
appear to be due to a prolonged clinical course with widespread
disease as a terminal event: in Anderson's series, the median
duration from date of diagnosis to death was only 4 months, and
many of Bosch's patients died in the immediate post-operative
period. This data supports the clinical impression that Western
patients (who in general present with symptoms of dysphagia or
odynophagia) have widespread disease at the time of diagnosis. In
theory effective systemic chemotherapy should have a major role to
play in their treatment. Until recently, there were few studies
involving the use of antineoplastic drugs in esophageal cancer. Over
the last 5-8 years however a number of single agent and combination
chemotherapy trials have been reported.[3] These studies initially
focused on patients with advanced disease. When objective
regressions were seen in this population, the same regimens were
used in a multimodality setting. The purpose of this paper is to
review the results of programs involving chemotherapy-surgery-
radiation, and chemotherapy followed by radiation. The toxicities of
radiation and of chemotherapy when used alone have recently been
reviewed and will only be briefly discussed unless additive toxicity
of combined therapy has been noted.[3,4]

TABLE I
EXTENT OF DISEASE
AUTOPSY DATA

Study	Patient number	Local only%	Distant only %	Local + Dist.
Anderson*	79	9	2	82
Bosch	82	27	7	50

*Autopsy performed a median of four months from diagnosis

Chemotherapy Surgery and Radiation

The largest experience with chemotherapy-containing multimodality programs in esophageal cancer has been with programs using chemotherapy prior to surgery, with or without post-operative radiation therapy. All studies reported to date can be characterized as single-arm Phase II trials, and involve patients with epidermoid carcinoma. Randomized studies have only recently begun. In general, reported trials have involved one to two cycles of chemotherapy given over 3-6 weeks prior to surgery. When the surgical procedure used has been identified it usually involved a single stage operation, with esophago-gastrostomy following an esophagectomy; many studies have only been reported in abstract form and the details of surgery have not been given. The colon has occasionally been used to re-construct the alimentary tract. A modified Ivor-Lewis procedure has been most commonly used; extrathoracic esophagectomy has also been employed. Because of potential synergistic pulmonary toxicity when chemotherapeutic agents, e.g. bleomycin or mitomycin C, have been given pre-operatively, close monitoring of the FiO_2 is mandatory; every effort should be made to keep it below 40%. When radiation therapy has been given post-operatively, it has, in general, been started 3-4 weeks following surgery. Nutritional support is commonly used in the Memorial Hospital studies, but total parenteral nutrition was avoided unless the patient was totally obstructed. Our preference has been to use enteral nutrition, with a naso-gastric tube, a motorized pump and a high calorie-high protein solution. This allows nutrition replenishment on an outpatient basis. Details of nutritional support in most other studies are not yet available.

In most reported studies, entrance requirements included renal, pulmonary, and hepatic function that was adequate to allow consideration of surgery and of high-dose cisplatin, which is the common denominator of almost every chemotherapy trial. The pre-operative staging used has in general involved radiographic and radionuclide studies that allow assessment of distant metastases and extent of local-regional tumor. Computerized tomography has now replaced invasive techniques such as mediastinoscopy, laparotomy, and azygous venography.[5] Bronchoscopy, to rule out asymptomatic invasion of the trachea or bronchus, is usually routinely performed in all patients in whom the primary tumor was less than 30 cms. from the incisor teeth.Thus, patients who are candidates for pre-operative programs have clinical stage $T_{1-2}N_xM_0$ epidermoid cancer of the esophagus, using the American Joint Commission On Cancer staging system.[6]

Results of Pre operative Chemotherapy-Trials

Two small trials using single-agent chemotherapy prior to surgery have been reported. In both studies, bleomycin was used. Fujimaki et al treated 19 Japanese patients with intramuscular bleomycin daily or every other day to a total dosage of 30 to 600 mg (planned total dose 300 mg).[7] Surgery was performed seven to ten days following completion of chemo-therapy. One patient developed significant bleomycin pulmonary toxicity. Of the 19 patients, nine had resectable disease, four of whom were still alive 2 to 5 years from the start of treatment. All ten of those with unresectable disease were dead within 1 year.

Wada et al used a similar regimen.[8] They reported some evidence of tumor regression in 11/18 patients.

Preoperative regimens using combination chemotherapy have now been reported. (Table 2) Two studies involving cisplatin, bleomycin and, later, vindesine were reported from Memorial Hospital. In the first, 34 patients with disease clinically limited to the local-regional area were treated with cisplatin and a bleomycin infusion.[9] A single course of chemotherapy was given prior to surgery, which was performed 3 weeks after treatment was started. In the Memorial trials, assessment of antitumor response was performed by evaluating serial barium esophagrams and pathologic findings at surgery; details of the response criteria have been reported.[9] Of the 34 patients entered into the preoperative arm of the study, 14% had partial responses to cisplatin and bleomycin; an additional 44% had minor regressions. All patients underwent exploration, with 76% having resectable disease. The operative mortality was 11%. Following surgery, a second cycle of chemotherapy, identical to the first, was given for those with T_3 or N_1 tumor. RT was given at 3200 rads of radiation in 400 rad doses twice a week for 4 weeks, beginning immediately after the completion of the first course of postoperative chemotherapy. One year of maintenance chemotherapy with cisplatin and bleomycin was planned but proved impractical. The study was begun in 1976 and completed in 1979; median survival for the whole group was 9.7 months; three patients (9%) lived for more than 3 years.

TABLE 2:Chemotherapy Prior to Surgery

Drugs	Pts Enter.	Resect. %	RxMort. %	Sur %*
Bleo	19	47	NS#	21+
DDP-Bleo	34	76	14.7	8.8^X
DDP-VDS-Bleo	34	82	8.8	23
DDP-VCR-Bleo-FU	10	100	NS	NS
DDP-VP-16-Bleo	6	NS	NS	NS
DDP-VDS-MGBG	5	80	20	NS
DDP-Mito-Bleo	15	73	45	NS

#=Not Stated, *=at time of last report,+=2-5 years post-treatment, ^{X} minimum follow-up 4.5 years

The conclusion of this trial was that preoperative chemotherapy with this type of regimen was possible, with no increase in operative morbidity or mortality. When compared to the historical control group of Memorial patients receiving preoperative radiation during the period from 1966 to 1976, the resection rate appeared to be at least as good and probably better. However, survival was not improved, probably because of the only modest activity of the two-drug combination.

In the second study, vindesine was added to the cisplatin-bleomycin combination after it had shown activity in a single-agent phase II trial.[10] The three agents (cisplatin-vindesine-bleomycin or DVB) were again given prior to surgery to a second group of 34 patients.[11] Only two courses of chemotherapy were planned in this trial, initially one before and one after surgery. After it was noted that in patients with metastatic disease the maximum degree of response was achieved after two courses of DVB, the protocol was amended to give both cycles preoperatively.[12] Surgery was then performed on day 56. Patients with T_3 or N_1 disease, or those with unresectable tumor, were then given 5500 rads, over 5 to 6 weeks, to the chest. Preoperatively, 30/34 patients had at least stage 2 disease as seen by barium esophagram. Following one to two cycles of induction chemotherapy, downstaging of the primary tumor was seen in ten patients; that is, radiographic and histologic review demonstrated sufficient tumor shrinkage to downstage the esophageal primary (T_0, T_{is}, or T_1, as compared to T_{1-2}). In three patients, no residual disease was found in the resected specimen. Two patients, both with resectable disease, died postoperatively, one from a pontine hemorrhage and one with respiratory failure. A third patient developed renal failure following her second course of postoperative chemotherapy. The operative mortality was thus 5.6%, and the overall treatment-related mortality was 9%. Major but nonfatal postoperative complications were seen in ten patients. Three had pulmonary problems; six had transient cardiac arrhythmias. Only one patient had an anastomatic leak. The minimum followup for the 34 patients entered into the DVB trial is 36 months, and the median is 51 months; the median survival for the whole group was 16.2 months. All six patients with unresectable disease died within 9 months. Of the 28 patients with resectable tumor, two died postoperatively, one died a drug-related death, and two died of other causes. Fifteen patients have died of recurrent disease. Eight patients remain alive, (24% of all patients, 28% of those with resectable disease).

Several additional reports involving preoperative treatment with combination chemotherapy have now been presented in abstract form. El-Akkad et al included a group of ten patients with local-regional disease (receiving two cycles of preoperative chemotherapy) among 33 patients who were treated with a combination of cisplatin, vincristine, bleomycin, and 5-Fluorouracil.[12] Six patients had major (>50%) tumor regression. In this small group, there appeared to be no increase in operative morbidity or mortality. Long-term survival data was not available.

Forestiere et al included six patients treated preoperatively among a group of 16 evaluable patients receiving a combination of cisplatin, bleomycin, and VP-16.[13] Two had partial responses, with tumor downstaging being seen in both. Kelsen et al, using a combination of cisplatin, vindesine, and methyl-glyoxal bis (quanylhydrazone) (DVM), treated five patients preoperatively. Two cycles of DVM were given prior to surgery.[14] Major responses were seen in three patients, including one histologically proven complete response. There was one operative mortality. The other four patients were still alive 9 to 19 months after starting therapy.

Kukla et al have reported, in abstract form, the results of a trial using preoperative chemotherapy including cisplatin, mitomycin, prednisone, and bleomycin.[15] Two cycles of chemotherapy preceded surgery. Of 15 patients entered into the study, 11 (73%) had resectable disease. Five of these 11 patients died postoperatively, for a prohibitively high 45% operative mortality. Four of these deaths were felt to be due to chemotherapy-induced pulmonary toxicity.

PREOPERATIVE CHEMOTHERAPY AND RADIATION

Several trials have now looked at the use of concurrent chemotherapy and radiation prior to attempted resection. The theoretical advantages of this approach are first, that the drugs used will act as radiation sensitizers, and second, that the chemotherapy will also be effective against disease outside the radiated port. Presumably the agents used should have one or both of these properties.

Werner discussed the results of a combination of methotrexate and radiation.[16] This study, which was performed at the Groote Schuur Hospital in South Africa during the early to mid

1970s, involved 93 patients with potentially operable esophageal cancer. These were selected from a total of 491 newly diagnosed patients. The treatment plan included three doses of methotrexate 100 mg/m^2 given at seven-day intervals; this was followed by 2000 rads of radiation to the esophagus and periesophageal areas. Radiation was given in five-daily fractions (400 rads per dose). Surgery, involving an esophagectomy and esophagogastrostomy, was planned on day 21 after the completion of radiation. Following recovery from surgery, an additional 3600 rads of radiation was given.

Of the 93 patients entered into the study, 55 (59.1%) went to surgery after receiving methotrexate and radiation. At least some of the other patients refused surgery because of a symptomatic improvement in dysphagia. The resection rate was not stated. Operative mortality was 14.5%. Interestingly, in 27% of cases, there was no histologic evidence of residual disease in the resected specimen. For the 55 patients undergoing surgery, the average duration of survival was 26 months. For those refusing or not undergoing exploration, average survival was 22.6 months. The authors comment that the quality of survival appeared to be better for the chemotherapy-radiation group.

Fujimake and colleagues treated 76 patients with bleomycin and radiation prior to exploration[7]. Bleoymcyin at 7.5 mg was given, initially daily and then twice weekly, during a 3-week period of radiation (total radiation dosage was 3000 rads). Surgery was performed seven to ten days after completion of radiation. An additional group of 19 patients was given bleomycin alone. Of the whole group of 95 patients, 58 (61%) had resectable disease, 10/19 receiving chemotherapy alone, and 48/76 receiving both bleomycin and radiation. Pulmonary toxicity was seen in seven patients, three of whom died postoperatively. Four additional patients died of other operative complications (overall operative mortality 7%). At the time of their report, 8 of the 27 patients at risk for 3 or more years were still alive.

Four studies have been reported in final or in abstract form in which a 5 Fluorouracil (5FU) infusion plus mitomycin C or cisplatin was given with concurrent RT as pre-operative therapy. The three pilot trials were performed at Wayne State. In the first study, Franklin et.al. treated a group of 55 patients with mitomycin C 10mg/M^2 and 5FU 1000 mg/M^2 as a continuous infusion.[17] Radiation therapy of 3000 Rads was given from days 1-21. Thirty patients were treated with curative intent (Group I) and the remaining 25 received palliative therapy (Group II). At least 9 Group II patients also underwent exploration with or without resection, so that the difference in approach between the two groups is unclear. Of the 30 Group I patients, 76.6% had resectable disease. There was a 30% operative mortality (7/23 patients); at least one additional patient died suddenly pre-operatively and may have had a treatment-related death. The median survival of the whole group was 49 weeks. At the time of the latest follow up report, 5 patients (16.6%) were still alive.

Two subsequent follow-up studies were performed by the same group, substituting cisplatin for mitomycin C. The treatment regimen was otherwise unchanged. Steiger et al reported, as part of a larger review of surgery following chemotherapy plus RT, the results of cisplatin-5FU-RT in a group of 31 patients with local-regional disease.[18] Five of these patients died prior to surgery. 21/26 remaining patients underwent esophagectomy. The median survival of the operative group receieving cisplatin-5FU was not given. Teichmann et. al., reporting from the same institution, presented the results of the same regimen in a group of 21 patients.[19] The resection rate was 71%. The treatment related mortality was again substantial (27%); median survival for the whole group was 18 months.

Following the Wayne State pilot studies, the Southwest Oncology Group (SWOG) and the Radiation Therapy Oncology Group (RTOG) performed a large Phase II trial using cisplatin, a 5 FU infusion, and concurrent RT.[20] The only change in the treatment plan was a lower dose of cisplatin (75mg/M^2 instead of 100 mg/M^2). Preliminary results show that of 110 patients completing pre-operative therapy, 22% did not undergo surgery. Of the 86 patients who were explored, 9% died post-operatively. The resection rate was not given; the number of patients dying from treatment related but non-surgical causes (eg drug toxicity) was not stated. Survival data are not yet available.

Severe pulmonary toxicity in patients receiving both chemotherapy and radiation prior to surgery was also noted by Adelstein et.al.[21] A small group of 8 patients was given cisplatin and 5FU plus 3000 rads of RT prior to surgery; 7 patients also received methotrexate. Despite careful control of the FiO_2, 5 patients developed severe respiratory distress; 3 died. These investigators were continuing their study without RT.

CHEMOTHERAPY AND RADIATION

A number of patients will either refuse surgery, will have medical contraindications to surgery (such as severely limited pulmonary reserve), or will have extensive local-regional disease that is considered unresectable. Since radiation therapy alone has been unsatisfactory, there has been increasing interest in the use of combined chemotherapy and radiation. The results of a number of these trials are summarized in Table 3.

Kolaric et al explored the use of Bleomycin, Adriamycin, and finally a combination of the two, plus radiation therapy, in three sequential studies. In each trial, a control arm received chemotherapy alone.[22-24] As can be seen from Table 3, the numbers of patients in each group was rather small. For each trial, the objective response rate and survival was better for the chemotherapy-radiation arm. Toxicity, however, was on occasion substantial.

TABLE 3: Chemotherapy Followed By Radiation

DRUGS	RT(rads)	PATIENTS	SURVIVAL
Bleo	5-7000	24	55%(1yr)
Adria	4500-5200	15	NS
Bleo-Adria	3600-4000	15	27%(1yr)
Bleo	5-6000 rad	40	6.2mo (median)
Randomized Trial			
-	5-6000 rad	37	6.4mo (median)
DDP-Bleo	5500 rad	9	22%(5yr)
DDP-VDS-Bleo	5500 rad	11	27%(2yr)
MTX-Bleo-VCR-5FU	5000 rad	26	11mo (median)
DDP-MTX-5FU	6000 rad	9	7 mo

Bleo=Bleomycin, Adria=Adriamycin,DDP=Cisplatin, VDS=Vindesine, VCR=Vincristine,5FU= 5Flurouracil, MTX=Methotrexate (Modified from Seminars in Oncology)

The Eastern Cooperative Oncology Group (ECOG) recently reported the results of a randomized trial comparing radiation in a dose of 5000 to 6000 rads given over 5 to 6 weeks with the same radiation schedule, plus bleomycin at 15 mg given intravenously each day of radiation.[25] At a total dosage of 210 mg, bleomycin was stopped. Ninety-one patients were entered into this study, 77 of whom were evaluable. While toxicity was acceptable, survival was poor; there was no difference in either median or long-term survival for either radiation or radiation plus bleomycin (median survivals were 6.4 and 6.2 months, with four long-term survivors on each arm).

Coonley et al and Kelsen et al treated a total of 20 patients with local-regional disease with either Cisplatin-Bleomycin or with cisplatin-vindesine-bleomycin.[26-27]. The objective tumor response rates seen were similar to those of the larger group treated preoperatively (22% for cisplatin-bleomycin and 55% for cisplatin-vindesine-bleomycin). Radiation was well tolerated by most patients. Of the 20 patients treated, five were long-term survivors (two with cisplatin-bleomycin, three with cisplatin-vindesine-bleomycin).

Marcial et al used a combination of methotrexate, bleomycin, 5-fluorouracil, and vincristine prior to 5000

rads of radiation.[28]
Twenty-six patients were entered into this trial. There was one
drug-related death. Objective tumor shrinkage was seen in 55% of
patients after chemotherapy. Following radiation therapy, 66% had
complete remissions; however, how this was defined was not clear.
The median survival for the whole group was 11 months.

Abitol et al treated a small group of nine patients with 5-
fluorouracil, cisplatin and methotrexate plus 5000 rads of
radiation.[29] Seven patients had esophageal cancer, and two had
gastric cardia lesions. Objective responses were seen in 89%. The
median survival for the whole group was 7 months.

Berenzweig et al treated a group of five patients with a
combination of cisplatin, methotrexate, bleomycin, and methyl
glyoxal bis (guanyl/hydrazone) (MGBG) prior to radiation.[30] They
were part of a larger group of 18 patients receiving this
chemotherapy. The median survival for this group was 8 months.
Marantz et al treated 24 patients with locally advanced,
inoperable cancer with cisplatin-bleomycin followed by RT (4000
rads in 4 weeks) and concurrent 5FU [31]. Objective responses were
quantitated to both chemotherapy alone and to RT-5FU. Surgery was
then offered to selected patients. The overall response rate was
61%. Four complete responders underwent exploration; in two
patients, no residual viable tumor was found. There were two
treatment related deaths (one drug and one operative mortality).
Long term survival data were not yet available.

CONCLUSIONS

Recent reviews have confirmed that the outlook for patients treated
with surgery or radiation therapy alone is extremely poor. It has
been hoped that, for patients with disease clinically limited to the
esophagus and periesophageal tissues, the prognosis would be
improved if multimodality therapy was employed. This review
suggests that, although there are some encouraging preliminary
studies, there is as yet no clear evidence that a combination
approach is superior to conventional therapy.

Initial studies with combined modality programs used
radiation prior to or following surgery. These results have recently
been summarized; they do not appear to be superior to surgery
alone[32] The development of drug combinations with activity in the
30% to 60% range has expanded the combined-modality approach to
include chemotherapy. Since esophageal cancer is frequently
widespread at diagnosis, the use of induction chemotherapy is
theoretically attractive; a simultaneous attack on both the primary
tumor and on metastatic disease can be employed. The combination

of chemotherapy followed by surgery had demonstrated its usefulness in testicular and ovarian cancers. In those two solid tumors, drug regimens of a high degree of activity have been developed, and surgical debulking followed by additional chemotherapy seems a firmly established concept. In esophageal cancer, the same approach is under study. It is clear, however, that chemotherapy combinations in esophageal cancer are currently much less effective; in testicular cancer, 60%-complete remission rates are commonly reported, and in esophageal cancer, histologically proven complete responses are rare. Clearly, much more work needs to be done in this field, although preliminary data suggests that even with currently available regimens, such as cisplatin-vindesine-bleomycin, a modest improvement in survival may be obtained. The use of concurrent chemotherapy and radiation, prior to surgery, is also under study. Factors that need to be addressed here are whether radiation adds to the regimen and whether or not the combination leads to unacceptable operative morbidity and mortality. The pilot studies from Wayne State, for example, have a 27% to 30% treatment-related mortality, which is substantially more than the number of patients still alive at the time of their final report.[19] The preliminary data from the SWOG and RTOG studies, in which over a fifth of patients were not able to undergo surgery, in addition to at least a 9% treatment related mortality, also suggests substantially toxicity.

In summary, although the preliminary results are encouraging, the available data do not yet support the routine use of preoperative chemotherapy alone or in combination with radiation. A number of investigational trials are currently underway. Hopefully in the next 2 to 4 years, the role of chemotherapy in local-regional esophageal cancer will be more clearly defined.

REFERENCES
1. Anderson, L., Lad, T., Autopsy Findings in Squamous Cell Carcinoma of the Esophagus, Cancer 50: 1587-1590, 1982.
2. Bosch, A., et al, Autopsy Findings in Carcinoma f the Esophagus, Acta Radio Oncol 18: 103-112, 1979.
3. Kelsen, D., Chemotherapy of Esophageal Cancer, Semin Oncol ll: 159-168, 1984.
4. Hancock, S., Glatstein, E., Radiation Therapy of Esophageal Cancer, Semin Oncol ll: 144-158, 1984.
5. Haluorsen, R., Thompson, W., Computed Tomographic Evaluation of Esophageal Carcinoma, Semin Oncol ll:113-126, 1984.
6. American Joint Committee on Cancer, "Esophagus" Manual For Staging of Cancer, second edition JB Lippincott, Co., Philadelphia, 1983, pp. 61-66.
7. Fujimaki M, et al: Role of preoperative administration of bleomycin and radiation in the treatment of esophageal can-

Esophageal Cancer / 251

cer. Jpn J Surg 5:48, 1975

8. Wada T, Matoumoto Y, Amano T: Chemotherapy of esophageal cancer with bleomycin. Prog Antimicrob Anti-cancer Chemotherop 2:696, 1970

9. Kelsen DP, Bains M, Hilaris B, et al: Cisplatin-based preoperative chemotherapy of esophageal carcinoma in adjuvant therapy of cancer III, in Salmon S, Jones S (eds): New York, Grune and Stratton, Inc., 1981, pp 495-502

10. Kelsen DP, Bains MS, Cvitkovic E, et al: Vindesine in the treatment of esophageal carcinoma: A phase II study. Cancer Treat Rep 63:2019-2021, 1979

11. Bains M, Kelsen DP, Beattie EJ, et al: Treatment of esophageal carcinoma by combined preoperative chemotherapy. Ann Thorac Surg 34:521-528, 1982

12. El-Akkad S, Amer M, Kerth W: Combined chemotherapy, surgery and radiation therapy for esophageal cancer. Proceed 13th International Cancer Cong 40, 1983 (abstr)

13. Forestiere A, Pateg H, Hankins JR, et al: Cisplatin, bleomycin and VP-16 in combination for epidermoid carcinoma of the esophagus. Proc ASCO 2:123, 1983 (abstr)

14. Kelsen DP, Coonley C, Hilaris B, et al: Cisplatin, vindesine, and methyl-glyoxal bis (quanylhydrazone) combination chemotherapy of esophageal cancer. Pro ASCO 2:128, 1983 (abstr)

15. Kukla L, Lad T, McGuire, W, et al: Multimodality therapy of squamous carcinoma of the esophagus. Proceed ASCO AACR 22:449, 1981 (abstr)

16. Werner D: The multi-disciplinary approach in the management of squamous carcinoma of the esophagus: The Groote Schuur Hospital Experience. Front Gastroint Res 5:130-135, 1979

17. Franklin R, Steiger Z, Vaishampayan G, et al: Combined modality therapy for esophageal squamous cell carcinoma. Cancer 51:1062-1071, 1983

18. Steiger Z, Franklin R, Wilson R: Eradication and palliation of squamous cell carcinoma of the esophagus with chemotherapy, radiotheray, and surgical therapy. J Thorac Cardiovasc Surg 82:713-719, 1981

19. Leichmann L, Steiger Z, Seydel L: Combined preoperative chemotherapy and radiation for cancer of the esophagus. Sem Oncol 11:00-00, 1984

20. Leichman, L, Seydel, H., Steiger, Z., Pre-operative Adjuvant Therapy for Squamous Cell Cancer of the Esophagus: SWDG and RTOG Trials, Proc Asco 3:147, 1984 (abst).

21. Adelstein, D., et. al., Postoperative Respiratory Failure After Pre-Operative Chemotherapy and Mediastinal Radiation Therapy for Esophageal Cancer Pro Asco 3:135, 1984 (abst.)

22. Kolaric K, Maricic Z, Dujmovic L, et al: Therapy of advanced esophageal cancer with bleomycin, irradiation and

combination bleomycin with irradiation. Tumori 62:255-262, 1976

23. Kolaric K, Maricic Z, Roth A, et al: Adriamycin alone and in combination with radiotherapy in the treatment of inoperable esophageal cancer. Tumori 63:485-491, 1977

24. Kolaric K, Maricic Z, Roth A, et al: Combination of bleomycin and Adriamycin with and without radiation in the treatment of inoperable esophageal cancer. Cancer 45:2265-2273, 1980

25. Earle J, Gelber R, Moertel C: A controlled evaluation of combined radiation and bleomycin therapy for squamous cell carcinoma of the esophagus. Int J Radiat Oncol Biol Phys 6:821-826, 1980

26. Coonley C, Bains M, Kelsen DP, et al: Cisplatin-bleomycin in the treatment of esophageal carcinoma: A final report. Cancer 54: 2351-2355, 1984.

27. Kelsen DP, Hilaris B, Coonley C, et al: Cisplatin, vindesine and bleomycin chemotherapy of local-regional and advanced esophageal cancer. Am J Med 75:645-652, 1983

28. Marcial V, Velez-Garcia F, Cintron J, et al: Radiotherapy preceded by multi-drug chemotherapy in carcinoma of the esophagus. Cancer Clin Trials 3:127-130, 1980

29. Abitbol A, Straus M, Franklin G: Infusional chemotherapy and cyclic radiation therapy in inoperable esophageal and gastric cardia carcinoma. Am J Clini Oncol 6:195-201, 1983

30. Berenzweig M, Vogl S, Camacho F, et al: Esophageal squamous cancer chemotherapy with methyl-glyoxal bis (quanylhydrazone), methotrexate, bleomycin, and diamminedichloroplatinum. Proc ASCO 2:125, 1983

31. Marantz,A Schmilovich, A Santos, J et al Combined Therapy of Inoperable Locally Advanced Carcinoma of the Esophagus Proc. ASCO 3: 135, 1984. (abstract)

32. Kelsen, D Bains, M Hilaris, B et. al. Combined Modality Therapy of Esophageal Cancer Semin in Oncology 11: 169-177, 1984.

Primary Chemotherapy in Cancer Medicine, pages 253-258
© 1985 Alan R. Liss, Inc.

PREOPERATIVE CHEMOTHERAPY IN LOCALIZED CANCER OF THE
ESOPHAGUS WITH CIS-PLATINUM, VINDESINE AND BLEOMYCIN:

P. Schlag, R. Herrmann, D. Fritze, H. Buhr,
Ch. Herfarth and G. Schettler,
Div. of Surgical oncology,
Ruprecht-Karls-Universität, Heidelberg,
Germany.

The poor prognosis of patients with squamous cell
carcinoma of the esophagus is well recognized. About 40 %
of the patients have unresectable tumors at the time of
diagnosis. But even for those with localized disease
(who are potentially curable) 5 year survival rates are
well under 20 % (Giuli 1980, Linder 1982).
Preoperative radiotherapy neither increases resectability-
rate nor survival time. This is conclusively demonstrated
by the EORTC-Trial No 40762, in which surgery alone was
compared with preoperative radiotherapy plus operative
treatment (Gignoux 1984).
In an attempt to improve the poor results we initiated a
study with preoperative chemotherapy followed by surgery
in localized esophageal cancer. This trial is based on
various phase II studies suggesting that cis-platinum
containing regimes have a remarkable activity in squamous
cell carcinoma of the esophagus (Kelsen 1978 and 1981).
The aim of our study was:
1. To examine, if preoperative chemotherapy with cis-
platinum, vindesine and bleomycin (DVB) could be given safely without adversely influencing the out-come of surgery.
2. To assess antitumor activity of DVB-chemotherapy
administered preoperatively to patients with localized,
potentially resectable cancer of the esophagus.
3. To find out wether reduction of tumor size by preoperative DVB-chemotherapy would result in an increase of
resectability-rates.

Eligibility criteria included histologically confirmed
squamous cell carcinoma of the esophagus potentially
curable by surgery alone, exclusion of distant metastases
by CT-scan or sonography, age under 65 years, no prior
chemo- or radiotherapy, Karnofsky performance status above
70 %, normal hematologic and renal function (creatinin
clearance more than 70 ml/min) and normal pulmonary
function test.
The chemotherapy regimen used was similar to the one
reported by Kelsen (1981).
Day 1: cis-platinum 120 mg/m^2 i.v. with vigorous hydration
and mannitol induced diuresis
vindesine 3 mg/m^2 i.v.
Day 3: bleomycin 10 mg/m^2 i.v. push.
Day 3-6: bleomycin 10 mg/m^2 i.v. by continuous infusion.
The schedule was repeated on day 22, provided white blood
count and renal function were normal. Surgery was performed
3-4 weeks after the second cycle of chemotherapy.
So far 23 patients, 2 women and 21 men, have been
entered into this protocol. The median age was 53 years,
ranging from 35-64 years. Tumor localisation was the
upper third of the esophagus in 4 patients, the middle
third in 11 patients and the lower third in 8 patients.
A total of 42 preoperative DVB-chemotherapy-cycles were
administered. Four patients received one cycle, 2 patients
because of severe toxicity and 2 patients because of
tumor progression. The incidence and grade of the chemotherapy induced side effects are shown in table 1 and 2
according to the WHO-classification. The most common toxic
effects, as would be expected, were vomiting, nausea and
alopecia.

Table 1

Side Effects of Preoperative Chemotherapy
(number of patients)

	WHO-Grades				
	0	1	2	3	4
Nausea/Vomiting	0	5	2	11	1
Hair	0	2	6	15	0
Fever with Drugs	12	4	7	–	–
Diarrhea	16	2	5	–	–
Stomatitis	22	–	1	–	–

In one fourth of the patients preoperative chemotherapy
leads to severe haematological toxicity. Nephrotoxicity
was relatively low according to WHO criteria, but this
classification possibly underestimates the true transitory
functional impairment of the kidneys observed.
As mentioned, in 2 patients the severity of toxicity
necessitated the termination of chemotherapy following the
first cycle. There were no chemotherapy related deaths.

Table 2

Toxic Effects of Preoperative Chemotherapy

(number of patients)

WHO-Grades

	0	1	2	3	4
Leukocytes	10	3	5	3	2
Thrombocytes	17	2	–	2	2
Blood creatinine	17	4	2	–	–

The effect of chemotherapy was assessed preoperatively by
barium-swallow x-rays and by esophago-gastroscopy including
biopsy. Also, the course of the clinical condition and
the tumor-related symptoms were recorded. Actually, there
are no satisfactory response criteria for preoperative
chemotherapy in localized esophageal cancer. Therefore
we have used the following classification.
- "No change" was defined as a stable disease according to
  patients subjective or objective condition in comparing
  pre- and post-chemotherapy status.
- "Minor response" was defined as an improvement in the
  subjective symptoms in particular related to dysphagia
  whenever an objective tumor-regression could not be
  documented unequivocally by the methods described.
- "Major response" was classified as a clear cut
  measurable reduction documented by barium swallow and/or
  endoscopy.
- "Complete remission" was only assumed if the careful
  histological work up of the total operative specimen
  gave no evidence of residual tumor.

Using these criteria preoperative chemotherapy was
effective in 14 out of the 23 patients. This includes 1
patient with a complete remission; in the others there
were 4 patients with minor and 9 patients with major
response. In 5 patients no change was noted including the
2 patients in which preoperative chemotherapy had to be
terminated after the first cycle due to toxicity. It
should be emphasized, that among the 4 patients with preoperative tumor progression 3 did not receive bleomycin.
The reason for this transitory protocol modification was
the occurence of severe postoperative pulmonary problems
in the first patients treated. Bleomycin use however
was restarted for all the other patients after adaequate
anaesthesiologic attention was paid to the special
problems of this treatment. In particular this means the
restriction of oxygen concentration during anaesthesia
and the postoperative period to below 30 % and a careful
monitoring of fluid replacement (Allen 1981, Toledo 1982).
Depending on tumor-localisation total or subtotal
esophagectomy by right side thoracotomy was the operative
therapy of choice. Blunt mediastinal removal of the
esophagus was not used in this protocol. The intestinal
passage was reconstruced in all the cases by the mobilized
stomach with an intrathoracic anastomosis after subtotal

and a cervical anastomosis after total esophagectomy.
Two patients with tumor localisation in the upper third of
the esophagus refused operative treatment after major
response during preoperative chemotherapy. In these cases
radical surgery would have included total esophagectomy
with laryngectomy. In 18 patients tumor resection was
possible in 11 patients curatively and in 7 patients
palliatively. An inoperable situation was found in 3 cases.
At the moment it is difficult to judge if the relatively
high rate of resectability is due to selection of the
patients or to the preoperative chemotherapy used. The
latter is possibly supported by the fact, that curative
resection in the group with response to chemotherapy are
more frequent than in the non-responders.

Table 3

Response to Preoperative Chemotherapy and

Operative Procedure

	Curative Resections (n= 11)	Palliative Resections (n= 7)	Explorative Procedures (n= 3)	Surgery Refused (n= 2)
Progression	1	1	2	-
No Change	1	3	-	-
Minimal Response	2	2	1	-
Major Response	6	1	-	2
Complete Remission	1	-	-	-

Our results indicate that 2 cycles of preoperative DVB-chemotherapy do not adversely influence the operative procedures. Even including the 2 patients lost in the beginning of this study by an adult respiratory distress syndrom (ARDS), the total postoperative mortality (4/21) is comparable to that reported in the literature (Giuli 1984).

So far it is too early to draw any conclusion regarding the long term survival of our patients. The follow up period is too short to make a relevant analysis wether preoperative chemotherapy improve patients survival in comparison to surgery alone.
At this time the results of preoperative chemotherapy in esophageal cancer obtained in this study, can be summarized as follows:
1. The data confirm the efficacy of DVB-chemotherapy in esophageal carcinoma.
2. The use of 2 cycles DVB preoperatively is feasible under appropriate precautions and does not compromize surgical treatment.
3. The resectability of esophagus-carcinomas may be improved following preoperative chemotherapy.
4. Side effects of this treatment modality must not be underestimated.

Primary Chemotherapy in Cancer Medicine, pages 259–282
© 1985 Alan R. Liss, Inc.

COMBINATION OF CYTOSTATICS AND RADIATION - A NEW TREND IN
THE TREATMENT OF INOPERABLE ESOPHAGEAL CANCER

Krsto Kolarić

Central Institute for Tumors and Allied Diseases,
Zagreb

The poor prognosis and low curability rate of esophageal cancer are well known today. Neither new surgical procedures nor supervoltage radiation have significantly improved
long-term therapeutic results and survival rates of these
patients (Pearson, 1969; Gunnlangsson et al. 1970; Rambo et
al. 1975; Davies et al. 1978). The main contributing factors
to these low survival rates are delayed diagnosis and physical weakness with malnutrition. Delayed diagnosis usually
means a very advanced tumor process. Current surgical literature reports metastasizing lymph nodes of the mediastinum
in approximately 75% of these patients (Gunnlangsson et al.
1970; Rambo et al. 1975). Physical weakness is common because of inadequate nutrition due to esophageal obstruction
and the patient's advanced years. The 5-year survival rate
of operable cases averages 9% (1-19%) and 6% (2-14%) for
those treated with supervoltage radiation (Linder 1976;
Wieland et al. 1977) which produce a moderate response in
30-50% of patients treated, with a high given dose of 6,000
-7,000 cGy. Recently, 5-year survival rate reportedly has
increased up to 30% after preoperative radiation (Nakayama
et al. 1967; 1974). It is important however to emphasize
that only approximately 25% of patients are in operable
condition when the diagnosis is established. These statistics clearly suggest that today the majority of patients
with esophageal cancer are subject to only palliative treatment. Chemotherapy of esophageal cancer, as a palliative
measure, is still in the investigational phase and the antitumor activity has been observed with only a few single-
agent drugs, mainly antitumor antibiotics (Shastri et al.
1971; Terashima 1973; Tancini et al. 1974; Kelsen et al.

1978). Although the results of American and Japanese authors are controversial, Bleomycin so far proves to be most
effective (Okamoto 1971; Asakawa et al. 1973; Ravry et al.
1973; Nabeya et al. 1974). There have been sporadic reports
on appreciable responses obtained with Methotrexate, 5-Flu-
orouracil, Cis platinum and Vindesine (Roussel 1978; Desai
et al. 1979; Kelsen et al. 1981). Furthermore, it must be
pointed out that the number of chemotherapeutic trials for
patients with esophageal cancer is insignificant, so that
for the time being there are only few published data from
controlled studies (Desai et al. 1979; Kolarić et al. 1976,
1977, 1980, 1984). For these reasons we still do not have a
generally accepted attitude towards cytostatic treatment of
this advanced type of cancer.

Reports on combination chemotherapy until 1981 did not
show any treatment advantage over cytostatic drugs used a-
lone (Bleomycin + Adriamycin, Kolarić 1980; cis DDP + Bleomycin, Kelsen 1978, Ravry 1980). The first encouraging results recently appeared in the literature with the combination of cis DDP, Vindesin and Bleomycin (55% response rate,
Kelsen 1982), or with cis DDP, Bleomycin and Methotrexate
(50% response rate, Vogl 1982). In 1984 two reports (Benedik-
ian 1984, Desai 1984) observed a high response rate (66% for
5-FU + Adriamycin + cis DDP + VP-16 and 70% - cis DDP +
Bleomycin + Methotrexate + Mitomycin C) in advanced squamous cell esophageal cancer. The number of combination
chemotherapy trials is still very low and no controlled
studies have been published.

In search of new palliative methods which would increase
therapeutic results, we have performed several randomized
studies in sequential manners using cytostatics alone or in
combination with radiation. Before starting clinical studies
we have in vitro tested (V-79 lung hamsters cells - Hella
cells - L mice cells) interaction of Bleomycin and Adriamycin with radiation (Bistrović et al. 1976, 1978, 1980; Nagy et al. 1983). All the results showed potentiation of
cell killing effect, when the cells were exposed to cytostatics before or during the radiation. This finding was a
rationale for combining Bleomycin or Adriamycin with radiation in our following clinical studies.

Between 1976-1980 115 patients with advanced inoperable
esophageal cancer entered these studies, but only 103 completed the treatment program and were evaluated. The first
study (A) included 39 patients who received Bleomycin alone
or in combination with radiation. The second study (B) consisted of 33 patients treated with Adriamycin alone or com-

bined with radiation. The third study (C) included 31 patients and this group of patients was treated with the combination of Bleomycin and Adriamycin or a combination of
these cytostatics with radiation.

As illustrated in table 1, about three quarters of the
tumors were localized in the middle part of the esophagus.

TABLE 1

Localization of Tumors in Esophagus

	Number of Patients	Upper third	Middle third	Lower third
Study A	39	6	29	4
Study B	33	4	24	5
Study C	31	-	19	19
Total	103	10	72	21

Esophagoscopy was performed prior to the treatment and tumor
tissue samples were sent for histopathologic analyses. Table
2 lists the histopathologic types of tumors. In all three
studies squamous cell carcinoma was the most prevalent with
71% of cases in study A, 73% in study B and 74% in study C.
Before the start of treatment, all patients had routine
blood tests, functional liver and kidney tests, a chest X-
ray with tomography of the mediastinum and an esophagogram
which was repeated every 3 weeks during treatment and once
a month in the follow-up period. In order to evaluate the
effect of the treatment, a control esophagoscopy was performed at the end of the treatment.

Detailed data on the type of the treatment program and
drugs and radiation dosage are given in table 3.

In study A, 15 randomly selected patients received Bleomycin alone, and 24 the combination of Bleomycin and radiation. In study B 18 patients were treated with Adriamycin
alone and 15 with the combination of Adriamycin and radiation. In study C, 16 patients received a combination of
Bleomycin and Adriamycin, and 15 a combination of Bleomycin
and Adriamycin plus radiotherapy. The patients were irradi-

TABLE 2

Pathohistology of Tumors

	Number of patients	Squamous cell	Anaplastic	Adenocarcinoma	Microcellular	Scirrhous	Unclassified
BLM	15	11 ⎫ 71%	1	-	-	1	2
BLM+RAD	24	17 ⎭	3	1	-	-	3
ADM	18	13 ⎫ 73%	2	2	-	-	1
ADM+RAD	15	11 ⎭	1	1	-	-	2
BLM+ADM	16	12 ⎫ 74%	-	-	2	-	2
BLM+ADM+RAD	15	11 ⎭	2	-	-	-	2
Total	103	75	9	4	2	1	12

BLM = Bleomycin

RAD = Radiation

ADM = Adriamycin

TABLE 3

Treatment's Schedules

Study A

Bleomycin   15 mg/m² body surface i.v. twice a week
                      - total dose 200-350 mg
Bleomycin+Radiation   10 mg/m² body surface i.v. twice a week
                      (total dose 180-250 mg) simultaneously
                      with radiation (3,800-4,400 cGy Beta-
                      tron, Siemens)

TABLE 3

Treatment's Schedules

Study B

| Adriamycin | 40 mg/m² body surface i.v. daily, 2 days - total 6 cycles with a rest period of 3 weeks between cycles |
| Adriamycin+Radiation | 40 mg/m² body surface i.v. daily, 2 days - 3 cycles simultaneously with radiation (3,800-4,400 cGy Betatron, Siemens) |

Study C

Bleomycin + Adriamycin	15 mg/m² body surface i.v. daily, day 1, 4 40 mg/m² body surface i.v. daily, day 2, 3 Total 5-6 cycles applied with 3 weeks rest periods between cycles
Bleomycin + Adriamycin	15 mg/m² body surface i.v. daily, day 1, 4 30 mg/m² body surface i.v. daily, day 2, 3
Irradiation	3,600-4,000 cGy (42 MeV Betatron, Siemens) 2 cycles of chemotherapy given simultaneously with radiation and 3rd cycle 1 month after radiation was completed

ated with fast electrons (42 MeV Betatron; Siemens) in two opposed thoracic fields focused strictly to the tumor lesion, the overall radiation dose having been 3,600-4,000 cGy. The total dose of Bleomycin was limited to 200-350 mg and that of Adriamycin to 550 mg/m² of body surface. In combined treatment modalities the total Bleomycin and Adriamycin dose was reduced by half.

All the toxic side effects were regularly checked, especially the leukocyte and platelet counts in addition to ECG controls in study B and C.

With regard to the criteria for the evaluation of treatment results, esophagography was the leading objective method. Cases of complete esophagus restitution with peristaltics were classed into the complete remission group. Esophagus restitution by more than 50%, as compared with the X-ray prior to treatment, was put down as partial remission. Cases of complete and partial remissions were also verified by endoscopy and their duration had to be at least 1 month.

Furthermore, it should be mentioned that all the patients were in a poor physical condition (68 patients Karnofsky scale grade 50-100, 35 patients grade 30-40) because of malnutrition; actually, about one half of the patients had to undergo total parenteral nutrition prior to the start of treatment. All these patients constituted, as a matter of fact, a bad risk group for chemotherapy or chemoradiotherapy.

The results for 103 evaluable patients who completed the treatment programs are reviewed in table 4.

TABLE 4

Results of Treatment

	Number of patients	Complete remission (100%)	Partial remission (> 50%)	Response rate
Bleomycin	15	1	3	4/15 (26%)
			$p<0.01$	
Bleomycin + Radiation	24	6	9	15/24 (62%)
Adriamycin	18	1	5	6/18 (33%)
			$p<0.05$	
Adriamycin+ Radiation	15	4	5	9/15 (60%)
Bleomycin + Adriamycin	16	-	3	3/16 (19%)
			$p<0.01$	
Bleomycin + Adriamycin + Radiation	15	3	6	9/15 (60%)

In study A out of 15 patients treated with Bleomycin only, 4 responded to treatment with a response rate of 26%. There was 1 complete and 3 partial remissions. Combining Bleomycin with radiation was given in 24 patients. Fifteen patients responded to treatment, so that in this approach the response rate was 62%. Out of these there were 6 complete and 9 partial remissions. In study B, 18 patients were treated with Adriamycin alone and 6 responded to treatment with a response rate of 33%, 5 partial and 1 complete response were obtained. Nine responders were noted in 15 patients treated with the combination of Adriamycin and radiation achieving a response rate of 60% with 4 complete and 5 partial responses. In study C, there were only 3 partial responders out of 16 patients treated with a combination of Bleomycin and Adriamycin and the response rate obtained was 19%. In combined treatment using these two drugs and radiation, 3 complete and 6 partial responses were observed out of 15 patients treated. 60% of patients responded to this treatment approach. Statistical significance in treatment results existed in all three studies but only between chemotherapy alone and combined treatment modalities (study A, $p < 0.01$; study B, $p < 0.05$; study C, $p < 0.01$).

Concerning the median remission duration in months, it is evident that in all the three studies cytostatic treatment alone produces remissions of very short duration, i.e. Bleomycin 2.6, Adriamycin 3.2 and the combination of Bleomycin and Adriamycin 4.2 months. In combined treatment modalities median remission duration was noticeably longer, 14 months in the group treated with Bleomycin plus radiation, 13 months in Adriamycin plus radiation treatment, and 11 months in Bleomycin plus Adriamycin plus radiation modality. All the remissions were obtained in squamous cell carcinomas, except 7 responses in other pathohistologic types.

There was an evident difference in the survival rate of patients who responded to treatment and those who did not.

In all three studies none of the patients in the non-responders' group survived a year, whereas 25, 17 and 33% of responders, respectively, treated with Bleomycin or Adriamycin alone or in combination, survived 1 year. Combined treatment showed a higher percentage of 1-year survivors, i.e. 73% in study A, 67% in study B and 44% in study C. 2-year survivors were observed only in combined treatment modalities, 40% in study A, 44% in study B and 33% of responders in study C. The end results, i.e. 5-year survival rate in all three combined modalities ranged from

22-27% of responding patients (average 24% - 8/33). No one of
5-year survivors showed recurrence of disease and we consider them practically cured.
   Toxic side effects of treatment are presented in table
5 and 6.

TABLE 5

Toxic Side Effects and Complications of Treatment

Study A

	Bleomycin (15 patients)		Bleomycin+Radiation (24 patients)	
	n	%	n	%
Temperature	5	33	7	29
Oral ulcera	4	27	8	33
Hyperpigmentation	6	40	10	42
Hyperkeratosis	5	33	9	38
Alopecia	3	20	4	17
Pulmonary fibrosis	1	7	3	13
Esophagobronchial fistula	1	7	4	17

Study B

	Adriamycin (18 patients)		Adriamycin+Radiation (15 patients)	
	n	%	n	%
Alopecia	18	100	14	93
Nausea-vomiting	8	44	8	53
Leukopenia	2	11	5	33
Thrombocytopenia	-		-	
ECG changes	1	6	1	7
Potentiation of radiation dermatitis	-	-	1	7
Esophagobronchial fistula	-	-	2	13

TABLE   6

Toxic Side Effects and Complications of Treatment

Study C

	Bleomycin + Adriamycin		Bleomycin + Adriamycin + Radiation	
	patients	%	patients	%
Alopecia	16	100	14	93
Nausea	12	75	14	93
Vomiting	10	62	12	75
Leukopenia	4	25	6	40
	(1,800-3,000)		(1,000-2,500)	
Thrombocytopenia	0		1	7
			(35,000)	
ECG changes	2	12	3	20
Cardiac failure	0		0	
Fever	4	25	3	20
Hyperkeratosis	0		0	
Skin pigmentation	0		0	
Decreased pulmonary vital capacity	3	19	4	33
X-ray interstitial pulmonary changes	1	6	1	7
Oral ulcera	4	25	3	20
Retrosternal pain	-	-	8	53
Esophagobronchial fistula	-	-	4	27
Rupture of the aorta	-	-	1	7

Approximately one third of the patients given Bleomycin alone experienced temperature, oral ulcera, hyperpigmentation of the skin and hyperkeratosis. Similar toxicity was encountered in patients receiving radiation and Bleomycin. However, this group of patients tended to suffer more from pulmonary fibrosis and esophagobronchial fistulas.

In study B alopecia caused by Adriamycin was present in almost all patients in both treatment modalities. Nausea and vomiting occurred in approximately 50% of patients whereas myelosuppression was more severe after treatment with both Adriamycin and radiation. ECG changes were similar in both therapeutic regimens. For 1 patient in the combined group, radiation dermatitis was particularly severe, almost to the point of skin necrosis. Two esophagobronchial fistulas also occurred in this group.

In study C all toxic side effects were more pronounced. Alopecia was involved in almost all patients. Gastrointestinal disturbances in terms of nausea and vomiting were present in two thirds of patients and were somewhat more evident in the combined treatment group. In de same group myelosuppression was also more intensive. ECG changes were observed in 12% of the patients in the chemotherapy group and in 20% in the combined treatment group. It should also be noted that one half of the patients in the combined treatment group manifested retrosternal pain and difficulties in swallowing after an exposure of 1,000-1,500 cGy. We explain this phenomenon by irridiation mucositis. In study C, combined treatment was much more aggressive. This was particularly reflected in the enhanced physical exhaustion of the patients associated with loss of body weight at the end of such a treatment. Body weight dropped on the average by about 15% as compared with the weight before the start of treatment, so that responders achieved their initial body weight 1-2 months after completed treatment. In the same group of patients there were four esophagobronchial fistulas and one rupture of aorta. It is very difficult to avoid these serious types of complications which occurred mostly in combined treatment modalities, bearing in mind the localization of the tumor in the middle third of the esophagus and its intimate contact with the aorta and the bronchii.

By analyzing the results of our three sequential randomized studies, we arrive at the conclusion that Adriamycin does have antitumor activity on inoperable esophageal cancer and that it is not any less effective than Bleomycin. This has not been proven before, and Nygard has very recently (1983) reconfirmed antitumor activity of Adriamycin in squamous cell esophageal cancer. It is, however, very important to mention that remissions achieved with Bleomycin or Adriamycin alone were mostly partial and quite short, averaging 2-3 months in duration. In study A and B the therapeutic results were significantly improved when Bleomycin or Adriamycin were combined with radiation. With these palliative methods of treatment, response rates were over 60% with a median remission duration of 11-14 months. Also the survival of these patients was significantly prolonged. In combined approach toxic side effects were severe but tolerable for patients. The superiority of the combined treatment approach was also evident in study C, i.e. the combination of Bleomycin plus Adriamycin and radiation was much more effective than Bleomycin plus Adriamycin alone. With regard to remission quality, it should be noted that combined treatment achieved more complete remissions as well, which was not the case in the treatment of patients receiving chemotherapy alone.

The analysis of the dependance of treatment results on age, sex and tumor localization in the esophagus afforded no conclusions as to the possible dependance of therapeutic response on these factors. This conclusion was evident in all three studies.

On the other hand, an analysis and comparison of the results of these studies warrants the conclusion that combination of Bleomycin and Adriamycin did not prove to be more effective in antitumorigenic terms than treatment with either of these cytostatics alone. Similarly, the combination of Bleomycin and Adriamycin with radiation does not at all improve the results achieved by applying any of these cytostatics in combination with radiation.

One of our recent trials was focused on testing the therapeutic results obtained by two combined approaches, which also included, along with Bleomycin or Adriamycin, 5-Fluorouracil a cytostatic drug already known to possess as a single agent or in combination, a moderate antitumorigenic activity in esophageal cancer (Desai et al. 1979; Hellerstein et al. 1983). The combination of 5-Fluorouracil with radiation has also produced good results, particularly in the treatment of esophageal cancer, rectal adenocarcinoma, and anal squamous cell carcinoma (Byfield et al. 1980; Sischy et al. 1980; Franklin et al. 1983).

The trial included a total of 61 patients with inoperable esophageal cancer and with no clinical signs of distant metastases. There were 58 men and 3 women, aged 32 to 75 years (mean age 67). In all patients the pathohistologic

diagnosis of the disease was confirmed by esophagoscopic
tissue samples. The patients had not been previously treated
with chemotherapy or radiotherapy. Patients older than 75
were not included in the trial, and neither were patients
with a performance status (Karnofsky score) of < 40. Other
criteria included normal bone marrow (leukocyte and throm-
bocyte count), liver, heart and kidney function. Along with
these examinations all the patients underwent - before and
after treatment - esophagoscopy, barium meal esophagography
and lung X-ray with tomography of the mediastinum.

Fifty-six randomly assigned patients completed the therapy schedule and could be evaluated. The clinical characteristics of the patients are reported in table 7. The table shows that a 10% or more loss of body weight was established in 32, and a loss of less than 10% in 24 patients.
The site of most tumors was the middle third of the esophagus; fewer tumors were sited in the lower third (18 cases),
and only 2 in the upper third. The length of the filling
defect segment of the esophagogram was also recorded, since
this was thought to constitute one of the signs of tumor
extent. Thus, in 84% of patients the tumor-involved segment
of the esophagus was found to exceed 5 cm, and in 16 patients it even exceeded 8 cm. In terms of pathohistologic
findings, squamous cell carcinoma was found to predominate
(53 patients), and 3 patients had adenocarcinoma. Before
randomization the patients were stratified in terms of body
weight loss (< 10% vs. > 10%).

Treatment modality A included 5-Fluorouracil (10 mg/kg
body weight, i.v., 8-h drip, twice a week) and Bleomycin
(10 mg/m² body area, i.v., twice a week) simultaneously
with radiation (overall dose 3,400-4,000 cGy; 1,000 cGy a
week) - two opposed fields focused on the tumor process in
the esophagus and the area of the mediastinum. The patients
were irradiated with a 42 MeV Betatron (Siemens). Treatment
modality B comprised the same schedule for 5-Fluorouracil
with Adriamycin instead of Bleomycin at the dose of 30 mg/
m² body area, i.v., on days 1, 2, 23 and 24. The technique
and dose of radiation were the same as in modality A.

The results for all 56 evaluable patients are shown in
table 8. Of the 28 patients treated with 5-Fluorouracil,
Bleomycin and radiation, an objective remission was obtained
in 21, with 11 complete and 10 partial remissions (response
rate 75% - 21/28). When the response to this treatment modality was analyzed in relation to the loss of body weight as
a prognostic factor, a higher regression rate (85% - 11/13)
was observed in the group with a < 10% loss of body weight

TABLE 7

Patient Characteristics

	No. of patients	5-FU+ BLM+ rad.	5-FU+ ADM+ rad.
Patients entered in the study	61	31	30
Patients evaluable	56	28	28
Mean age	57	60	58
Male	55		
Female	3		
Weigt Loss			
< 10%	32	15	17
> 10%	24	13	11
Location of the Tumor in Esophagus			
Upper third	2	1	1
Middle third	36	20	16
Low third	18	7	11
Filling Defects (X-Ray)			
< 5 cm	9	6	3
5-8 cm	31	16	15
> 8 cm	16	6	10
Pathohistology			
Squamous cell	51	25	26
Adenocarcinoma	3	2	1
Anaplastic (squamous cell) carcinoma	2	1	1

TABLE 8

The Results of the Treatment

Treat-ment moda-lity	Weight loss	Complete response (100%)	Partial response (> 50%)	Sta-ble dis-ease (0-50%)	Pro-gres-sion	Response rate
5-FU +	< 10%	8 (61%)	3	2	0	11/13 (85%)
BLM +	> 10%	3 (20%)	7	3	2	10/15 (67%)
rad.	Total	11 (39%)	10 (36%)	5	2	21/28 (75%)
5-FU +	< 10%	1	7	3	0	8/11 (73%)
ADM +	> 10%	1	9	2	5	10/17 (59%)
rad.	Total	2 (8%)	16 (57%)	5	5	18/28 (64%)

$p < 0.05$ (only in complete responses)

as compared to the > 10% group. where 67% of patients (10/ 15) responded to therapy. Nevertheless, the difference was not statistically significant ($p > 0.05$). However, there were more complete remissions (8 vs 3) in the group with the lower body weight loss. Modality B - 5-Fluorouracil, Adriamycin plus radiation - produced 18 remissions, 2 complete and 16 partial ones (response rate 64% - 18/28). In this modality, the loss of body weight did not affect treatment results. The comparison of the overall response in groups A and B showed an almost identical response, i.e., 75% in group A and 64% in group B ($p > 0.05$). However, the quality of the response differed, with 11 cases (39%) of complete remission in group A as compared to only 2 (8%) in group B. The difference was statistically significant ($p < 0.05$).

In analyzing the results of our trial, we were also interested in whether the patients' age had any bearing on the chemotherapeutic response. The same response rates were obtained with both modalities for patients under and over 55 years of age (67 vs 71%; $p > 0.05$). The review of the overall response in relation to the loss of body weight showed a response in the < 10% group in 79% (19/24), and in the > 10% group in 63% of patients (20/32). The difference

was not statistically significant (p > 0.05).
The length of the filling defect (on the esophagogram
as related to the therapeutic result was also analyzed. A
statistically significant difference was found only between
the < 5 cm group (8/9 - 89%) and the > 8 cm filling defect
group (8/16 - 50%), i.e., the patients with a smaller tumor
mass responded better to therapy.

The duration of the remissions was considerably longer
in the modality A group (6-18+ months; mean, 12+ months)
than in the modality B group (3-10+ months; mean, 6.8+months).
Since the average follow-up of all patients was 18 months,
we also recorded the survival. Thus, 21 patients out of 28
treated by modality A (75%) survived 12 months; the same
survival period was observed in 5 of 28 patients (18%) treated by modality B. The survival of 18 months was more indic-
ative: the rate was 64% (18/28) in the modality A group,
whereas no patient treated by modality B survived that long.
The toxic side effects are shown in table 9.

TABLE 9

Toxic Side Effects and Complications of the Treatment

	5-Fluorouracil + Bleomycin + radiation (28 patients)	5-Fluorouracil + Adriamycin + radiation (28 patients)
Alopecia	0	26
Mucositis with retrosternal pain	16	18
Leukopenia (grade I-II)	4	3
Thrombocytopenia (grade I)	–	1
Skin erythema	2	–
Fever	10	–
Fistula (esophagus-tracheal)	2	–
Rupture of aorta	–	1 (death)
Hematemesis	1	–
ECG changes	–	4
Lung fibrosis with cardiac failure	1 (death)	–

In the modality A group, the most pronounced side effect was mucositis with retrosternal pain, which occurred 10 to 20 days after the start of therapy. Attempts to reduce this side effect with antacids and a mushy diet did not produce a noticeable effect. Fifteen to 20 days after the completion of therapy mucositis symptoms disappeared spontaneously. Leukopenia was less pronounced, whereas a febrile condition (due to the administration of Bleomycin) appeared in 10 patients. A tracheobronchial fistula developed in 2 cases (10 and 25 days, respectively, after completion of therapy). A palliative gastrostomy was performed in these cases. One and a half month after therapy a pronounced pulmonary fibrosis with cardiac failure developed in one case. The patient died of cardiac failure 3 months after the completion of therapy.

With regard to toxic side effects in the group treated by modality B, 26 of the 28 patients developed alopecia (from Adriamycin). Eighteen patients had a pronounced mucositis which disappeared spontaneously 20 to 30 days after the end of therapy. Bone marrow suppression was very mild; we also had one death due to the rupture of the aorta and hemorrhage. Four patients showed ECG alterations towards the end of therapy (ventricular extrasystole in two cases, tachycardia in one, and atrial fibrillation with absolute arrhythmia in one). The control examination, 2 to 3 months after the end of treatment, showed these changes to have disappeared.

Comparison of the results of this trial with our earlier reports concerning combined approaches in the treatment of esophageal cancer showed that the addition of 5-Fluorouracil to Bleomycin and radiation improved the therapeutic results, particularly in terms of a higher rate of complete remissions with practically no difference in the severity of side effects. The statement was not true for the group of patients in whom the same drug was administered along with Adriamycin and radiation.

Our ongoing pilot trial in chemoradiotherapy of esophageal cancer includes combination of 4-epi-doxorubicin and radiation. Namely, one of the recent Adriamycin analogues, 4-epi-doxorubicin (4-epi DX) has proved very effective, particularly in solid tumors. Preclinical and clinical trials of 4-epi DX have shown this cytostatic drug to possess an antitumorigenic spectrum matching more or less that of Adriamycin, while the toxic side effects are substantially less pronounced, particularly in so far as bone marrow, gastro-intestinal and cardiotoxicity are concerned. Very recently, Young (1984) reported the data of 4-epi DX activity in squamous cell head and neck tumors. Out of 24 evaluable patients, 5 partial remissions and 6 minor regressions were observed.

Since until now interaction of 4-epi-doxorubicin and radiation was not investigated, analogously, we have also studied the interference of this new compound with radiation on V-79 hamsters lung cells (Kolarić et al. 1984). When exposed to 4-epi-doxorubicin, the cells were approximately 8 times more sensitive to radiation, and their life span was shortened. These results encouraged us to perform a pilot clinical study combining 4-epi-doxorubicin + radiation in inoperable squamous cell esophageal cancer.

During 1984, 17 patients (15 males and 2 females) between the ages of 36-75 years entered the study (mean age 62 years). All the patients suffered from inoperable tumors (without distant metastases) and had not been previously treated. In 11 patients tumor was localised in the middle third of esophagus, while in the remaining group, it was localised in the lower or upper third. The tumors were pathohistologically confirmed in all the patients (squamous cell carcinomas). The same laboratory and clinical investigations before and during treatment, as well as treatment and toxicity criteria, were applied. Patients older than 75 years, furthermore, patients with heart, liver or kidney failure, were excluded from the study.

Patients were irradiated using two opposed thoracic fields (42 MeV Betatron-Siemens), with a daily dose of 200 cGy, e.g. 1,000 cGy weekly. The total radiation dosage was 3,400 - 3,800 cGy. Simultaneously with radiation, 4-epi-doxorubicin was administered in the daily dose of 50 mg/m^2, days 1, 2 and 22, 23. The drug was injected into the tube of a running infusion.

All 17 patients completed the treatment program and were evaluable. The results showed a clear cut antitumor activity and synergistic action of 4-epi-doxorubicin + radiation combination. Out of 17 evaluable patients, 6 complete and 7 partial remissions were achieved with a response rate of 76% (13/17). Furthermore, 4 patients showed a minor regression (stable disease), and no progression was observed. In 3 out of 6 patients with complete remission the endoscopic finding was even pathohistologically negative. The median remission duration was 6+ months, but in complete responders 11+ months, during average observation period of 14 months.

Analysing some prognostic factors (age, weight loss and

performance status) which could influence therapeutic results, we found that only performance status < 60 (Karnofsky score), was a poor risk factor. Namely, out of 6 patients
who were in this group, only 2 responded with partial regression.

Toxic side effects were expressed mainly in the form of
radiation mucositis and retrosternal pain in 60% of patients,
which occured 10-12 days after the start of treatment. Attempts to reduce this side effects with antacids and a
mushy diet produced a moderate effect. Fifteen to 20 days
after the completion of therapy mucositis symptoms disappeared completely. Leukopenia was less pronounced (3 patients)and no thrombocytopenia was observed. Tracheobronchial fistula, which occured in about 20% of patients in such
a type of treatment, were not observed. Regarding cardiotoxicity, no one case of heart failure was noticed. In one
patient ventricular extrasystoles were temporarily expressed
in ECG records during the treatment. The control examination of the patient 3 months after the end of treatment
showed these changes to have disappeared.

It is necessary to stress that the results we have observed with 4-epi-doxorubicin + radiation treatment have
again reconfirmed the advantage of combined approach in the
treatment of esophageal cancer. Here we think on the results
we have earlier achieved with Bleomycin + radiation (63% response), Adriamycin + radiation (60%) and the combination of
Bleomycin, 5-Fluorouracil + radiation (74%). In this respect
synergistic antitumor activity of 4-epi-doxorubicin + radiation offers a new perspective and possibilities in the
treatment of locoregionally spread esophageal tumors.

Other reports on trials including cytostatics with radiation in the treatment of inoperable esophageal cancer
also suggested the advantages of such a schedule. Here, it
is necessary to mention that Nabeya (1971) and Asakawa
(1973) have first reported on better results using combination of Bleomycin and radiation in esophageal cancer, but
in small series of patiens. Furthermore, Byfield et al.
(1980) achieved a complete clinical remission in 5 of 6 patients, by administering 5-Fluorouracil in a continuous drip
with concurrent radiation. The very small number of patients
in this trial certainly limits the value of the results.
The latest report by Franklin et al. (1983) on the preoperative administration (in 18 patients) of 5-Fluorouracil and
Mitomycin C with radiation (3,000 cGy) showed - at subsequent esophagectomy - a complete cure in 6 patients, i.e.,
no tumor process in the resected part of the esophagus.

However, 3 patients had intramural, and 9 transmural but resectable tumors. Furthermore, very recently Marantz (1984)
reported favourable results using combination of Bleomycin +
cis Platinum + radiation. An objective response was observed
in 61% of patients (13/22) with 19% of complete responses.
Leichman (1984), using preoperatively 5-Fluorouracil + cis-
Platinum combined with 3000 cGy of radiation, found 22% of
patients with no cancer at the surgery (19/86). In contrast,
negative results have also been reported with regard to the
combined modality approach in the treatment of inoperable
esophageal cancer. Roussel et al. (1983) reported a controlled EORTC trial in which the combination of standard Methotrexate and radiation doses did not prove to be superior to
radiation alone. The ECOG trial (Earl et al. 1980) focused
on radiation alone and in combination with Bleomycin did not
yield encouraging results about the advantage of the combined approach.

Although the combination of cytostatic drugs and radiation is superior to chemotherapy alone in the treatment of
esophageal cancer, the still insufficient number of controlled clinical radiotherapy and radiochemotherapy trials does
not allow a definitive view regarding the value of chemoradiotherapy as compared to radiotherapy alone. Nevertheless,
chemoradiotherapy offers a higher response rate (60-80%),
higher proportion of complete responses (up to 40%), longer
remission duration, lower radiation dosage (3,200-4,000 cGy)
and consequently better tolerance of treatment. It is still
not solved the question whether such an approach could pro-
longe the survival of patients. Two controlled clinical
trials focused on this approach, are ongoing. An international cooperative group led by Wu Huang from Peking is
evaluating a randomized study involving radiation alone as
one approach, and radiation - Adriamycin as another (Wu
Huang et al. 1983). Another current EORTC randomized trial
plans to evaluate radiation alone, and radiation with the
concomitant administration of cis-Platinum. These trials may
provide a more specific answer in the near future, as to the
actual value of chemoradiotherapy in inoperable esophageal
cancer.

The summation of all our past clinical trials focused on
the treatment of inoperable esophageal cancer warrants, in
our opinion, the conclusion that combined approach has so
far proved to be one of the optimal treatment modalities,
particularly if it involves 5-Fluorouracil, Bleomycin and
radiation.

SUMMARY

The prognosis of patients with squamous cell carcinoma
of the esophagus remains dismal, in spite of technical advances in both surgery and radiation therapy. Chemotherapy
as a palliative approach is still in the investigational
phase and the very moderate antitumor activity has been observed with only a few single agents (Bleomycin, Adriamycin,
Cis Platinum, 5-Fluorouracil, Vindesine). In an attempt to
improve therapeutic results, cytostatic agents, which inter-
acts with radiation, are now combined with radiotherapy. In
a sequential manner several controlled clinical studies were
performed in more than 250 patients, using antitumor drugs
alone or in combination with radiation. The results of these
studies showed superiority of combined approach, either in
remission rate or remission duration. Combination of Bleomycin + radiation achieved a response rate of 62%, Adriamycin + radiation 60%, while both drugs combined with radiation showed the same response rate but higher toxicity. By
adding 5-Fluorouracil to Adriamycin/Bleomycin + radiation
therapy, 64% and even 75% responses were observed compared
to only 30-40% with cytostatics alone. With combined approach a median remission duration of 16 months was reached.
An ongoing clinical trial, based upon in vitro proved synergism of 4-epi-doxorubicin and radiation, showed very promising results. Namely, this new analogue of Adriamycin, when
combined with radiation, resulted in 6 complete and 7 partial remissions out of 17 patients entered the study (13/17
- 76%). Furthermore, 4 patients showed a minor regression
(< 50%), and no progression was observed. The advantages of
chemoradiotherapy in esophageal cancer could be summarized
as follows: higher response rate (60-80%), higher proportion
of complete responses (up to 45%), longer remission duration,
lower radiation dosage (3,200-4,000 cGy) and consequently
better tolerance of treatment (less morbidity). The longer
follow up will show, whether combined approach could increase 5-year survival rate of these patients.

REFERENCES

Asakawa,H., Kowada, K., and Watarai, J. (1973): Radiotherapy in conjunction with bleomycin therapy for esophageal
carcinoma. Documentation (Nippon-Kayaku, Tokyo).
Bedikian, A. (1984): Phase II evaluation of 5-Fluoro-
uracil, Adriamycin, Cis Platinum and Vepesid in patients
with esophageal cancer. ASCO, Abstracts C-571, Toronto.
Bistrović, M., Maričić, Z.,Kolarić, K. (1976): Interac-

tion of Bleomycin and radiation in combined treatment of L-mice cells. Int. J. Cancer 18: 540-544.

Bistrović, M., Nagy, B., Maričić, Z., Kolarić, K. (1978): Interaction of Adriamycin and radiation in combined treatment of L-mice cells. Europ. J. Cancer 14: 411-414.

Bistrović, M., Nagy, B., Maričić, Z. (1980): The repair of radiation injury in L-cells treated by Adriamycin. Europ. J. Cancer 16: 333-338.

Byfield, J.E., Barone, R., Mendelsohn, J., Frankel, S., Quinol, L., Sharp, T., Seagren, S. (1980): Infusional 5-Fluorouracil and X-ray therapy for non-resectable esophageal cancer. Cancer, 45: 703-708.

Davies, H.L., Von Hof, D.D., Rozencweig, M., Handelsman, H., Soper, W.T., Muggia, F.M. (1978): Gastrointestinal cancer; in Staquet, Randomized trials in cancer, pp. 147-230 (Raven Press, New York).

Desai, D., Gelber, R., Ezdinli, E., Falkson, G. (1979): Chemotherapy of advanced esophageal carcinoma. ASCO/AARC Proc., 374.

Desai, P.B., Advani, S.H., Dinshaw, K.A (1984): Preliminary experience in chemotherapy of advanced esophageal cancer - a report of 70 patients treated with Cis Platinum + Bleomycin + Methotrexyte + Mitomycin C combination. ASCO, Abstracts C-516, Toronto.

Earl, J.D., Gelber, R.D., Moertel, C.G., Hahn, R.G. (1980): A contolled evaluation of combined radiation and bleomycin therapy for squamous cell carcinoma of the esophagus. Int. J. Radiat. Oncol. Biol. Phys. 6: 821-826.

Franklin, R., Steiger, Zw., Vaishampayan, G., Asfaw, I., Rosenberg, J., Loh, J., Hoschner, J., Miller, P. (1983): Combined modality therapy for esophageal squamous cell cancer. Cancer 51: 1062-1071.

Gunnlangsson, G.H., Wychulis, A.R., Roland, C., Ellis, F.H. (1970): Analysis of the records of 1657 patients with carcinoma of the esophagus and cardia of the stomach. Surgery Gynec. Obstet. 130: 997-1005.

Hellerstein, S., Rosen, S., Kies, M., Tsang, T., Shaw, J. (1983): Diamminedichloroplatine and 5-fluorouracil combined chemotherapy of epidermoid esophageal cancer. ASCO Proc. 497.

Kelsen, D.P., Ahuja, R., Hopfan, S., Bains, M.S., Kosloff, C., Martini, M., McCormack, P., Golbey, R.B. (1981): Combined modality therapy of esophageal carcinoma. Cancer 48: 31-37.

Kelsen, D.P., Cvitkovic, E., Bains, M., Shils, M., Howard, J., Hopfan, S., Golbey, R.B. (1978): Cis-Dichlorodiammineplatinum (II) and bleomycin in the treatment of esophageal cancer. Cancer Treatment Rep. 62: 1041-1046.

Kelsen, D.P., Bains, M., Hilaris, B., Chapman, R., Mc Cormack, P., Alexander, J., Hopfan, S., Martini, M. (1982): Combination chemotherapy of esophageal carcinoma using Cisplatin, Vindesine and Bleomycin. Cancer 49: 1174-1177.

Kolarić, K., Maričić, Z., Roth, A., Dujmović, I. (1976): Therapy of advanced esophageal cancer with bleomycin, irradiation and combination of bleomycin and irradiation. Tumori 62: 255-262.

Kolarić, K., Maričić, Z., Roth, A., Dujmović, I. (1977): Adriamycin alone and in combination with radiotherapy in the treatment of inoperable esophageal cancer. Tumori 63: 485-491.

Kolarić, K., Maričić, Z., Roth, A., Dujmović, I. (1980): Chemotherapy vs. chemoradiotherapy in inoperable esophageal cancer. Oncology 37, supp. 1: 77-82.

Kolarić, K., Maričić, Z., Roth, A., Dujmović, I. (1980): Combination of bleomycin and adriamycin with and without radiation in the treatment of inoperable esophageal cancer-A randomized study. Cancer 45: 2265-2273.

Kolarić, K., Roth, A., Dujmović, I. (1980): Bleomycin infusion combined with radiotherapy in the treatment of inoperable esophageal cancer. Tumori 66: 515-621.

Kolarić, K., Roth, A., Dujmović, I. (1984): The value of two combined chemoradiotherapy approaches in the treatment of inoperable esophageal cancer. Tumori 70: 69-75.

Kolarić, K. (1984): The role of 4-Epi-Doxorubicin in the treatment of gastrointestinal tumors. International Symposium on Advances in Antracyclin Chemotherapy - Abstracts, Milano.

Leichman, L., Seidel, H.G., Steiger, Z. (1984): Preoperative adjuvant therapy for squamous cell cancer of the esophagus. ASCO, Abstracts C-575, Toronto.

Linder, F. (1976): Tumoren der Speiseröhre. Therapiewoche 26: 318-326.

Marantz, A., Schmilovich, A., Santos, J., Muro, H., Hunis, A., Chacon, D. (1984): Combined therapy of inoperable locally advanced carcinoma of the esophagus. ASCO, Abstracts C-525, Toronto.

Nabeya, K. and Tagikawa, H. (1974): Clinical evaluation of bleomycin for the treatment of esophageal cancer. Abstr. XIth Int. Cancer Congress, Florence.

Nakayama, K. and Kinoshita, Y. (1974): Cancer of the gastrointestinal tract. II. Treatment localised and advanced. J. Am. med. Ass. 227: 178-189.

Nakayama, K., Orihata, H., Yamaguchi, K. (1967): Surgical treatment combined with preoperative concentrated irradiation for esophageal cancer. Cancer 20: 778-788.

Nygard, K. (1983): Irradiation, Bleomycin, Adriamycin and surgery in the treatment of squamous cell esophageal cancer. II Int. Congr. for Diseases of the esophagus. Abstracts, S-1, Rome.

Okamoto, T. (1971): Treatment of esophageal cancer with bleomycin. Proc. 7th Int. Congr. Chemother., vol. 2, pp. 639-642.

Pearson, J.G. (1969): The value of radiotherapy in the management of esophageal cancer. Am. J. Roentg. 105: 500-514.

Rambo, V., O'Brien, P.H., Clinton, M., Stroud, M.R., Parker, E.F. (1975): Carcinoma of the esophagus. J. Surg. Oncol. 7: 355-365.

Ravry, M., Moertel, C.G., Schut, A.J., Hahn, R.G., Reitmeier, R.J. (1973): Teatment of advanced squamous cell carcinoma of gastro-intestinal tract with bleomycin. Cancer Chemother. Rep. 57: 493-495.

Roussel, A. (1978): L'association methotrexate - radiotherapie dans le traitement du cancer de l'oesophage. XIIe Int. Cancer Congress, Buenos Aires, Abst. 149.

Roussel, A., Jacob, J.H., Ollivier, J.M. (1983): Radiotherapy alone and associated with chemotherapy in the treatment of inoperable esophageal cancer. EORTC symp. on treatment of advanced gastrointestinal cancer, Proc. 1.

Sischy, B., Remington, J., Sobel, S.H. (1980): Treatment of carcinoma of the rectum and squamous carcinoma of the anus by combination chemotherapy, radiotherapy and operation. Surg. Gynecol. Obstet. 151: 369-371.

Shastri, S., Slayton, R.E., Wolter, J., Perlia, C.P., Taylor, S.G. (1971): Clinical study with bleomycin. Cancer 28: 1142-1146.

Tancini, G., Bajetta, E., Bonadonna, G. (1974): Terapia con bleomicina da sola o in associazione con methotrexate nel carcinoma epidermoide dell'esofago. Tumori 60: 65-71.

Terashima, L. (1973): Combination therapy of bleomycin with radiation. Documentation (Nippon-Kayaku, Tokyo).

Vogl, S.E., Greenwald, E., Kaplan, B.H. (1981): Effective chemotherapy for esophageal cancer with Methotrexate, Bleomycin and Cis-Diamminedichloroplatinum. Cancer 48: 2555-2558.

Wieland, C. and Hymmen, U. (1977): Strahlentherapie und Behandlungsergebnisse des Oesophaguskarzinoms. Strahlentherapie 153: 719-725.

Wu Huang, T., Friedman, M., Beretta, G., Kolarić, K. (1983): Radiation alone vs. radiation plus adriamycin treatment in unresectable esophageal cancer - A randomized prospective study (in progress - personal communication Peking).

Young, C.V., Magee, M.J., Wittes, W.E. (1984): Phase II assessment of Epirubicin in head and neck cancer. International Symposium on advances in antracyclin chemotherapy. Abstracts, Milano.

Primary Chemotherapy in Cancer Medicine, pages 283-293
© 1985 Alan R. Liss, Inc.

PREOPERATIVE CHEMOTHERAPY IN PATIENTS WITH GASTRIC CANCER

H.O. Klein, M.D.

Medical Clinic, University of Cologne
5000 Köln 41, F.R.G.

The incidence rate of gastric cancer is decreasing in
Europe and in the United States. However, the outcome of
patients afflicted by this type of cancer is still poor
(Moertel 1982). In recently reported large series of cases
the resectability rate was between 60 and 65%. But only 50
to 55% of the patients could be resected curatively. The
operative mortality for subtotal resections is about 10% and
for total gastrectomy around 20%. The survival rate of curatively resected patients at 5 years lies between 40 to 60%.
Adjuvant chemotherapy (postoperatively) is of no importance.

Therefore, there is a need to explore new modalities of
treatment. Such an approach is the preoperative chemotherapy in patients with gastric cancer.

The following theoretical advantages of preoperative
chemotherapy may exist (Table 1).

Most important for the concept of preoperative chemotherapy are observations concerning kinetics of tumor cells.
The proliferative activity of stomach cancer cells is in
comparison with normal gastric mucosa cells high (Gross and
Klein 1981) (Table 2). The DNA content of gastric cancer
cells is normally between hyperdiploidic and tetraploidic
values. Rarely, there are so-called mosaic tumors, i.e.
tumors with several DNA stem lines (Böhm and Sandritter
1975, Stich and Steel 1962, Wiendl 1975).

Studies using animal models have demonstrated that
within 24 hours following removal of the primary tumor there

is an increase in the labelling index of distant tumor foci which lasts from 7 to 10 days (Gunduz et al. 1979). There is also a decrease in tumor doubling time and a measurable increase in tumor size which becomes apparent about 1 week following tumor removal. The enhanced tumor growth is probably the result of the amplification of the so-called growth fraction.

TABLE 1.

Theoretical Advantages of Preoperative Cytostatic Chemotherapy in Gastric Cancer

- increased rate of operability
- increased rate of curative resection
- reduced spread and seeding of viable tumor cells during operation
- precise evaluation of therapeutic results after chemotherapy by following surgery
- better accessibility of cytostatic drugs to micrometastases due to an unimpaired vascular system
- unperturbed cell kinetics of tumor population
- information on the efficacy of cytostatic drugs on different histologic types of gastric cancer in primary and metastases

In other animal experiments Fisher and coworkers (1983) compared postoperative cytostatic treatment, given on the day when the labelling index of metastases was on peak or on the day when the labelling index had returned to the preoperative level, with preoperative chemotherapy. It was found that tumor growth was more retarded and survival significantly more prolonged when cytostatic treatment was given prior to the surgical removal of the primary tumor. This means that such a treatment procedure inhibited the spread and seeding of viable tumor cells during operation.

Furthermore, cell kinetics are also of importance with respect to the development of resistant tumor cell populations by mutation (Goldie and Coldman 1979). In order to reduce the birth rate of tumor cells, which may be enhanced in distant metastases after removal of the primary tumor, preoperative chemotherapy seems to be justified.

Parameters of Cell Kinetics

	Normal Gastric Mucosa	Gastric Cancer	Normal Gastric Mucosa adjocent to Cancer	Early Gastric Cancer
Mitotic Index (%₀)	1,0 - 1,4	1,2 - 5,0	1,7	
H^3 Labelling Index (%)	7 - 16	9 - 41	23	
Median Cell Cycle Time (Hrs.)	24 - 122	72 - 204		4 - 15 Days
DNA Synthesis Time (Hrs.)	7 - 10	11 - 23		
Duration of Mitosis (Hrs.)	0,6 - 1,1	0,3 - 1,2		
Duration of G_2 Phase	1 - 4	2 - 12		
Birth Rate of Cells (per 1000 Cells/Hrs.)	3 - 16	3,5 - 24,3		

(Klein et al.,1981)

Table 2: Proliferative activity of stomach cancer cells in comparison with normal gastric mucosa cells.

A further advantage of preoperative chemotherapy is that the efficacy of cytostatic drugs on different histologic types of gastric cancer can be judged accurately in the primary tumor and metastases. Japanese investigators (Kawashima et al. 1979, Okada et al. 1979, Okada et al. 1981) showed that 5-FU, mitomycin C and neocarcinostatine are effective in gastric cancer especially in lymphnode metastases. The effectiveness of 5-FU begins with dosages of more than 5 g administered over a period between 14 to 20 days. 5-FU is effective in papillary, tubular and differentiated adeno as well as in signet ring cell carcinoma. Preoperative chemotherapy was performed mostly orally but also intraarterially and only rarely intravenously.

There are few clinical investigations concerning preoperative chemotherapy in gastric cancer (Table 3). The only randomized trial is one of Jinnai and Higashi (1976). They used mitomycin C in a dosage and schedules outlined in Fig. 1. The authors found that patients with stage III disease had a survival advantage at 5 years with respect to

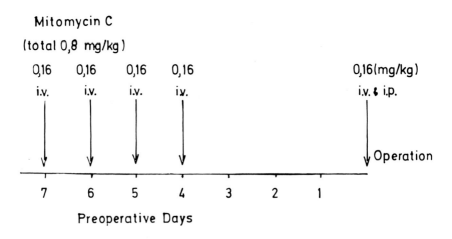

Fig. 1:Schedule of preoperative adjuvant chemotherapy for gastric cancer (Jinnai and Higashi, 1976).

TABLE 3.

Trials with Prechemotherapy in Gastric Cancer

Authors	Randomized Trial	Treatment Protocol	No. of Patients	Survival Rates at 5 Years
Jinnai and Higashi (1976)	Yes	MMC (i.v)	not stated	for patients with stage III } 21,4% control group / 41,4% P CTH group / no difference for patients with stage I + II
Fujimoto et al. (1976)	No	MTX + 5-FU + VLB + MMC (i.a.)	control n = 99 / P CHT n = 62	for patients with neoplastic invasion of the gastric serosa } 23,7% control group / 32,2% P CHT group
Nishioka et al. (1982)	No	P CHT: 5-FU (oral) post CHT: MMC + 5-FU (i.v.) MMC + 5-FU (i.v.)	control n = 222 / P and Post CHT n = 64 / Post CHT n = 59	P + Post CHT group 53% / Post CHT group 49% / Control group 40% } ns
Stephens et. al. (1984)	No	F A M + BCNU (i.a.)	27	11/13 patients with potentially curable disease are free of disease between 1 and 5 years

MMC = Mitomycin C   5-FU = 5-Fluorouracil   FAM = 5-FU, Doxorubicin,   P CHT = prechemoth.
MTX = Amethopterin   VLB = Vinblastin   Mitomycin C   Post CHT = postchem.
ns = not significant

patients in the control group (Fig. 2). There was no difference with respect to survival for patients with stage I and
II disease. In a study of Stephens and co-workers (1984)

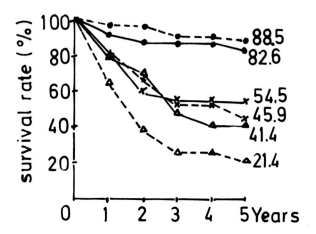

Fig. 2: Survival rates after surgery combined with preoperative adjuvant chemotherapy for gastric cancer (Jinnai and
Higashi, 1976)

———————————— combined with chemotherapy

— — — — — — — — control

• stage I   x stage II   Δ stage III

combination chemotherapy with FAM (5-FU, ADM, MMC) + BCNU
was used. In 13 patients with potentially curable disease
11 are free of disease between 1 and 5 years after preoperative chemotherapy. In the other trials of Fujimoto and co-
workers (1976) and Nishioka and co-workers (1982) - trials
which were not randomized - there were only small differences between the control group and patients treated preoperatively or pre- and postoperatively with respect to
survival.

In our own group we perform a trial in patients with
advanced inoperable gastric cancer using a sequential high
dose chemotherapy with the FAMeth-protocol (Klein et al.
1984). An update of the results is given in Fig. 3 and 4:
52 out of 86 patients (61%) came in remission whereby 10

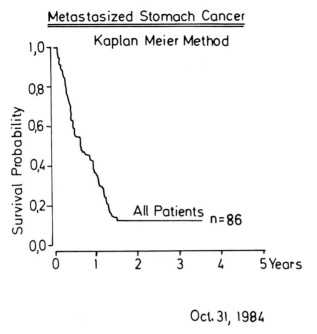

Fig. 3: Survival curve of all patients with metastasized stomach cancer treated by the FAMeth-protocol.

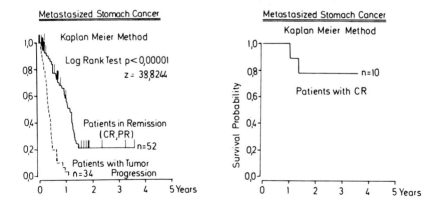

Fig. 4: Survival curves of patients with metastasized stomach cancer treated by the FAMeth-protocol.

patients had a complete response. The median survival for
responders is about 15 months and for all patients about 9
months (Figs 3 and 4   ). Patients in complete remission
are all off chemotherapy: 78% live free of disease between
15 months and 3½ years (Fig. 4).
Initially, it was intended that all patients being clinically in complete remission should undergo a confirmative
operation. Besides this issue we also wanted to know how many patients would accept a confirmative operation and what
are the kind and rate of side effects of such a procedure?
Twelve patients were considered to be clinically in complete remission. Only three of these twelve accepted a
second look operation. In two of them there was still evidence of tumor. The third was free of any disease. The
characteristics of these patients are listed in Table 4.
The major reasons of the nine patients who rejected a second look operation were fears of a high mortality rate and
severe postoperative side effects.

However, as outlined in Table 4, there were no major
side effects postoperatively if cytostatic chemotherapy was
administered only. In one other patient who was treated
preoperatively by radiotherapy and cytostatics, an incurable
anastomotic leak was observed after total gastrectomy and
splenectomy (patient no. 1, Table 4). Stephens and co-
workers (1984) reported a postoperative mortality rate of
11% in patients who had preoperative chemotherapy (FAM +
BCNU). This rate is not higher than observed after gastroc-
tomy without prior chemotherapy (Moertel 1982).

In conclusion, from a theoretical point of view preoperative chemotherapy seems to have some advantages in
patients with advanced gastric cancer. However, a review of
the literature reveals only four clinical trials. All
showed an improvement of survival for those patients who
were preoperatively treated with cytostatic drugs. But only
one trial was randomized. Preoperative chemotherapy in gastric cancer seems relatively well tolerated and does not
increase perioperative mortality. To assess the importance
of preoperative chemotherapy, prospective randomized trials
with more effective cytostatic protocols than have been
used prevously should be performed.

Metastasized Stomach Cancer

Patients	Sex	Age (Y)	K-I* (%)	Pre-Chemotherapy		CHT**	RT***	Operation	Post-Chemotherapy		Postop. Side-Effects
				Status	Histology				Localisation of		
									Primary Tumor	Metastases	
P.S.	♂	43	80	metast. Corpus-Ca. inop.(Laparotomy)	Undiff. Adeno-Ca.	Florafur-BCNU 6 Cycles	20 Gy on Stomach	Gastrectomy+ Splenectomy	Corpus	Lymphnodes	Anastomotic Leak
SchW.	♂	63	70	metast. Corpus-Ca. inop.(Laparotomy)	Anapl.-Ca., mono-cellular Mucus Production	HD-MTX-HD-5FU-ADM 3 Cycles	∅	Gastrectomy+ Splenectomy	Corpus	Lymphnodes (Micrometastases)	∅
J.G.	♀	62	80	metast. Cardia-Ca. inop.(Laparotomy)	Undiff. Adeno-Ca.	HD-MTX-HD-5FU-ADM 10 Cycles	∅	Gastrectomy+ Splenectomy	∅	∅	∅
B.A.	♂	44	90	Gastrectomy, Relapse inop.	Signet Cell-Ca.	HD MTX-HD 5FU-ADM 12 Cycles	∅	Inoperability due to Infiltration in Lymphnodes+Pancreas	Removed by first Operation	Lymphnodes	∅

* K-I = Karnofsky-Index   ** CHT = Chemotherapy   *** = Radiotherapy

Table 4: Characteristics of patients with metastasized stomach cancer treated preoperatively by chemotherapy or chemotherapy and radiotherapy.

References

Böhm N, Sandritter W (1975). DNA in human tumors: a cyto-
photometric study. Curr Top Pathol 60:151.
Fisher B, Gunduz N, Saffer EA (1983). Influence of the interval between primary tumor removal and chemotherapy on
kinetics and growth of metastases. Cancer Res 43:1488.
Fujimoto S, Akao T, Itol B, Koshizuka I, Koyano K (1976). A
study of survival in patients with stomach cancer treated
by a combination of preoperative intra-arterial infusion
therapy and surgery. Cancer 37:1648.
Goldie JH, Coldman, AJ (1979). A mathematic model for relating the drug sensitivity of tumors to their spontaneous
mutation rate. Cancer Treatm Rep 63:1727.
Gross R, Klein HO (1981). Ergebnisse und Perspektiven der
zytostatischen Behandlung des fortgeschrittenen Magenkarzinoms. Therapiewoche 31:5384.
Gunduz N, Fisher B, Saffer EA (1979). Effect of surgical removal on the growth and kinetics of residual tumor. Cancer
Res 39:3861.
Jinnai D, Higashi H (1976). Extended radical operation with
preoperative chemotherapy for gastric cancer. In Hirayama
T (ed): "Cancer in Asia", Baltimore: Univ Park Press, pp
111-119.
Kawashima Y, Kitade F, Osawa N, Sekimoto T, Okada K, Ando T,
Chikamori M, Yagi A, Yamada S, Sakuramoto K, Kato Y, Yasui
H, Okajimo K (1979). Preoperative administration of antineoplastic agents against gastric cancer, IV: clinical
evaluation of combined chemotherapy with mitomycin C and
5-fluorouracil. Gan To Kagaku Ryoho 6:363.
Klein HO, Dias Wickramanayake P, Schulz V, Mohr R, Oerker-
mann H, Farrokh GR (1984). 5-fluorouracil, adriamycin and
methotrexate: a combination protocol (FAMeth) for the
treatment of metastasized stomach cancer. In Kimura K,
Fujii S, Ogawa M, Bodey GP, Alberto P (eds): "Fluoro-
pyrimidines in Cancer Therapy", Elsevier Science Publish-
ers BV, pp 280-287.
Moertel CG (1982). The stomach. In Holland JF and Frei III
E (eds): "Cancer Medicine", Philadelphia: Lea and Fiebiger,
2nd edition, pp 1760-1774.
Nishioka B, Ouchi T, Watanabe S, Umehara M, Yamane E, Yahata
K, Muto F, Kojima O, Nomiyama S, Sakita M, Fujita Y, Maji-
ma S (1982). Follow-up study of preoperative oral administration of an antineoplastic agent as an adjuvant chemotherapy in stomach cancer. Gan To Kagaku Ryoho 9:1427.
Okada K, Kitade F, Mabuchi A, Osawa N, Yasuda M, Kawashima

Y, Yagi A, Yamada S, Sakuramoto K, Okajima K, Kita R, Sumida T, Kasagawa O (1979). Preoperative administration of antineoplastic agents against gastric cancer. V Clinical evaluation of combined chemotherapy with neocarzinostatin (NCS) and 5-fluorouracil (combined NF therapy). Nippon Gan Chiryo Gakkai Shi 14:834.

Okada K, Kitade F, Kawashima Y, Yagi A, Yamada S, Sakuramoto K, Okajima K (1981). A comparative study of preoperative combined chemotherapy with mitomycin C and 5-fluorouracil (MF therapy), and neocarzinostatin and 5-fluorouracil (NF therapy) against gastric cancer. Nippon Geka Gakkai Zasshi 82:34.

Stephens FO, Johnson AW, Crea P (1984). Preoperative "basal" chemotherapy in the management of cancer of the stomach. Med J Aust 140:143.

Stich HF, Steel HD (1962). DNA content of tumor cells. III Mosaic composition of sarcomas and carcinomas in man J nat Cancer Inst 28:1207.

Wiendl HJ (1975). Zur Frühdiagnose des Magenkarzinoms. Gastroskopische, histologisch-zytologische und zytophotometrische Untersuchungen. In Maurer G (ed): "Praktische Chirurgie", Heft 89, Stuttgart: Enke.

Primary Chemotherapy in Cancer Medicine, pages 295–300
© 1985 Alan R. Liss, Inc.

PANCREATIC CANCER: A NEW TARGET FOR ADJUVANT THERAPY AND
CHEMOTHERAPY

Franco M. Muggia, Alec Megibow, Harold O.
Douglass, Jr.
Rita and Stanley H. Kaplan Cancer Center of
NYU Medical Center and The Gastrointestinal
Tumor Study Group

Only the exceptional patient presenting with pancreatic
cancer is considered for surgical resection. This situation
has not been substantially altered even with the introduction of diagnostic techniques such as computerized tomography (CT) which may allow earlier diagnosis of pancreatic
lesions. Diagnosis is rendered difficult because of the
desmoplastic reaction and fibrosis commonly accompanying
pancreatic cancer which may delay diagnostic signs until
obstruction of major ducts or of the vascular supply occurs. Another powerful reason, however, is the nihilism
which still prevails in approaching this disease. We review here certain aspects which render pancreatic cancer
a new target for chemotherapy and which stimulate new
adjuvant trials.

Chemotherapy of Advanced Pancreatic Cancer

Phase II studies in pancreatic cancer chemotherapy have
lagged behind those of other common malignancies. The
Gastrointestinal Tumor Study Group has performed a number
of Phase II studies (Table 1) and compared these results
in terms of survival to a combination of streptozocin,
mitomycin and 5 Fluorouracil (SMF). Current studies include: epirubicin following early leads (4); ifosfamide including uroprotection with mesna, and platinum analogs.
Several refinements are taking place in these studies: 1)
patients entering Phase II trials will not have received
prior chemotherapy; 2) CT scans will be used in evaluating
response; and such responses will be reviewed by group
radiologists.

TABLE 1

GITSG Single Drug Studies in Pancreatic Cancer

Drug	Responses/Total	Ref
Doxorubicin	2/15	1
Methotrexate	1/25	1
Actinomycin D	1/28	1
ICRF-159	2/24	2
Beta-2-deoxyguanosine	2/25	2
Dianhydrogalactilol	1/26	2
Chlorozotocin high, low	3/30, 0/27	3
Maytansine	0/48	3

Awaiting publication and/or completion: cisplatin, triazinate, AZQ

Other leads in the chemotherapy of this disease include studies by other Cooperative Oncology Groups and Centers (Table 2). More recent studies by the Southwest Oncology

TABLE 2

Other Phase II Studies in Pancreatic Cancer

Drug	Responses/Total	Group (Ref)
MeCCNU	3/34	ECOG (5)
BCNU	0/20	Mayo (6)
Vindesine	1/15	MSKCC (7)
AMSA	0/27	SEG (8)
AMSA	0/31	SWOG (9)
Metoprine	0/24	MSKCC (10)

Group with Methyl-glioxal bis-guanylhydrazone (MGBG), and dihydroxyanthracenedione have been carried out on untreated patients in comparison with combination chemotherapy consisting of SMF plus doxorubicin. A review of sequential advanced disease studies by SWOG indicated that 31 of 222 patients survived more than 1 year (11). These patients include 14/80 on SMF, 7/77 on MF, 1/22 on MGBG, 3/33 on SMF + doxorubicin and 6/10 receiving the last two regimens sequentially. At Memorial Sloan-Kettering Cancer Center

single agent studies with etoposide are proceeding. Taken
all together this experience suggests an advantage for combination chemotherapy over single agents which was not apparent for 5FU and BCNU versus 5FU (5). However, continued
exploration of single agents in the most favorable circumstances (i.e. no prior treatment) is justified to provide
building blocks for more effective regimens.

Other leads to be pursued include: 1) combinations with
cisplatin to exploit synergism between it and other chemotherapeutic drugs. The Mayo Clinic has reported preliminary
favorable results in combination with doxorubicin and 5FU
yielding 5 responses, 3 of them complete out of 21 patients
(12). 2) hormonal therapy with progestins, estrogens or
antiestrogens alone or in combination with drugs to follow
laboratory leads showing synergistic cytotoxicity against
pancreatic cancer cell lines (13). 3) biochemical modula-
tion of 5FU with leucovorin and other metabolite/antimeta-
bolite approaches (14) have not yet been extended to pancreatic cancer but have proven to be of interest in other
gastrointestinal cancers and 4) intraperitoneal therapy.
The latter is currently being explored by GITSG and offers
attractive possibilities in a disease with common intraperitoneal and hepatic spread, and in an effort to exploit
synergism inherent in some drug combinations. However, no
information is yet available on the concentrations x time
exposure of a primary pancreatic tumor. We turn now to approaches in localized stages.

Treatment of locally Unresectable Disease
    Landmark studies by the GITSG established superiority of
5FU plus radiation alone in surgically staged patients with
disease confined within a 20x20 cm field. No improvement was
obtained when doxorubicin was combined with radiation, and
the current GITSG trial is superimposing maintenance with
SMF following the initial 5FU plus radiation, and comparing
it with SMF alone. Use of chemotherapy by itself in this
trial will prove informative on the responsiveness of these
earlier stages of disease, and also will indicate whether
chemotherapy is to prove a suitable alternative to combined
modality in this circumstance.

Experimental combined modality treatments will continue
to hold some appeal in locally unresectable pancreatic cancer. Several trials utilizing experimental forms of radiation have been conducted: These include radiation to possi-

ble secondary sites, neutron irradiation, intraoperative
radiation, interstitial radiation, and hyperfractionation.
Chemotherapy has been included in some of these trials
both by the systemic, the intraperitoneal or the intraarterial route. Preliminary experience with extended irradiation following intraarterial 5FU has been described: 3 partial responses out of 15 evaluable patients were obtained
in a pilot study at the University of Wisconsin (15). At
the Mayo Clinic, trial of intraperitoneal radiocolloids as
well as 5FU and external radiation has been instituted.
These studies should provide information on the interaction
between these various therapeutic modalities.

Adjuvant Chemotherapy

If chemotherapy has an impact in the treatment of pancreatic cancer, it would be more likely to indicate benefit
in earlier stages of disease. However, trials in resectable
pancreatic cancer are difficult to carry out because of the
rarity of this condition. Results of GITSG study 9273 have
recently been updated (16). This trial is the only study
comparing a combined modality adjuvant treatment (5FU +
radiation) with the usual observation following resection.
An additional cohort receiving adjuvant therapy following
closure of the control arm has now been compared with the
randomized cohorts. The 1 year survival fraction is .50,
.67, and .70 out of 22, 21, and 32 patients respectively
in the randomized control, randomized treatment and directly assigned treatments arms. The 2 year survival fractions
are .18, .43, and .61, respectively. This study has stimulated additional adjuvant approaches.

An intergroup study including major US cooperative
groups has just been activated. It compares two treatment
arms: The arm of the previously cited adjuvant trial, and
a "sandwich" chemotherapy-radiation approach. This latter
treatment consists of one cycle of SMF followed by radiation and simultaneous 5FU on first 3 and last 3 days as in
the other arm, and then followed by 2 additional cycles of
SMF. This approach is partially based on the kinetic and
spontaneous mutation theories of drug resistance predicting
greater success of chemotherapy when applied at the earlier
possible time. Efforts at improving systemic therapy are
particularly important since 40% of recurrences in the adjuvant treatment arm actually occurred outside the radiation port.

Future Prospects

The results of the GITSG adjuvant study have also stimulated interest on the chemotherapy of pancreatic cancer.
In addition, combination versus single agent trials suggest
some efficacy of the standard drugs when used in combination. Whether this combination proves as efficacious as
combined modality in the early stages is also being tested.
Finally, there is hope that new drugs of greater efficacy
will be detected through Phase II studies which include new
procedures of evaluation such as CT scanning on previously
untreated patients. Epirubicin and ifosfamide are two such
drugs that are being studied by these methods of evaluation.

New roles for chemotherapy need to be assessed in this
disease, and one needs to discard outmoded cynicism. Con-
version of unresectable to resectable disease by preoperative therapy needs to be considered. Supplementing systemic
and local treatment by intraperitoneal therapy is also undergoing preliminary evaluation. Study of these measures
should be based on sound theoretical considerations, on the
natural course of the disease, and on initial indications
of the ability of chemotherapy to alter it.

References

1.Schein PS, Lavin PT, and Moertel CA (1978). Randomized
   Phase II clinical trial of adriamycin in advanced measurable pancreatic carcinoma: A GITSG report. Cancer 42:19- .
2.Gastrointestinal Tumor Study Group: Kaplan RS (1978). Phase
   II trial of ICRF-159, beta-2-deoxyguanosine and galactitol
   in advanced measurable pancreatic carcinoma. Proc. AACR &
   ASCO 19:335.
3.Gastrointestinal Tumor Study Group: Levin, B, Stablein DM.
   Phase II trials of maytansine, low dose chlorozotocin and
   high dose chlorozotocin as single agents against advanced
   measurable adenocarcinoma of the pancreas. Cancer Treat.
   Rep. (To be published).
4.Wils JA, Green MD, and Muggia FM (1984). Treatment of pancreatic carcinoma: a role for chemotherapy. In: Advances
   in Anthracycline Chemotherapy: Epirubicin. G. Bonadonna
   (Ed.), Masson Italia; Milano, pp. 119-127.
5.Douglass HO, Lavin PT, and Moertel CG (1976). Nitrosoureas:
   Useful agents in the treatment of advanced gastrointestinal cancer. Cancer Treat. Rep. 60:769-   .
6.Kovach JS, Moertel CG, Schutt AJ, et al. (1974). A controlled study of combined 1, 3-bis(2-chlorethyl)1-nitrosourea

and 5-Fluorouracil therapy for advanced gastric and pancreatic cancer. Cancer 33:563.

7. Magill GB, Cheng EW, Currie VE (1981). Chemotherapy of pancreatic ca with vindesine. Proc ASCO 22:458.

8. Omura GA, Bartolucci NA, Lessner HE, and Hill GJ (1984). Phase II evaluation of amsacrine in colorectal, gastric, and pancreatic carcinomas: A Southeastern Cancer Study Group Trial. Cancer Treat. Rep. 68:929-930.

9. Rivkin SE, Stephens RL, Natale RG, O'Bryan R, Chen TT, Baker LH, Balcerzak SP, Ihamasr M, Legha SS, Oishi N, Coltman CA Jr. (1984). Phase II trial of Amsacrine in pancreatic carcinoma: A Southwestern Oncology Group Study. Cancer Treat. Rep. 68:1411-12.

10. Sternberg CN, Magill GB, Sordillo PP, Cheng EW, Kemeny N. (1984). Phase II evaluation of metoprine in advanced pancreatic adenocarcinoma. Cancer Treat. Rep. 68:1053-54.

11. Bukowski RM 1984). Characteristics of long term survivors receiving chemotherapy for pancreatic adenocarcinoma in Southwest Oncology Group (SWOG) studies. Proc ASCO 3:149.

12. Moertel C, Fleming T, O'Connell M, Schult A, and Rubin J. (1984). A phase II trial of combined intensive course of 5FU, adriamycin and cisplatin in advanced gastric and pancreatic carcinoma. Proc. ASCO 3:137.

13. Benz C (1984). Endocrine responsiveness of human pancreatic carcinoma. Clin. Res. 32:412A.

14. Machover D, Schwarzenberg L, Goldschmidt E, et al. (1982). Treatment of advanced colorectal and gastric adenocarcinomas with 5FU combined with high dose folinic acid: a pilot study. Cancer Treat. Rep. 66:1803-1808.

15. Ramirez G, Wiley A, Wirtanen G, Davis TE (1980). A combined modality approach to the treatment of unresectable carcinoma of the pancreas in Int. Congress on Diagnosis and Treatment of Upper Gastrointestinal Tumors./ M. Friedman, M. Ogawa & D. Kisner (Eds), Excerpta Medica-Int. Congress Series 542, pp. 488-492.

Primary Chemotherapy in Cancer Medicine, pages 301–315
© 1985 Alan R. Liss, Inc.

CHEMOTHERAPY (5-FLUOROURACIL, ADRIAMYCIN AND CISPLATIN)
PRECEDING IRRADIATION IN LOCALLY ADVANCED UNRESECTABLE
CARCINOMA OF THE PANCREAS: A PHASE II STUDY.

D.J.Th. Wagener, W.J. Hoogenraad, H. Kruisselbrink, P. Schillings, S.P. Strijk, Th. Wobbes
and S.H. Yap
Department of Internal Medicine, Division of
Medical Oncology, St. Radboud University Hospital, Nijmegen, The Netherlands

The prognosis of patients with carcinoma of the pancreas is poor, as illustrated in the first figure (Fig. 1).
Specific survival curves show a distinct difference between
survival rates of patients with resections compared to
those treated by any other method operative or not. However
only a small percentage of patients with carcinoma of the
pancreas has resectable cancer.

We analyzed all patients with a carcinoma of the pancreas who were treated in our hospital from 1968 to 1982.
These patients were staged according to the Vermont Tumor
Registry System (1),in which Stage I disease is defined as
tumor confined to the pancreas, Stage II as tumor with in-
growth in surrounding tissue or positive regional lymph
nodes and Stage III disease as a tumor with metastases

TABLE 1

Stage of Pancreatic Cancer

	I	II	III
Kruisselbrink (1983)	6 (9%)	35 (53%)	25 (38%)
Leadbetter (1975)	21 (10%)	71 (36%)	104 (53%)

As shown in Table 1, only 6 patients (9%) had stage I disease and these all underwent a Whipple operation. The ma-

jority of the patients (53%) had stage II disease and 38% of the patients had stage III disease. In the study of Leadbetter et al. (1), 10% of the patients were diagnosed with stage I disease, 36% with stage II and 53% with stage III disease.

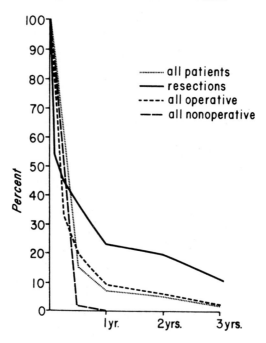

SURVIVAL
CANCER OF THE PANCREAS

Fig. 1.: Survival rates according to management (Gray, L.W., Crook, L.N, Cohn Jr., I.: Carcinoma of the pancreas, in: Seventh National Cancer Conference Proceedings, pp. 503-510. New York, American Cancer Society, 1973).

The study I want to discuss today is confined to patients with locally advanced tumor (stage II), which constitutes about 40-50% of the total group of patients with cancer of the pancreas. In order to put our results in proper perspective we would like to briefly review the results of chemotherapy and irradiation as published in the literature.

Single-Agent Therapy

5-Fluorouracil is the most thoroughly investigated drug in the treatment of advanced pancreatic cancer. Response rates have been reported ranging from 0-67%. In reviewing collected series, Carter and coworkers reported a response rate of 28% (2) (Table 2). However, the most current trials record a response rate of 20% or less.

TABLE 2

Single Agent Therapy in Pancreatic Cancer

	Number of Responders/Patients	Response Rate %
5-fluorouracil	60/212	28
mitomycin-C	12/ 44	27
streptozotocin	8/ 22	36
adriamycin	2/ 15	13
epi-adriamycin	7/ 26	27
ifosfamide	4/ 21	19

In the same collected series, mitomycin-C resulted in 12 responses in 44 patients (2). Among the chloroethyl-nitrosureas, which were evaluated in a small patient series, only streptozotocin, a naturally occuring nitrosurea, produced tumor regression in 31 to 50% of cases; this has been exploited in recent combination chemotherapeutic regimens (3, 4, 5).

Among other groups examining single-agent therapy in pancreatic cancer, the American Gastrointestinal Tumor Study Group has undertaken a series of phase II studies of individual anticancer agents (6). Of the group treated with

adriamycin, 15 of 25 patients received the drug as initial
therapy; 2 of these 15 previously untreated patients a-
chieved a partial response (13%). The median survival of
all previously untreated cases was 12 weeks. None of the
previously treated cases responded. Epi-adriamycin was also
recently tested in the EORTC Gastrointestinal Tumor Group
(7). Of the 26 patients treated, two patients achieved a
complete remission and five patients a partial response.
The median duration of the response was 7 months and the
median survival 9 months. When the activity of ifosfamide
in pancreatic cancer was recently examined (8), 4 out of 21
patients showed a response. The duration of the four responses was 7,8, 8+ and 10 months.

Combination Chemotherapy Studies

Even with the small number of active single agents available, there has been continued interest in combination chemotherapy. Initially, the combinations of streptozotocin,
mitomycin-C and 5-fluorouracil (SMF) (9) appeared to be the
most promising, as well as that of the FAM-scheme, consisting of 5-fluorouracil, adriamycin and mitomycin-C (10).
Tables 3 and 4 summarize the results of the most important
trials using these combinations.

TABLE 3

SMF (Streptozotocin, Mito-C, 5-FU) in Pancreatic Cancer

No. of Patients	Resp. (%)	Median Resp. Duration (Months)	Author	
23	43	10	WIGGANS 1978	(9)
22	32	9.5	ABERHALDEN 1977	(11)
56	34	8	BUKOWSKI 1983	(12)
66	4	4	OSTER 1982	(13)

TABLE 4

FAM (5-FU, ADM, Mito-C) in Pancreatic Cancer

No. of Patients	Resp. (%)	Median Resp. Duration (Months)	Author	
27	37	12	SMITH 1979	(10)
15	40	13+	BITRAN 1979	(14)
56	9	7	OSTER 1982	(13)
11	0		KLAPDOR 1982	(15)

Bukowski described a multicenter randomized trial comparing SMF to MF and obtained response rates of 34% for SMF and 8% for MF (12). The median duration of response for SMF-treated patients was 8 months. It should be noted that no survival advantage could be observed. The results of the Cancer and Acute Leukemia Group B, described by Oster et al. (13), were particularly disappointing since they were unable to confirm the earlier reports indicating substantial activity for the SMF and FAM regimens. Likewise, in a small, randomized trial conducted by Klapdor et al. (15), not only were there responses observed among 11 patients treated with FAM, but the side effects were also more severe compared to 5-FU plus BCNU. At the last ASCO-meeting, Cullinan et al. (16) also presented disappointing results with FAM. They compared treatment with 5-FU, 5-FU and adriamycin, and FAM and observed no meaningful difference in palliation as measured by symptomatic response, improved performance status or weight gain. The survival curves for all three treatment arms essentially overlap (median 5 months).

Radiation Therapy

Of the various irradiation techniques now used (external beam irradiation by supervoltage equipment, irradiation with fast neutrons, interstitial and intra-operative therapy), external beam irradiation is the most accepted. This method of irradiation has been advocated for both the palliative and potentially curative management of unresectable carcinoma of the pancreas. Most oncologists currently use

this technique in combination with 5-fluorouracil chemotherapy. This technique has evolved from a variety of studies, the most important of which is that of the Gastrointestinal Study Group (17). This group confirmed the value
of this approach in a three-armed, prospectively randomized
study comparing high-dose radiation therapy (6000 cGy)
alone with high-dose radiation plus 5-FU versus standard-
dose (4000 cGy) radiation therapy plus 5-FU. Since both
radiation groups that were given 5-FU did equally well in
terms of survival (Fig. 2), while the high-dose radiation
arm had substantial toxicity, the standard dose arm has
emerged as the standard of reference in the management of
this disease.

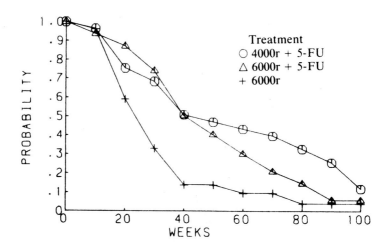

Fig. 2.: Survival measured from date of surgery.

Materials and Methods

Beginning in 1980, patients in our hospital with locally
advanced pancreatic cancer were treated with combination
chemotherapy followed by irradiation.

Before going into the details, I would like to make
some remarks about the problems encountered with evaluation
of the response in patients with locally advanced pancre-

atic tumor. Although we have at our disposal such new techniques as computerized tomography and ultrasonography, the determination of response remains unreliable. In fact, we appear to be dealing with an unmeasurable disease. For this reason the response must be defined according to the WHO guideliness for unmeasurable disease (18). A complete response (CR) is therefore defined as the complete disappearance of all known disease. A partial response (PR) is defined as an estimated decrease in tumor size of 50% or more, and no change (NC) is defined as no significant change. This includes stable disease, estimated decrease of less than 50%, and lesions with an estimated increase of less than 25%. Dicrease progression is defined as an appearance of any new lesion not previously identified, or an estimated increase of 25% or more in existent lesions. The results must have been observed for a minimum of 4 weeks after initiation of treatment. Some investigators do not mention the response at all in their publications. Instead, only survival, which is the clearest indication of efficacy, is used in the evaluation of treatment.

The chemotherapy used in our hospital is the FAP regimen, consisting of 5-fluorouracil, adriamycin and cisplatin (FAP-5). We choose this treatment-scheme because of promising results using this schedule in the treatment of stomach cancer (19). The dose and schedule of the chemotherapeutic component are described in Table 5.

TABLE 5

FAP - REGIMEN

Drug	Dose mg/m^2	Route	Day 1 2 3 4 5
5-FU	300	i.v.	x x x x x
ADM	50	i.v.	x
CDDP	20	i.v.	x x x x x

The course was repeated on day 21. The definite treatment schedule was determined after we had treated three patients (see Table 6). The first two patients were evaluated after 6 cycles, and then given another two FAP courses with an interval of 6 weeks. In patient 1, progression was seen after 8 cycles and the treatment was stopped. In patient 2 there was still a partial response after 8 cycles and we then gave the patient 3 FAM courses. After this treatment the tumor showed slight progression and the treatment was therefore completed with irradiation as described by the Gastrointestinal Tumor Study Group (17). This consisted of a split-course of 4000 cGy in combination with 5-FU (500 mg/m^2) on days 1-3 of the two irradiation periods. This treatment was well tolerated by the patient and the definite protocol was defined as 6 FAP cycles followed by irradiation of 4000 cGy (split-course) in combination with 5-FU. Patients were evaluated for response by physical examination, computerized tomography, ultrasonography and for the first four patients, also by laparotomy.

TABLE 6

FAP Followed by Irradiation Combined with 5-FU

Age	Sex	Resp.	Duration Resp. (Months)	Survival (Months)	Treatment (Cycles)
1.37	M	NC	9	11	6 + 2
2.61	F	PR	17	29	6 + 2 + 3 FAM+RT
3.60	M	NC	13	19	6 + 3 FAM+RT
4.50	F	NC	13	17	6 + RT
5.61	M	PR	18	18	6 + RT
6.61	F	PR	24	27	6 + RT
7.55	F	NC	8	11	5 + RT
8.63	M	NC	8	10	4 refused
9.44	F	PR	7	8	5
10.41	M	NC	5+	5+	5 under

Median duration of response: 11 months (range 5+ - 24)

Median duration of survival: 13.5 months (range 5+ - 29)

Results

As shown in Table 6 four out of 10 patients achieved a partial remission after chemotherapy. Six patients showed stable disease. After 6 cycles of chemotherapy, patient 6 had achieved clinically a complete remission (Figs 3, 4, 5, and 6 and 7).

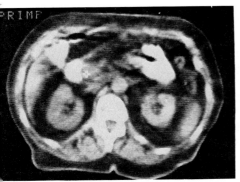
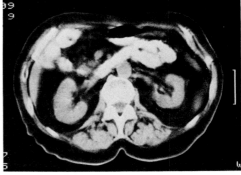

Fig. 3: CT-scan before chemo-   Fig. 4: CT-scan after 6
       therapy.   cycles of FAP.

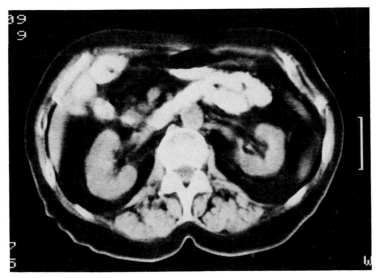

Fig. 5: CT-scan after 6
cycles of FAP

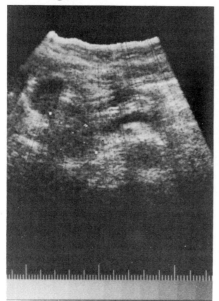
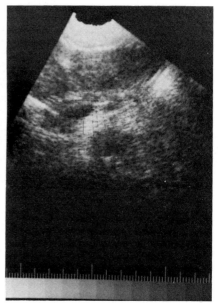

Fig. 6: Ultrasound before   Fig. 7: Ultrasound after
        chemotherapy. Tumor   6 cycles of FAP.
        indicated by white
        spots.

The decision was made to operate upon this patient in order
to investigate the feasibility of a Whipple procedure. However, it appeared shat some lymph nodes were still positive,
indicating the unreliability of our clinical methods. The
histology of the lymph nodes was drastically changed in
comparison to the structure before treatment (Figs. 8 and
9) due to the cytotoxic effects of the chemotherapy.

        Although the pathologist determined that the cells
were all non-viable, it is the policy of our surgeon that
a positive lymph node is a contra-indication for intensive
surgery. The operation was therefore terminated and the patient was irradiated according to the protocol.

        The median duration of response for the whole treat-
ment group was 11 months. The median survival was 13.5
months with a range from 5+ - 29 months.

        Discussion

The results of this study compare favorably with the experience of others using Whipple resection (20), neutron beam
(21), particle therapy (22), external beam (17) and external beam and implant therapy (24) (Table 7).

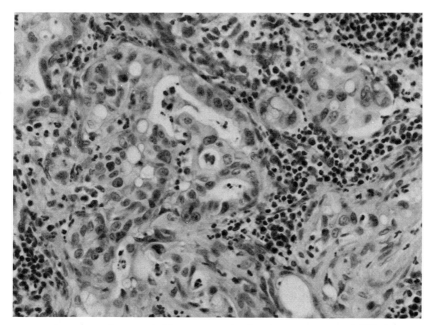

Fig. 8: Histology of the tumor before treatment (400x).

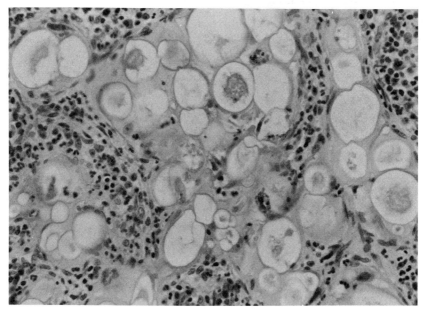

Fig. 9: Histology of the tumor after chemotherapy (400x).

TABLE 7

Results of Treatment for Carcinoma of the Pancreas

author		treatment	no. of pts	median survival (months)
Tepper	(20)	Whipple	145	12
Kaul	(21)	neutrons	31	9
Castro	(22)	helium nuclei	41	9
Moertel	(17)	ext. beam	25	5.3
Whittington	(23)	ext. beam	36	7.5
Shipley	(24)	implant + ext. beam	12	11
current series		FAP + ext. beam	10	13.5

TABLE 8

Combined Modality Treatment for Locally Advanced Pancreatic Cancer

author		no. of pts	radio-therapy	chemo-therapy	median survival (months)
Moertel	(17)	28	4000 Rads + 5-FU		9.7
		31	6000 Rads + 5-FU		9.3
Newall	(25)	11	6000 Rads	FAM (post-X)	10
Schein	(26)	26	4500 Rads (split)	FAM (1 cycle pre-X 6 cycles post-X	13+
Whittington	(23)	19	6300-7000 Rads	varying 5-FU comb.	12
current series		10	4000 Rads (split) + 5-FU	FAP (pre-X)	13.5

The survival of patients in the current series also compares favorably with patients treated with radiotherapy and chemotherapy, as described in the literature (Table 8). Whether the promising results of our treatment scheme are due to the chemotherapy given prior to the irradiation is not known. The study is still too preliminary to draw such conclusions. However, they are encouraging and we intend to continue this study.

References

1. Leadbetter A, Foster RS, Haines CR (1975). Carcinoma of the pancreas. Am J Surg 192:356.
2. Carter SK and Comis RL (1975). Adenocarcinoma of the pancreas, prognostic variables and criteria of response. In: Cancer Therapy: Prognostic factors and criteria of response, Chapter 3, 327. Editor: MJ Staquet. Raven Press, New York.
3. Dupriest RW, Hungtinton M, Massey WH, Weiss AJ and Fletcher WS (1975). Streptozotocin therapy in 22 cancer patients. Cancer 35:358.
4. Stolkinsky DC, Sadoff L, Braunwald J and Bateman JR (1972). Streptozotocin in the treatment of cancer. Cancer 30:61.
5. Broder LE and Carter SK (1974). Streptozotocin: Clinical brochure. Therapy evaluation program, National Cancer Institute, Dupriest RW, Hungtinton M, Massey WH, Bethesda MD.
6. Schein PS, Lavin PT, Moertel CG et al (1978). Randomized phase II clinical trial of adriamycin in advanced measurable pancreatic carcinoma. A Gastrointestinal Tumor Study Group report. Cancer 42:19.
7. Wils J, Bleiberg H, Blijham G et al (1983). Phase II trial of 4-epi-adriamycin in metastatic pancreatic carcinoma (Abstract). Fourth EORTC-NCI Symposium on New Drugs in Cancer Therapy. Brussels.
8. Loehrer PJ, Williams SD, Einhorn LH and Estes NC (1984). A phase I-II trial of ifosfamide and N-acetylcysteine in advanced pancreatic cancer. Proc Amer Soc Clin Oncol 3:149.
9. Wiggans G, Woolley PV, MacDonald JS, Smythe TA, Ueno W and Schein PS (1978). Phase II trial of streptozotocin, mitomycin-C and 5-fluorouracil (SMF) in the treatment of advanced pancreatic cancer. Cancer 41:387.
10. Smith FP, Macdonald JS, Woolley PV, Hoth DF, Smythe TA, Lichtenfeld B, Levin B and Schein PS (1979). Phase II evaluation of FAM, 5-fluorouracil (F), adriamycin (A) and mitomycin-C (M) in advanced pancreatic cancer. Proc Amer Soc

Clin Oncol 20:415.
11. Alberhalden RT, Bukowski RM, Groppe CW, Hewlett JS and
Weick JK (1977). Streptozotocin and 5-fluorouracil with and
without mitomycin-C in the treatment of pancreatic adenocarcinoma. Proc Amer Soc Clin Oncol 18:301.
12. Bukowski RM, Balcerzak SP, O'Bryan RM, Bonnet JD and
Chen TT (1983). Randomized trial of 5-fluorouracil and mitomycin-C with or without streptozotocin for advanced pancreatic cancer. Cancer 52:1577.
13. Oster MW, Theologides A, Cooper MR, Rafla S, Hutchinson
JL, Holland JH, Anbar D and Perry MC (1982). Fluorouracil
(F) + adriamycin (A) + mitomycin (M) (FAM) in advanced pancreatic cancer. Proc Am Soc Clin Oncol 1:90.
14. Bitran JD, Desser RK, Kozloff MF, Billings AA and
Shapiro CM (1979). Treatment of metastatic pancreatic and
gastric adenocarcinomas with 5-fluorouracil, adriamycin and
mitomycin-C (FAM). Cancer Treatment Reports 63:2049.
15. Klapdor R, Lehmann U, Kloppel G, Schreiber HW and Greten
J (1982). Palliative treatment of pancreatic carcinoma with
5-FU + BCNU and FAM: a prospective randomized study. Diges-
tion 25:43.
16. Cullinan S, Moertel C, Fleming T, Everson L, Krook J,
Schult A, Ceoria IL (1984). A randomized comparison of 5-FU
alone, 5-FU + adriamycin and 5-FU + adriamycin + mitomycin-C
(FAM) in gastric and pancreatic cancer. Proc ASCO 137.
17. Moertel CG, Frytak, S, Hahn RG et al (1981). Therapy of
locally unresectable pancreatic carcinoma: a randomized
comparison of high dose (6000 Rads) radiation alone, moderate dose radiation (4000 Rads + 5-fluorouracil), and high
dose radiation + 5-fluorouracil. Cancer 48:1705.
18. WHO Handbook for reporting results of cancer treatment.
WHO, Geneva 1979 (Offset publication no. 48), p. 16.
19. Wagener DJTh, Yap SH, Wobbes Th, Burghouts JThM, van
Dam FE, Hillen MFP, Hoogendoorn GJ, Scheerder H, van der
Vegt SGL. Phase II trial of 5-fluorouracil, adriamycin and
cis-platin (FAP) in advanced gastric cancer. Cancer Chemotherapy and Pharmacology (in the press).
20. Tepper V, Mardi G, Suit H (1976). Carcinoma of the pancreas: Review of MGH experience from 1963 to 1973: Analysis
of surgical failure and implications for radiation therapy.
Cancer 37:1519.
21. Kaul R, Cohen L, Hendrickson F, Awscholonn M, Hiegsa
AF, Rosenberg I (1981). Pancreatic carcinoma: Results with
fast neutron therapy. Int J Radiat Oncol Biol Phys 7:173.
22. Castro JR, Quivey JM, Lyman JT, Chen GTY, Phillips TL,
Tobias CA and Alpen EL (1980). Current status of clinical

particle radiotherapy at Lawrence Berkeley Laboratory. Cancer 46:633.
23. Whittington R, Solin L, Mohiuddin M, Cantor RI, Rosato FE, Biermann WA, Weiss SM and Pajak TF (1984). Multimodality therapy of localized unresectable pancreatic adenocarcinoma. Cancer 54:1991.
24. Shipley WU, Nardi GL, Cohen AM, Ling CC (1980). Iodine-125 implant and external beam irradiation in patients with localized pancreatic carcinoma. Cancer 45:709.
25. Newall J, Wernz J, Gouge T, Muggia F (1982). Locally inoperable pancreatic cancer: A combined modality protocol - toxicity and survival. Proc Amer Soc Clin Oncol 1:97.
26. Schein PS, Smith FP, Dritschillo A, Stablein DC and Ahlgren JD (1983). Phase I-II trial of combined modality FAM (5-fluorouracil, adriamycin, and mitomycin-C) plus split course radiation (FAM-RT-FAM) for locally advanced gastric and pancreatic cancer: A Mid-Atlantic oncology program study. Proc Amer Soc Clin Oncol 2:126.

Primary Chemotherapy in Cancer Medicine, pages 317–338
© 1985 Alan R. Liss, Inc.

CHEMOTHERAPY AS INITIAL MANAGEMENT OF PATIENTS WITH
OPERABLE COLORECTAL CANCER

A. Papaioannou, M.D., A. Polychronis, M.D.,
G. Plataniotis, M.D., M. Tsamouri, M.D.
J. Kozonis, M.D., J. Nomicos, M.D.

Mount Vernon Hospital, Mt. Vernon, NY, U.S.A.,
Evangelismos Hospital, Athens, Greece

INTRODUCTION

Excluding skin cancer, colorectal carcinoma (CRCa) is
the most frequently encountered malignant neoplasm in the
United States. In men, only lung cancer and in women, only
breast cancer cause more deaths than CRCa. Despite greater
public awareness, the availability of screening tests and
better surgical treatment, CRCa continues to kill almost
exclusively because of uncontrolled systemic dissemination,
more than 50% of those manifesting the disease (Welch and
Donaldson 1974). It therefore appeared likely that improvements in end results in this disease may be forthcoming only
if, in addition to detecting the disease earlier, better
means were discovered for its systemic control. The lack of
truly effective systemic agents at the time this study was
initiated was obvious and new avenues of treatment approach
appeared to be imperative.

To better understand the reasons for deciding on the
particular design of the study which is reported today, it
is necessary that we briefly review some of the scientific
notions prevailing at the time the protocol was under discussion by our group in 1976. There were at least three
considerations which influenced the design: a)many theoretical considerations along with some experimental and clinical
studies suggesting that chemotherapy might become more
effective if given before operation rather than after it, as
all adjuvant protocols called for at that time; b)a great
deal of dissatisfaction with the results of single-agent
postoperative adjuvant chemotherapy in colorectal carcinoma

and c)a considerable amount of theoretical, experimental and some clinical evidence pointing to the value of anticoagulation in the treatment of cancer. We shall discuss each of these considerations briefly.

A. The Value of Preoperative Chemotherapy (PrCh)

The theoretical considerations that render administration of chemotherapy advisable before rather than after surgery have been previously presented in detail (Papaioannou 1981 and 1984; Papaioannou et al., 1985). Briefly here, we should discuss the kinetic considerations prevailing at the time this study was designed and summarize the other advantages of PrCh.

1. Norton and Simon (1977) suggested that the highest chemosensitivity point of tumors obeying Gomberzian kinetics
is at the time of their maximal growth rate which is at the inflexion point of the Gomberzian curve. This point corresponds to approximately 37% of the maximal tumor size and roughly occurs just before the diagnosis is clinically made. Although the Norton-Simon hypothesis has not gained acceptance since that time, a newer kinetic theory (Goldie and Coldman 1979) based on the spontaneous development of chemoresistant clones, expected to occur by random mutation during the natural history of any tumor, places the maximal chances of chemotherapeutic success (and the lowest point of chemoresistant clones) exactly at the same point, namely, at or just before the diagnosis is clinically made. On the basis of both these kinetic considerations, it therefore appears advisable to initiate systemic chemotherapy at the first moment the diagnosis is made.

2. An important advantage of PrCh is the practical "in vivo"
   assessment of tumor chemosensitivity, possibly better than
in any "in vitro" test. Tumor response to chemotherapy is a phenomenon with many and highly complex components (Watson 1981), only a small part of which can be measured in any "in vitro" chemosensitivity test. Correlations of clinical tumor response to recurrence were truly predictive following PrCh in patients with osteogenic sarcoma (Frei III 1982) but only partially so in patients with stage III breast cancer (Papaioannou et al., 1983). At any rate, if the tumor is initially resected as is currently done almost universally, the opportunity to assess the "in vivo" chemosensitivity is

lost and treatment is continued blindly in the form of post-operative adjuvant chemotherapy for months or years until a recurrence becomes clinically evident. It is only then that the clinician appreciates the hardly justifiable iatrogenic patient inconvenience or outright suffering and depression and the waste of human and financial resources. In addition, the possibility of reduction in patient survival exists if appropriate therapy is not instituted at the earliest possible point in time when such treatment is more likely to be suc-cessful (Schabel 1975). In the same context, hormonal agents and the manipulation of the immune system can also be tested if the primary tumor is not resected.

3. The smaller the neoplastic focus, the more effective the chemotherapy, since the likelihood for the neoplastic cells to be better oxygenated, to divide more actively and to accumulate fewer metabolites inhibiting the efficacy of the chemotherapeutic agents is greater at this stage.

4. If the operation precedes chemotherapy, as is currently routinely practiced, the most important micrometastatic burden, possibly present to some extent in all solid tumors, is given an opportunity to increase in size. This is partic-ularly so under the conditions of immunosuppression and other factors at work in the perioperative period.

5. The immunosuppression induced by chemotherapeutic agents is not an obstacle to their use before operation. Following the initial drug-induced immunosuppressive phase, immunity not only recovers but in fact exceeds its strength present before chemotherapy. This phenomenon, known as "immunological overshoot" can be exploited clinically by timing the operative procedure durign this phase. Thus, chemotherapy may be used initially as a cancericidal agent and later as a nonspecific immunostimulant. The immuno-suppressive effects of trauma, anesthesia, etc., may thus, at least partly, be counteracted.

6. Metastases are known to form from cell variants pre-existing in the primary tumor. If these cells enter into the circulation with intact metastatic potential during surgical manipulations, they would be more likely to form new metastases, particularly in the state of postoperative hypercoagulability and immunosuppression, both of which favor the establishment of new metastases. If, however, the potential of these cells is diminished or eliminated by

preoperative chemotherapy, this possibility is reduced.

7. The presumed postoperative micrometastatic enhancement
   resulting from the resection of the primary, for whatever
of the above-discussed reasons, may be reduced or completely
prevented, if indeed the micrometastatic disease is more
effectively dealt with through PrCh.

8. When primary tumors are treated by PrCh, their size and
   vascularity are reduced and their resectability is
improved. After PrCh, operations are made easier and the
saving of blood and operative time may be appreciable.

Experimental evidence attesting to the efficacy of preoperative chemotherapy has existed for at least 25 years
(Brock 1959) but, somehow, has not been given due consideration by oncologists. The table below summarizes some of the
available experimental data (Table 1). In addition, Karrer

TABLE 1   Experiments on PrCh

Tumor Model	Contr. Group	Excision + Postop ChemoRx	PrCh + Excision	Reference	
Shay Chloro-leukoma	0%	15%	80%	Brock	1959
Spont.Metast. AdenoCa.	0%	0%	70-80%	Bogden etal	1959
B16 Melanoma	0%	38-43%	50.5-87.9%	Pendergrast etal	1979
Lewis Lung	–	50%	90%	Schabel	1979
Transpl.Met. AdenoCa	–	13%	67%	Schabel etal	1979
B16 Melanoma	0%	26%	80%	Osteene Wilson	1980

(1967), testing a great variety of treatment schedules,
using the Lewis lung tumor, showed a linear dose response
curve when chemotherapy was begun two days before amputation
of the tumor-bearing extremity and it was continued for five
days thereafter. Likewise, Fisher and his coworkers (1979)
observed an advantage in delaying the removal of the primary
tumor to treat the metastatic disease first, by a variety of
chemoimmunotherapy regimens.

Clinical studies supportive of the PrCh concept in CRCa
did not exist in 1976. However, there were two clinical
trials in breast cancer which were relevant to this question.

In retrospect, they both support the theoretical conclusions
at which Norton-Simon (1977) and Goldie and Coldman (1979)
arrived, namely, that efficacy of the adjuvant chemotherapy
is probably greatest at or about the time the diagnosis is
made. The first study is one of the earliest large-scale
collaborative trials in the U.S., testing Thiotepa given
during mastectomy and in the first two postoperative days.
Although, initially, differences between control and treated
groups were not observed, ten years later, premenopausal
patients with four or more positive nodes given Thiotepa had
a 20% survival advantage over untreated controls (Fisher et
al., 1968). The second study is a Scandinavian cooperative
trial using a 6-day course of Cyclophosphamide on alternate
patients, starting the day of mastectomy. Radiotherapy
followed on all patients except in one institution where
chemotherapy was delayed by 2-4 weeks to have radiotherapy
completed. Treated patients had a statistically significant
survival advantage over controls which was maintained for
over 12 years. Interestingly however, those patients whose
chemotherapy was delayed, lost this survival advantage,
suggesting that the approximately 3-week delay in institut-
ing chemotherapy was responsible for the loss of chemotherapeutic effectiveness. We have suggested (Papaioannou 1981)
the most likely explanation for this observation is that
immediately after the resection of the primary tumor, micrometastases become more vulnerable to chemotherapy because
their growth rate is accelerated, usually for a short period
of time only, as many experimental observations have shown.
This immediate postoperative period may well be a more
advantageous point to give chemotherapy than 2-4 weeks later,
as is usually practiced today. The loss of efficacy of
chemotherapeutic treatment, if given three weeks after
mastectomy, as in the Scandinavian trial, strongly supports
this notion. On the basis of this experience, we also tried
preoperative chemotherapy in a variety of gastrointestinal
tumors, using different treatment schedules, as a pilot
study. Adverse effects of PrCh were not observed during
this pilot work (Avgoustis et al., 1977) and we were, therefore, encouraged to proceed with the present controlled trial.

B. The Choice of Chemotherapy Regimen

    Postoperative adjuvant chemotherapy using single agents
for colorectal cancer had been disappointing a decade ago
despite sound experimental evidence strongly suggesting that

it would be effective if used when tumor burden is low (for review, see Schabel 1975). Meaningful differences were not observed in any of the early large-scale trials using FUDR (Dwight et al., 1973), Thiotepa (Dickson et al., 1971), short-term 5-Fluorouracil in two treatment schedules (Higgins et al., 1976 and Higgins et al., 1978), or 5-Fluorouracil over one year (Craig et al., 1979). Only in Duke's C patients with rectal cancer in the latter study was a statistically significant increase in the disease-free interval and in survival noted, but this was not known in 1976 at the start of our study. In contrast, interest had been increasing in the many theoretical advantages of combination chemotherapy and there were some initial encouraging reports (Carter 1976, Possey and Morgan 1977, Buroker et al., 1978). Thus, the opinion prevailed that, by combining most agents known to have some activity (from 15% to 20%) in advanced disease, results were likely to improve. The nitrosoureas, although effective, were not included in our protocol because they are highly immunosuppressive and their use in the preoperative regimen would have precluded operation for at least six weeks.

C. The Value of Anticoagulation in the Treatment of Cancer

Evidence abounds as to the efficacy of anticoagulants in interfering with the growth of tumors. The interested reader is referred to relatively recent, excellent reviews (Hilgard and Thornes 1976, Wood 1971, Zacharski et al., 1979). Experimentally, it has been shown repeatedly that agents which will interfere in any way with clot formation will have an antitumor effect, e.g., Heparin (Agostino and Clifton 1963), Warfarin, Urokinase and Streptokinase (Thornes 1974), Aspirin (Gassic et al., 1972), Dextran (Suemasu 1970), Dipyridamole and its derivatives (Ambrus et al., 1975) and agents inducing hypofibrinogenemia (Williams and Maugham 1972). Conversely, conditions which enhance coagulation increase the incidence of experimental metastases, e.g., epsilon amino caproic acid, induction of hyperfibrinogenemia, activation of Factor XII (Agostino 1970) and administration of endotoxin which stimulates tissue factor activation in leukocytes (Lerner et al., 1971). Radioisotope-labelled fibrinogen is taken up by many types of malignancy and its reduction by anticoagulation is associated with a more favorable course of the tumor (Schaffer 1964). The inhibition of tumor growth by anticoagulation in these models may be due to either a direct effect of the coagulation inhibition or to potentiation of immune or other host mechanisms. It has been postulated that the formation of clots at the periphery of the tumor may enhance tumor growth by facilitating attachment of tumor cells to the endothelium, by providing nutrients or growth stimulants or serving as a structural lattice upon which tumor cells can proliferate, or even providing protection against host defense mechanisms (Hilgard and Thornes 1976; Wood 1971).

The possibility of a relationship between the local formation of fibrin and the growth of human tumors has been entertained since 1878 when Billroth described the existence of tumor cells within a thrombus in human beings and related this to the development of metastasis. A variety of histochemical, immunologic and radioisotopic techniques have permitted detection of fibrin in human tumors but the true meaning of these thrombi has not been systematically studied. Several studies have shown, however, that by interfering with tumor homeostasis, anticoagulants can affect the natural history of tumors as well as patient survival. Thornes for example (Thornes 1972 and 1974) showed that the demands on chemotherapeutic agents in controlling the disease, decreased to approximately 25% once Warfarin therapy was initiated. He also reported that patients with advanced malignancies of similar histological types, given Warfarin in addition to chemotherapy, had a 40.6% two-year survival, contrasted to a 17.8% survival of the control group who were treated by chemotherapy alone (p $<$ 0.01). Many other cases have been reported of patients benefiting from a variety of anticoagulants or fibrinolytic agents with their having primaries at different sites, e.g., ovary, breast, lymphoma and leukemia (Thornes et al., 1972), promyelocytic leukemia (Drapkin et al., 1978), squamous cell carcinoma of the lung (Elias et al., 1973; Elias et al., 1975). It should be noted that regression of some of these tumors was possible, even if they were highly resistant to chemotherapy. Some observers have struck a negative note (Edlis et al., 1976; Rohwedder and Sagastume 1977) in the sense of not seeing any benefit. However, to our knowledge, there have been no reports where acceleration of tumor growth by treatment with anticoagulants was observed. Likewise, Waddell (1973) indicated suggested benefit by treatment with Warfarin in patients with pancreatic carcinoma, and Reis et al., (1968) with Stage II and III carcinoma of the uterine cervix. Also, Williams and Maugham (1972) reported regressions in patients with cancer of the breast, lung and colon, who received Ancrod therapy which is known to induce hypofibrinogenemia. An impressive study, although with a limited number of patients, was that of Hoover et al., (1978) using Warfarin as an adjuvant to amputation for osteosarcoma. Another line of evidence suggesting the efficacy of anticoagulants in malignancy comes from prospective large-scale studies of patients receiving anticoagulants prophylactically against cardiovascular disease, whose subsequent incidence of malignancy was considerably lower than that of their counterparts serving as controls (Michaels 1964; Michaels 1974).

Our own choice of using heparin rather than any other anticoagulant was influenced by the ability of heparin to induce lymphocytosis (Jance et al., 1962) and by work done in Dr. Chirigos' laboratory at the National Cancer Institute. The latter workers demonstrated that the tumoricidal function of macrophages is enhanced by polyanions and, more specifically, by heparin, through a mechanism most likely mediated by interferon production (Shultz et al., 1977). At the time, therefore, it appeared to us that heparin might be used as a dual agent, namely, with antitumor activity due to its anticoagulant properties, as well as a nonspecific stimulator of host resistance against cancer. It also appeared reasonable to achieve maximal anticoagulation prior to initiating chemotherapy and to maintain it throughout its course. Sludging and the well-known slow and inefficient circulation in the center of tumors might be overcome by heparin, thus enhancing delivery as well as efficacy of concomitantly administered chemotherapy. For these reasons, we initiated full anticoagulation one day before, during the five days of chemotherapy administration, and for one day following its cessation.

On the basis of all these considerations and in the absence of satisfactory alternatives, we decided to use a multi-agent regimen with short-lasting immunosuppressive properties, before and after operation and to compare it with the same regimen given after operation alone, so that observed differences could be attributable to the different timing of administration of the regimen. The addition of heparin in the second group was designed to study the possible enhancement of the effects of chemotherapy by anticoagulation.

PATIENTS AND STUDY METHODS

This study was instituted in November, 1976 on a prospective basis, to test the value of PrCh with or without anticoagulation by heparin in CRCa. The study was closed at the end of 1979.

Patient Selection. Considered candidates for the study were all patients admitted to the B Surgical Unit of Evangelismos Hospital with histologically proven or strongly suspected by historical,physical, endoscopic and radiological data as having carcinoma of the colon or rectum. The patient had to be physically fit (Karnofski's index 80% or more) and be no older than 75 years of age. Anemic patients were transfused to hematocrit 40% prior to chemotherapy or surgery. In addition to routine investigations and barium enema, preoperative workup included liver scan, alkaline phosphatase and γ GT. In addition, any other investigation deemed necessary on the basis of individual patient's symptoms was also done. Excluded were: a) patients whose cardiac status precluded long-term administration of Adriamycin; b) those whose workup was highly suggestive of metastatic disease in the liver or elsewhere; c) those who, despite negative workup,were found to have metastatic liver disease or peritoneal implants at operation; and d) those with history of another treated malignant neoplasm other than in the skin; e) patients 76 years or older.

Protocol Design. Initially, this study was set up as two separate ones. The first was to test the value of PrCh with its own controls receiving postoperative chemotherapy alone; the second was to test the combination of PrCh plus heparin anticoagulation, again with its own controls receiving postoperative chemotherapy alone. As the accrual of patients was slow and a considerably greater proportion of patients in both control groups was found at operation to have clinically undetectable liver metastases and were therefore dropped from further consideration, adjustments had to be made. It was decided to join the two control groups and to unify the two studies into one with three arms. This has created the discrepancy in the number of patients in the control group being larger than each of the two other arms. Each patient signed an Informed Consent and was allocated prospectively to one of the three groups in succession. The three arms thus formed called for the following:

Group I
one cycle PrCh; operation with intraoperative chemotherapy;
11 cycles postoperative chemotherapy.
Group II
one cycle PrCh + heparin; operation with intraoperative
chemotherapy; 11 cycles postoperative chemotherapy.
Group III
    no PrCh; operation; 12 cycles postoperative chemothera-
py.
Chemotherapy Regimen. The preoperative cycle consisted of
the following drugs given iv: Day 1 - Oncovin 2 mg; Day 2 -
Adriamycin 40 mg. and 5-Fluorouracil 500 mg; Day 3 -
5-Fluorouracil 500 mg; Day 4 - 5-Fluorouracil 500 mg. and
Adriamycin 40 mg.

    Intraoperative chemotherapy consisted of 5-Fluorouracil
1,000 mg in 1,000 cc 5% dextrose in water, given as an iv
drip beginning one half-hour prior to exploration. The iv
continued throughout the entire duration of operation, and
for a total of approximately six hours, so as to cover about
two to three hours after the completion of operation.

    Postoperative cycles: Day 1 - Oncovin 2 mg; Day 2 -
5-Fluorouracil 1,000 mg and Adriamycin 40 mg. all iv;
Days 1-5 - Cyclophosphamide 150 mg (three tablets) daily by
mouth.

    Heparin was given as a continuous iv drip containing
12,500 units of sodium heparin in 500 cc saline which was
renewed every 12 hours, to maintain clotting time beyond
30 minutes. Anticoagulation began one day prior to administration of each preoperative cycle, it was continued
throughout the four days of chemotherapy and was extended one
day after its completion.

RESULTS

    Although not prospectively stratified, the three groups
had a comparable distribution of abdominoperineal resections
(APR's) and colectomies. Table 2 shows the distribution of
age and of operations done in each group.

TABLE 2   Type of Operation and Age Distribution

Group	APR	Mean age	Colectomy	Mean age	All Patients	Mean age
I	4	53	11	58.3	15	57.1
II	6	56.6	10	56.7	16	56.6
III	7	61	15	63.4	22	62.6

APR: Abdomino-perineal resection.

The three groups were not entirely comparable as far as stage of disease was concerned but the differences were not marked.   Table 3 shows their distribution in this regard.

TABLE 3   Disease-Stage Distribution

Group	A	B_1	%	B_2	%	C^*	%	%B_2+C
I	-	4	26.6	9	60	2	13.3	74.1
II	1	3	18.7	7	43.7	5	31.3	75
III	-	2	9	14	63.6	6	27.9	91

Header: Astler-Coller Classification

* All C_2 except one C_1 in Group I

Postoperative complications and deaths are shown in Table 4.

TABLE 4   Complications and Deaths

Group	Suture Leak	Infect. Complic.	Other	Postop Death
I	1	-	-	2
II	-	3	2	-
III	2	2	3	2

There were no complications attributable to chemotherapy. Second malignant neoplasms have not been encountered up to now in any one of the groups.

The gross appearance of the tumor, where this could be
adequately evaluated, e.g., the rectum, did not show any
measurable differences in size following PrCh. However, as
a rule, the tumor two weeks after PrCh would look less
bloody, friable and shiny and, in some instances, with
questionably better mobility of its base. We often referred to the tumor two weeks after PrCh as "tired" or
"beat-up", but we could describe nothing that could be
objectively measured and therefore relied upon. Likewise,
in the few instances that histologic sections from biopsy
specimens (before PrCh) were compared with those from the
resected specimens after one cycle of PrCh, no distinct
histological changes could be identified. However, viewed
collectively, some morphological differences were noted
between the two groups receiving PrCh and those who did
not. Table 5 depicts some of these differences and Table
6, the degree of tumor differentiation between the three
groups.

TABLE 5   Histological Characteristics

Group	Degree of	Necrosis	Fibrosis	Ulceration
Gr I - (neg)		5	3	
n15 + (pos)		10	12	3
(% pos)		66.6%	80%	20%
Gr II*- (neg)		3	4	
n16 + (pos)		11	11	2
(% pos)		78.5%	73.3%	12.5%
GrIII - (neg)		3	2	
n22 + (pos)		19	20	8
(% pos)		86.3%	90.9%	36.4%

* Only 14 specimens available for study.

TABLE 6   Degree of Tumor Differentiation

Group	High	Middle	Low
I (n15)	1	13	1
II* (n16)	–	13	1
III (n22)	1	17	4

*Only 14 specimens available for study.

The survival of all cases, their recurrences, deaths and the stage distribution of the disease in each patient are shown in Table 7 (see next page). Substantial differences in survival are not seen among the three groups and, on the basis of such small numbers, it would be inadvisable to draw any conclusions whatsoever insofar as survival is concerned. However, if only the cases that developed recurrences are considered separately, rather striking differences become apparent. All deaths but one in the control group occurred within two years from operation, whereas only one-half of those occurring in the groups receiving PrCh took place before the end of the second postoperative year. As shown in Table 8, these differences were statistically significant.

TABLE 8   Survival of Patients with Recurrence (in months)

Group	Surgery to Rec.	Recovery to Death (mean)	significance	Surgery to Death (mean)	significance
I	19.8	20.4	I vs III p < 0.05	40.2	I vs III p < 0.05
II	19.1	6.5	II vs III N.S.	25.7	II vs III p < 0.1
I&II	19.5	13.8	I&II vs III p < 0.1	33.3	I&II vs III p < 0.05
III	12.2	5.4		17.7	

N.S.: Not significant

OVERALL SURVIVAL AND RECURRENCES

TABLE 7
GROUP I
n=15
PRE+
POSTOP
CHEMORx

GROUP II
n=16
SAME AS I
+HEPARIN

GROUP III
n=22
ONLY
POSTOP
CHEMORx

YEARS

——— : Living & Well
- - - - : Living with Disease
D : Dead of Disease
L : Lost to Follow-up

DISCUSSION

This study to our knowledge is the first prospective effort to test PrCh in CRCa of man. At the time we embarked on this trial we had great hopes that multi-agent chemotherapy properly timed before operation would truly improve results in the treatment of solid tumors, and we therefore felt that the timing of chemotherapy should be the only variable to be studied. As previously pointed out, the trial was initiated as PrCh vs. postoperative Ch completely separately from the anticoagulation question for which a second study was set up. Likewise, hopeful that multi-agent chemotherapy would be effective we felt it would probably be unethical to use untreated controls. In retrospect, this of course was unrealistic and a drawback of the trial design. The addition of anticoagulation to PrCh in retrospect is another drawback of design, since two questions are asked in a trial where abundance of patient-accrual was not certain. We had initially hoped that we would be able to attract the interest of other surgical groups in the country, once the trial was begun and safety could be demonstrated. This also proved to be unrealistic and the fear of most surgeons to operate on a patient who had chemotherapy three or four weeks before, continues to exist to this day, particularly when a large bowel anastomosis is at stake. Thus we proceeded with the trial with patients from only one surgical service. Three years later, when the first evaluation of the study was undertaken, no differences between groups could be detected and the study was closed. With a small number of evaluable patients available, any conclusions are unsafe. We can therefore neither conclude that PrCh is effective nor ineffective means to deal with CRCa particularly in the face of apparently ineffective chemotherapeutic regimen. The latter was evidenced by the lack of substantial size reduction of the primaries and the absence of any impact on survival. The same essentially unsatisfactory results were obtained with multi-agent adjuvant postoperative chemotherapy regimens (Possey & Morgan 1977, Buroker et al. 1978) despite the theoretical advantage of this approach. It remains therefore difficult to interpret the ability of PrCh to increase the free-of-disease interval from surgery

to recurrence as well as the survival from recurrence to
death as it was significantly and consistently observed for
both groups receiving PrCh (Table 8). One possible explanation is that PrCh is more effective than that given postoperatively because it affects primarily micrometastases
which are presumably more vulnerable to PrCh (Schabel 1975).
There is reason to believe that this was in fact so from a
number of observations: a) the fact that small metastases
to the liver not detectable by liver scan were found only
in the control groups where PrCh was not given, b) the rapid
failures of three patients with Astler-Coller C2 lesions in
group II who did not appear to have disseminated disease at
operation but shortly thereafter died of uncontrollable
disease, c) the fairly quick dissemination and death from
another patient of group II, who at operation was found to
have a stage A lesion that proceeded to metastasize in six
months , killing the host in ten months, d) the lower incidence of combined B2 + C lesions in groups I and II compared
to group III as well as compared to other series not receiving any chemotherapy (Table 9).

TABLE 9   Disease Stage Distribution

Stage	Frequency Distribution				
	Astler-Coller (%)	Gr I&II		Gr III	
		Pts.	%	Pts.	%
A	0.3	1	3.2	–	0
B_1	13.6	7	22.5	2	9.0
B_2	46.6	16	51.6	14	63.6
C_1	4.0	1	3.2	–	0
C_2	35.5	6	19.3	6	27.1
B_2 + C	86.1	23	74.1	20	90.7

These observations then suggest that PrCh substantially downgrades the tumor. This brings up the question of whether or not PrCh could have had more permanent effects had it been continued for two to three cycles. Interruption of its impact to the natural history of the disease by inducing systemic immunosuppression and the other untoward effects of surgery may have accounted for the course of events seen in our study. This is quite conceivable and one line of investigation worthy of pursuing. A number of other questions may be raised. Could it be that the immediate postoperative period is more appropriate to institute chemotherapy than three weeks before operation? Currently the NSABP is repeating an encouraging Canadian study showing the most impressive results to date on long-term survival of patients with CRCa. This was accomplished through a short course of 5-Fluorouracil delivered through a portal catheter for seven days starting immediately after operation (Fisher 1984). Whether or not the timing rather than the route of administration is the important feature here remains to be investigated. One factor however that has not been taken into account on both studies is the possible antitumor effects of intraportal administration of heparin alone, for which neither study has provided a control group. If the observations of Schultz et al. (1977) are applicable to human macrophages, the intraportal administration of heparin may well have important antitumor properties not only by interfering with clotting in the tumor ambience but also as a continuous stimulant of the numerous resident macrophages in the liver.

The question of anticoagulation could also be addressed in different ways. Could heparin anticoagulation with each cycle and not only for the preoperative cycle be more efficacious? Could longer duration, possibly continuous anticoagulation be more effective? Could Coumadin or possibly fibrinolytic agents be more effective than heparin? All these are possibilities that will require individual study. Although it certainly appears that in our study the addition of heparin in the one preoperative cycle did not have any appreciable influence on survival, this cannot possibly condone the principle.

With the sound theoretical considerations and experimental and clinical evidence that exists in its favor, the true value of heparin anticoagulation should be studied again, possibly in a protocol where this will be the only variable. In conclusion, PrCh with or without heparin anticoagulation appears to prolong the interval between surgery to recurrence and the survival between recurrence and death. No impact on the percentage of surviving patients could be documented, but the numbers are small and no conclusions can be drawn. Further study of both PrCh and of anticoagulation appears to be justified.

SUMMARY

The evidence in support of the concepts of PrCh and of anticoagulation in the management of primary CRCa are briefly presented. The first study incorporating both these novel approaches to the treatment of CRCa with a minimum follow-up of 5 years is herein presented. Whereas no discernible differences on survival were documented on a long-term basis, when patient who ultimately recurred in each group were compared, a substantial and statistically significant prolongation of the free-of-disease interval from surgery to recurrence and of survival from recurrence to death are revealed. PRCa and anticoagulation appear to deserve further study, in the management of operable CRCa.

REFERENCES

Agostino D (1970). Enhancement of pulmonary metastasis following intravenous infusion of a suspension of ellagic acid. Tumori 56:29-35.

Agostino D and Cliffton EE (1963). Decrease in pulmonary metastases: Potentiation of nitrogen mustard effect by heparin and fibrinolysin. Ann. Surg 157:400-08.

Ambrus JL, Ambrus CM, Pickern J, Solder S, and Bross I (1975). Hematologic changes and thromboembolic complications in neoplastic disease and their relationship to metastasis. J Med 6:433-458.

Astler VB, Coller, FA (1954). The prognostic significance of direct extension of cancer of the colon and rectum. Ann Surg 138:846-51.

Avgoustis A, Stathopoulos G, Polychronis A, Papaioannou AN (1979). Preoperative chemotherapy of gastrointestinal tumors: A feasibility study in "Basic for Cancer Therapy 1". Vol V, pp 263-268, BW Fox (ed), Pergamon Press, London.

Billroth (1879) (Cited by Zacharski et al, 1979).

Bogden AF, Esher HJ, Taylor DJ, Gray JH (1974). Comparative study on the effect of surgery, chemotherapy and immunotherapy alone and in combination on metastases of the 13762 mammary adenocarcinoma. Cancer Res 34:1627-30.

Brock N (1959). Neue Experimentelle ergebnisse mit N-lost-phosphamidestern. Strahlentherapie 41:347-53.

Buroker T, Kim PN, Gropper C et al (1978). 5-Fluorouracil infusion with Mitomycin C versus 5-Fluorouracil infusion with methyl-CCNU in the treatment of advanced colon cancer: a SWOG study. Cancer 42:1228-33.

Carter SK (1976). Large bowel cancer: the current status of treatment. J. Natl. Cancer Inst. 56:3-10.

Dixon JW, Longmire WP, Holden WD (1971). The use of triethylene thiophosphamide: an adjuvant to surgical treatment of gastric and colorectal cancer: ten-year follow-up. Ann Surg 173:26-39.

Drapkin RL, Gee TS, Dowling MD, Arlin Z, McKenzie S, Kempin S, and Clarkson B (1978). Prophylactic heparin therapy in acute promyelocytic leukemia. Cancer 41:2484-2490.

Dwight RW, Humphrey EW, Higgins GA et al (1973). FUDR, an adjuvant to surgery in cancer of the large bowel. J Surg Oncol 5:243-9.

Easter. Cooperative Oncology Group Progress Report. February, 1983.

Edlis HE, Goudsmit A, Brindley C, and Niemetz J (1976). Trial of heparin and cyclophosphamide (NSC-26271) in the treatment of lung cancer. Cancer Treat Rep 60:575-578.

Elias EG, Sepulveda F, and Mink I (1973). Increasing the efficiency of cancer chemotherapy with heparin: "Clinical study." J Surg Oncol 5:189-95.

Elias EG, Shulka SK, and Mink I (1975). Heparin and chemotherapy in the management of inoperable lung cancer. Cancer 36:129-136.

Fisher B (Feb. 1984). NSABP protocol C-02. A clinical trial evaluating the prolapse valve portal vein infusion of 5-Fluourouracil and sodium heparin in patients with resectable adenocarcinoma of the colon.

Fisher R, Gerhardt M., Saffer E (1979). VII. Effect of treatment prior to primary tumor removal on the growth of distal tumor. Cancer 43:451-9.

Fisher B, Ravdin RG, Ausman RK, Slack NH, Moore GE, Noer RJ
and cooperating investigators. Surgical adjuvant chemotherapy in cancer of the breast; result of a decade of
cooperative investigations. Ann Surg 168:337-43.

Frei E III (1982). Clinical cancer research: An embattled
species. Cancer 50:1979-82.

Gasic GJ, Gasic TB, and Murphy S (1972). Antimetastatic
effect of aspirin. Lancet 2:932.

Goldie HJ, Coldman AJ (1979). A mathematical model for
relating the drug sensitivity of tumors to their spontaneous mutation rate. Cancer Treat Reports 63:1727-30.

Grage T, Hill,G, Cornell T et al (1979). Adjuvant chemotherapy in large bowel cancer: updated analysis of single-
agent chemotherapy. Adjuvant Therapy of Cancer II.
Jones SE, Salmon SE (Eds). Grune and Stratton, New York.

Higgins GA et al (1984). Efficacy of prolonged intermittent
therapy with combined 5-Fluorouracil and Methyl-CCNU
following resection for carcinoma of the large bowel.
Cancer 53:1-8.

Higgins GA, Humphrey E, Juler GL (1976). Oral adjuvant
chemotherapy in the surgical treatment of large bowel
cancer. Cancer 38:1461-7.

Higgins GA, Lee LE, Dwight RW, Keehn RJ (1978). The case of
adjuvant 5-fluorouracil in colorectal cancer. Cancer
Clin Trials 1:35-41.

Hilgard P and Thornes RD (1976). Anticoagulants in the
treatment of cancer. Eur J Cancer 12:755-762.

Hoover HC and Ketcham AS (1975). Decreasing experimental
metastasis formation with anticoagulation and chemotherapy.
Surg Forum 26:173-174.

Janse CR, Cronkite EP, Mather GC, Nielsen NO, Rai K,
Adamik ER and Sipe CR (1962). Studies on lymphocytosis:
II. The production of lymphocytosis by intravenous
heparin in calves. Blood 20:443.

Karrer K, Humphreys SR, Goldin A (1967).An experimental
model for studying factors which influence metastases of
malignant tumors. Int J Cancer 2:213-8.

Lerner RG, Goldstein R and Cummings G (1971). Stimulation of
human leukocyte thromboplastic activity by endotoxin.
Proc. Soc. Exp. Biol Med 138:145-148.

Lessner HE et al (1982). Adjuvant therapy for colon cancer.
A prospective randomized trial. Proc Am Soc Clin Oncol
1:351.

Michaels L (1964). Cancer incidence and mortality in
patients having anticoagulant therapy. Lancet 2:832.

Michaels L (1974). The incidence and course of cancer in patients receiving anticoagulant therapy. J Med 5:98-106.

Nissen-Meyer R, Kjelgren K, Melmoik B et al: Surgical adjuvant chemotherapy with one single 6-day cyclophosphamide course: 12-year follow-up. Advances in Medical Oncology. A. Canonico et al (Eds) Advances in Medical Oncology Research and Education. Pergamon Press, Oxford, Vol. 12:1177-79, 1971.

Norton L, Simon R (1977). Tumor size, sensitivity of therapy and design of treatment schedules. Cancer Treat Reports 61:1307-17.

Osteen RT, Wilson RE: The timings of surgery and chemotherapy in an animal tumor model. 33rd Annual Meeting of the Society of Surgical Oncology, San Francisco, May 14, 1980.

Panetiere FJ, Chen TT. Analysis of 626 patients entered on the SWOG large bowel adjuvant program. Adjuvant Therapy of Cancer III. Salmon SE, Jones SE (Eds) Grune and Stratton, New York 1981, pp. 339-46.

Papaioannou AN (1984). Systemic therapy as the initial step in the management of operable breast cancer. Surg Cl N Amer 64:1181-91.

Papaioannou A, Kozonis J, Polychronis A, Papageorgiou G, Lissaios B, Kondylis D, Vasilaros S, Papadiamantis J, Tsiliakos S, Razis D, Throuvalas N, Papavassiliou K, Sakelaris J, Tsarouhas CH and Collaborating Investigators of the Hellenic Breast Cooperative Group (HBCG). Shrinkage of Stage III, Primary Breast Cancer (BC) to Preoperative (Preop) Systemic Therapy (Rx). Presented at the 3rd EORTC Cancer Working Conference, April 28, 1983, Amsterdam, Abstract IX.

Papaioannou AN, Kozonis J, Polychronis A et al (1985). Preoperative chemotherapy. Advantages and clinical application in stage III breast cancer. Recent Results in Cancer Research. Senn, UJ and Metzer U (eds) Springer-Verlag, New York. In the press.

Papaioannou AN (1981). Perspectives in Cancer Research: Preoperative chemotherapy for operable solid tumors. Eur J Cancer 17:963-9.

Pendergrast WJ Jr, Futrell JW (1979). Biologic determination of tumor growth in healing wounds. Ann Surg 189:181-8.

Possey LE, Morgan LR (1977). Methyl CCNU versus Methyl-CCNU plus 5-fluorouracil in carcinoma of the large bowel. Cancer Treat Reports 61:1453-8.

Ries J, Ludwig H and Appel W (1968). Anticoagulants in the radiation treatment of carcinoma of the female genitalia. Med Welt 38:2042-2047.

Rohwedder JJ and Sagastume E (1977). Heparin and polychemotherapy for treatment of lung cancer. Cancer Treat Rep 61:1399-1401.

Schabel FM (1975). Concepts for systemic treatment of micrometastases. Cancer 35:15-24.

Schabel FM Jr (1979). Personal communication.

Schabel FM Jr, Griswold DP Jr, Corbett TH, Laster WR Jr, Dyker DJ, Rose WC (1974). Recent studies with adjuvant chemotherapy or immunotherapy of metastatic solid tumors of mice. Adjuvant Therapy of Cancer II. SE Jones and SE Salmon (ed), Grune & Stratton, New York, pp. 476-88.

Schaeffer JR (1964). Interference in localization of I^{131} fibrinogen in rat tumors by anticoagulants. Am J Physiol 206:573-579.

Schultz RM, Papamatheakis JD, Chirigos MA (1977). Interferon: An inducer of macrophage activation by polyanions. Science 197:674-6.

Suemasu K (1970). Inhibitive effect of heparin and dextran sulfate on experimental pulmonary metastases. Gann 61:125.

Thornes RD (1974). Oral anticoagulant therapy of human cancer. J Med 5:83-91.

Thornes RD (1972). Fibrin and cancer. Br Med J 1:110.

Waddell WR (1973). Chemotherapy for carcinoma of the pancreas. Surgery 74:420.

Watson JV (1981). What does "response" in cancer chemotherapy really mean? Br Med J II, 34-37.

Welch JP, Dowaldron GA (1974). Recent experiences in the management of cancer of the colon and rectum. Am J Surg 127:258-66.

Williams JRB and Maugham E (1972). Treatment of tumor metastases by defibrination. Br Med J 3:174.

Wood, S Jr (1971). Mechanism of establishment of tumor metastases. In Pathobiology Annual, HL Ioachim, Ed, p.281.

Zacharski LR, Henderson WG, Rickles FR, Forman WB, Cornell CJ Jr, Forcier RJ, Harrower HW, Johnson RO (1979). Rationale and experimental design for the VA cooperative study of anticoagulation (Warfarin) in the treatment of cancer. Cancer 44:732-41.

SECTION VIII
UROLOGICAL CANCER

Primary Chemotherapy in Cancer Medicine, pages 341-350
© 1985 Alan R. Liss, Inc.

PREOPERATIVE CHEMOTHERAPY IN THE TREATMENT OF GERMINAL
TUMORS

Christopher J. Logothetis, M. D.

Associate Internist/Associate Professor of Medicine
M. D. Anderson Hospital and Tumor Institute
6723 Bertner Avenue, Houston, TX   77030

Since the development of vinblastine and bleomycin combination chemotherapy in the early 1970s, a decade of experience of combining surgery with chemotherapy has been
accrued. The development of curative chemotherapy in the
treatment of advanced germinal tumors has completely altered
the role of local modalities (surgery, radiation therapy) in
the management of these tumors. The ability to cure patients
with advanced disseminated disease has placed surgery in an
adjuvant role to chemotherapy. Although surgery has now
clearly been delegated to a secondary role in the treatment
of advanced germinal tumors, only with appropriate multidisciplinary treatment can a high cure rate for patients
with advanced germinal tumors be achieved.

The purpose of this brief report is not to discuss the
relative merits of various chemotherapy regimens which have
initially been developed, or the more recent promising advances in newer chemotherapy regimens employing conventionally available chemotherapeutic agents at different dosages
and schedules. In order to understand the surgical experience at the M. D. Anderson Hospital, it is important that a
brief summary of the therapeutic advances over the last
decade be made.

The initial introduction of vinblastine and bleomycin
by Samuels et al, demonstrated the ability to cure patients
with advanced metastatic disease. Although the ability to
cure such patients was obvious, persistent residual mature
teratomas were frequent results of this effective chemotherapy and required surgical removal. It was apparent in

the early experience that those patients who had total eradication of their disease, demonstrated by reduction the
serum biomarkers to normal levels and total disappearance of
their disease, had an excellent survival with high likelihood
of cure. Among those patients who failed to achieve a complete remission, attempts at local therapeutic modalities
were often fruitless. Such patients rapidly disseminated
their disease postoperatively and reinforced the concept
that patients with advanced testis cancer, even if radiographically they appeared to be localized, most frequently
are disseminated at clinical diagnosis.

With the introduction of cisplatinum, and its subsequent
addition to velban and bleomycin (VB+P), conclusions about
surgery preceded by chemotherapy have been made. These have
been corroborated by multiple investigators. Conclusion of
these combined efforts are:

1) Patients achieving a complete remission do not subsequently need a surgical exploration in the absence of a
persistent radiographic defect.

2) Patients who have elevated serum biomarkers preoperatively following chemotherapy rapidly disseminate their
disease. Serum biomarker elevations, therefore are an indicator of persistent systemic disease. Such patients should
not be submitted to surgery, but should be the subject of
further modifications in chemotherapy.

3) The finding of a mature teratoma postchemotherapy
is frequently a good prognostic finding with only a small
fraction of patients relapsing following the resection of
the large volume teratomatous masses.

4) Although teratomatous relapses are unusual in the
experience of the Memorial Sloan-Kettering Hospital and at
the M. D. Anderson Hospital, in the Indiana University experience, recent reports suggest that 1/3 of such patients
will develop a later recurrence with eventual disseminated
disease.

5) Patients who are treated with primary seminomatous
tumors without serum alpha fetoprotein elevations at the
time of their clinical presentation, should not be the subject of surgical exploration despite the persistence of
radiographically demonstrable "disease". The inherent dif-

ficulty in appropriately sampling such masses because of the characteristic desmoplastic response of a seminoma to chemotherapy make surgery treacherous.

6) Patients with persistent viable disease found unexpectedly among those initially treated with chemotherapy occurs in approximately 33% and is a poor prognostic finding with the majority of such patients eventually disseminating their disease postoperatively.

The sum of these conclusions suggest that in the initial experience of VB and VBP, that the true biology of teratomatous masses can not be predicted by the pathological findings at surgical exploration and optimal chemotherapy must be delivered prior to surgical exploration.

The M. D. Anderson Hospital experience with postoperative chemotherapy in the VBP era has been previously reported. Our conclusions were: (1) Despite optimal preoperative chemotherapy, almost 1/3 of patients will have persistent viable disease at surgery. Such patients will frequently disseminate postoperatively, although, occasional patients had surgical salvage without postoperative chemotherapy. (2) Optimal preoperative chemotherapy can best be delivered in a flexible rather than fixed number of preoperative courses. (3) Postchemotherapy surgical explorations are not true cancer operations resulting in wide resection of persistent viable cancer, but are operations removing large volume teratomatous masses, and simply identifying persistent viable disease for the chemotherapist.

Since that report, we have introduced a combination of $CISCA_{II}/VB_{IV}$ [(cytoxan 1 gm/m^2, adriamycin 90 mg/m^2, cisplatin 120 mg/m^2), alternated with (vinblastine 3 mg/m^2, bleomycin 30 mg X 5)] with a 92% disease free survival for testis cancer patients and a 50% disease free survival for extragonadal patients. Of the one hundred patients treated with this regimen, 38 have been submitted to surgical exploration. Indications for surgical exploration at the M. D. Anderson Hospital required the delivery of two courses beyond the development of a stable serum biomarker mass or a complete radiographic remission. Those patients who have normalization of their serum biomarkers for 2 courses with a stable radiographic mass are then submitted to a surgical exploration. 32 Patients who have met the criteria for surgical exploration at our institution, all have been found to be free of viable disease. Nineteen (59%) of the patients were found to have mature teratoma, 2 patients were found to have growing mature teratomas, an entity which we previously described, and 11 (34%) had desmoplasia and fibrous debris, but no evidence of viable carcinoma or teratoma (table 1).

TABLE 1

Patients

Dixon-Moore Class	Total	Requiring Surgery	
		Number	Percentage
Seminoma (Dixon-Moore I)	4	2	50
Embryonal carcinoma (Dixon-Moore II)	32	6	19
Mature teratoma (Dixon-Moore III)	0	0	0
Teratocarcinoma (Dixon-Moore IV)	52	20	38
Choricocarcinoma (Dixon-Moore V)	7	2	29
Pure endodermal sinus tumor	5	2	40
Total	100	32	32

Analysis of these patients in order to determine if the clinical stage, as defined by the modified Samuels staging system (table 2), or primary histology influenced the frequency of surgery was performed. It was found that those patients with Stage III-B$_4$ (advanced abdominal) disease had most frequent surgical explorations but this did not achieve

TABLE 2

Stage*		Patients Requiring Surgery	
	Total	Number	Percentage
Clinical II	22	5	23
III-B$_1$	3	0	0
III-B$_2$	12	5	42
III-B$_3$	16	5	32
III-B$_4$	23	12	52
III-B$_5$	15	3	20
Extragonadal	9	2	22
Total	100	32	32

* Modified Samuels staging criteria.

statistical significance .   Similarly, those
patients with Dixon-Moore category IV tumors (teratocarcinoma,
or malignant teratoma intermediate) had a slightly higher
frequency of subsequent surgical exploration, but this also
did not achieve statistical significance.

The conclusion of the cyclic chemotherapy experiences
confirms that a flexible number of preoperative courses of
chemotherapy can result in the delivery of optimal preoperative chemotherapy. By delivering optimal preoperative
chemotherapy with CISCA$_{II}$/VB$_{IV}$, we have no relapse rate and
no viable carcinoma is found at surgery.

An interesting finding is the absence of relapse among
patients with mature teratoma. It is our belief that histological examination cannot always predict the metastatic
potential of mature teratoma. The diagnosis of a mature
teratoma without metastatic potential can be made only in

the presence of a pathologically apparent mature teratoma
which is stable on chemotherapy.

The six patients who did not meet the preoperative
surgical criteria at our institution are of interest (table
3). Four of these patients were explored because of persistent serum biomarker elevations despite optimal preoperative chemotherapy. Such patients were tabulated as chemotherapy failures and were submitted to surgical exploration
in an attempt at surgical salvage. Three of these 4 patients
had elevated serum alpha fetoprotein only, and 1 had an
elevated serum alpha fetoprotein and bHCG. In 2 of these
patients a small focus of endodermal sinus tumor, in 1 a
small focus of embryonal carcinoma was found. Each of these
3 patients with elevated serum alpha fetoprotein only at the
time of exploration remain alive and disease-free without
evidence of recurrence. The single patient with an elevated
serum alpha fetoprotein and bHCG subsequently relapsed and
succumb to his disease. It appears that occasional patients
with persistent localized endodermal sinus tumor can be
salvaged by surgical exploration despite the persistence of
viable disease. We speculate that this occurs because endodermal sinus tumor can sometimes adopt a clinical behavior
of a mature teratoma, and because it is an obligate secretor
of alpha fetoprotein can be detected in minute amounts. Subsequent surgical exploration in this setting of a tumor which
can be detected in small volume, and has characteristics of
local recurrence, offers a potential for surgical cure. The
single patient who had an elevated alpha fetoprotein and
bHCG disseminated in the characteristic and expected fashion
and succumb to his disease.

Two patients were explored, not because of persistent
viable disease clinically, but because of their inability to
tolerate optimal preoperative chemotherapy. One of these
patients had a large volume choricocarcinoma and embryonal
extragonadal tumor treated initially with cyclic chemotherapy
having an excellent response, and then subsequently submitted
to surgical exploration after failing cyclic chemotherapy
and achieving a transient CR with alternate chemotherapy.
Unfortunately, the patient could not tolerate more than one
preoperative course with normalization of his markers, this
patient was not found to have viable disease at surgical exploration, but he rapidly disseminated his disease postoperatively and succumb to metastatic tumor. The second patient
is a patient who did not tolerate his full course of cyclic

TABLE 3

Initial Clinical Stage	Histology of Primary	Indications for Surgery	Operative Histology	Survival Duration postsurgery (weeks)
III-B$_5$	Terato-carcinoma	Rising AFP + bHCG	Embryonal + teratoma + EST	10 Died of disease
Extragonadal, mediastinum	Endodermal sinus	Rising AFP	EST	102 Disease-free
III-B$_5$	Embryonal carcinoma	Rising AFP	Embryonal	55 Disease-free
Clinical stage II	Seminoma + elevated AFP	Rising AFP	EST	86 Disease-free
III-B$_5$	Terato-carcinoma	Poor tolerance	Immature T	11*
Extragonadal, pelvis + retroperitoneum	MTT + MTU	Poor tolerance	Scar	22+ Died of disease

+Patient failed to achieve a complete remission with 7 courses of cycle therapy, 2 courses chemotherapy results in a normalization of his serum biomarkers. The patient was later explored. *Patient developed a rectal abscess with course ≠2 and candidiasis with course ≠3. Early surgical exploration was performed. Two courses of postoperative therapy were delivered.

chemotherapy because of recurrent infections. This patient was submitted to surgical exploration with only one course beyond the development of a complete remission. At surgical exploration a minute focus of immature teratoma was found. This patient did not disseminate postoperatively, but did receive postoperative chemotherapy. These last 2 cases demonstrate the results of suboptimal preoperative chemotherapy and its inability in predicting the eventual outcome of such patients. We believe this is further validation of the concept of optimal preoperative chemotherapy.

Indications for postoperative chemotherapy at the M. D. Anderson Hospital are summarized in (table 4). In addition to these indications, we believe that the findings of a persistent elevated serum alpha fetoprotein to modest levels with a single radiographic site may indicate the finding of a persistent localized endodermal sinus tumor.

TABLE 4

A. Contraindications	B. Indications
1. Elevated serum markers[a]	1. Persistent radiographic/ clinical mass following adequate chemotherapy,[b] with normal serum markers in patients with non- seminomatous germinal tu- mors
2. Inadequate chemotherapy in the presence of a residual mass	
3. Poor surgical risk	
4. Pure seminoma (despite the presence of persistent radiographic mass)	
	2. Suspicion of a °growing teratoma°
	3. Suspicion of histological conversion of a pure seminoma
	4. Suspicion of unrelated dis- order (second malignancy, inflammatory process)

[a]Alpha-fetoprotein, beta human chorionic gonadotropin.
[b]Adequate chemotherapy: 2 courses of systemic chemotherapy beyond the development of a stable radiographic and marker negative mass.

In this unusual clinical circumstance, surgical exploration
with attempt at salvage for focal resistant disease may be
considered. In general, though, it is our belief that the
persistent local viable disease is a sign of persistent
systemic viable disease and such patients should not be com-
mitted to surgical exploration, but rather to attempt at
salvage with further chemotherapy.

Our experience with advanced metastatic germ cell
tumors and the ability to consistently cure such patients
with cyclic chemotherapy has lead us to reconsider our approach to stage II testis cancer. Among patients with stage
II testis cancer, current approaches include a retroperitoneal lymph node dissection followed by adjuvant chemotherapy,
or a retroperitoneal lymph node dissection followed by ex-
pectant observation, and upon the development of relapse if
such occurs, the introduction of aggressive chemotherapy.
Both such approaches results in a high cure rate. At the
M. D. Anderson Hospital we believe that one can predict the
metastatic potential of such patients preoperatively, and
that attempts should be made in such a population with a
high cure rate in reducing the frequency of double therapy
(chemotherapy plus surgery). Among patients with clinical
stage II disease, the likelihood of finding stage II-C (+ 5
nodes by the Memorial Sloan-Kettering criteria, or eruption
through the nodal capsule by the M. D. Anderson criteria)
is very high. Such patients most frequently relapse postoperatively. Therefore, the approach at our institution
has been to introduce primary chemotherapy with selective
postchemotherapy surgical exploration for persistent disease.
Our experience is small, but there is some suggestion that
we have reduced the ultimate frequency of surgery in a
population without compromising the high cure rate. Of 28
patients, 7 have been submitted to surgical exploration.
All of these 28 patients remain alive and free of disease.
It is important to note that the frequency of surgery for
those patients who have initial Dixon-Moore IV tumors (tera-
tocarcinomas) is much higher than those patients who have
primary embryonal carcinoma (malignant teratoma undifferentiated, or Dixon-Moore II).

Metastatic germinal tumors have offered the opportunity
for the oncologist to successfully treat patients with widely
disseminated disease. They have also provided validation of
the concepts of combination chemotherapy and in our own experience with cyclic noncross resistant chemotherapy. In

addition, the incorporation of local modalities (surgery,
radiation) to the treatment of disseminated disease is most
clear in these very complex tumors and offer guidelines
which may be applied to other tumor types.

Primary Chemotherapy in Cancer Medicine, pages 351–358
© 1985 Alan R. Liss, Inc.

THE ROLE OF SURGERY IN STAGE IIC AND III NONSEMINOMATOUS
TESTICULAR CANCER

U. Metzger[1], P. Iten[1], F. Bammatter[2], A.R. von
Hochstetter[3], D. Hauri[4], V. Hofmann[2], F. Largia-
dèr[1]
Depart. Surg.[1], Pathol.[3], Urol.[4] and Div. Med.
Onc.[2], University Hospital, Zurich, Switzerland

Abstract

   30 Patients with stage IIC and III nonseminomatous
testicular cancer underwent surgery for residual tumor after
induction chemotherapy (postinductive surgery). There were
no operative deaths and surgical morbidity was not influenced by preoperative chemotherapy.

   A complete surgical remission was achieved in 9 of 15
patients with mediastinal or pulmonary deposits and in 6 of
12 patients with retroperitoneal metastases.

   Alphafetoprotein (AFP) levels over 10^4ng/ml at diagnosis and persistently elevated AFP values preoperatively were
associated with failure of surgery to achieve complete remission (p < .05) and to achieve long-term survival even
after surgical complete remission. Fifteen of 17 patients
with radical surgery remained disease-free after a median
follow-up of 33 months. Six of the 13 relapsing patients
had elevated AFP levels prior to definitive surgery. In one
patient a contralateral testicular cancer was diagnosed 60
months after postinductive surgery. Of the 17 disease-free
survivors, 12 had no tumor, 4 had mature teratoma and only
one patient had mature teratoma with malignant foci in the
resected surgical specimen.

   We conclude that AFP levels at diagnosis, elevated AFP
prior to definitive surgery, achievement of complete surgical remission and histology of residual tumor are important prognostic factors determining long-term survival in
residual stage IIC and III nonseminomatous testicular cancer.

Introduction

During the last decade, surgery for advanced testicular cancer has changed its role as primary therapy to that of adjuvant therapy. The majority of patients with disseminated nonseminomatous testicular cancer will achieve complete remission with Platinum-based chemotherapy as primary treatment (Einhorn et al., 1979, Vugrin et al., 1981). If there is only moderate tumor bulk at presentation, 80-90% of patients will have no evidence of disease after systemic treatment. Those with more bulky tumor who obtain a partial remission should then have residual tumor completely resected by surgery. This effectively restages the patient, provides therapeutic benefit to many, and determines the need for additional chemotherapy (Vugrin et al., 1981, Donohue et al., 1984). This is the second report of our experience in the combined modality approach to patients with advanced disease. Initial experience among 15 patients has been published previously (Stahel et al., 1982). In this report, special attention is given to indications and surgical considerations in residual nonseminomatous testicular cancer patients.

Patients and Methods

30 Patients with stage IIC and III nonseminomatous testicular cancer underwent surgery for residual tumor after induction chemotherapy (postinductive surgery) at the University Hospital of Zurich between September 1976 and December 1984. The mean age at surgery was 29 years with a range from 18-42 years. All patients had a high orchiectomy followed - in the earlier years of the study - by retroperitoneal lymphadenectomy in 8. The extent of disease before chemotherapy was determined by ultrasound, cat scan of the abdomen and whole lung tomography or cat scan of the thorax. Marker determinations for serial monitoring were done according to the generally accepted criteria (Carter, 1983). At presentation, the tumors were staged according to the International Workshop on Staging and Treatment of testicular cancer (Cavalli, 1980). All surgical-pathological specimens were classified according to the WHO International Histological Classification of germ cell tumors (Mostofi and Sobin, 1977). Induction chemotherapy consisted of the standard Einhorn regimen with or without Adriamycin or Actinomycin D. The indications for postinductive surgery were persistent tumor masses after chemotherapy, either following first induction (26 patients) or following re-

lapse (4 patients). The mean interval from the last course of chemotherapy to surgery was 2,8 months with a range from 1-24 months. The medium follow-up after surgery is 33 months.

Results

The operative procedures are listed in Table 1. In 6 of 12 patients with residual retroperitoneal disease all gross tumor was resected. Complete surgical remission was achieved in 9 of 15 patients with mediastinal or pulmonary deposits. In order to remove all gross tumor, the left kidney of one patient had to be sacrificed; in another patient, residual inguinal and iliacal nodes were resected. The median duration of hospitalisation was 10,5 postoperative days (range 6-18 days). There were no major surgical complications requiring reoperation and no operative death in the entire series.

TABLE 1

Operative Procedures

	n	Surgical CR
• Retroperitoneal Lymph Node Dissection	12	6
• Lung Wedge Excision	9	6
• Lung Lobectomy	2	2
• Lung Cryosurgery	2	-
• Mediastinal Lymph Node Dissection	2	1
• Miscellaneous	3	2
	30	17

After a median follow-up of 33 months following post-inductive surgery, 7 patients died of recurrent disease, 6 patients are alive with disease and are currently under "salvage" chemotherapy and/or radiation treatment. Seventeen patients have no objective signs of relapse. In Tables 2 and 3 the survival status is depicted with regard to

TABLE 2

Survival Following Chemotherapy and Surgery

(Median Follow-up 33 mts.)

Initial Histology	n	NED	LWD	DD
Terato Ca	13	10	1	2
Embryonal Ca	9	5	2	2
Chorio Ca	1	-	1	-
Yolk Sac Tumor	2	1	1	-
Mixed	5	1	1	3

NED = No Evidence of Disease

LWD = Alive With Disease

DD = Died of Disease

TABLE 3

Survival Following Chemotherapy and Surgery

(Median Follow-up 33 mts.)

Initial AFP	n	NED	LWD	DD
$\geq 10^4$ I.E./ml	4	-	-	4
$\leq 10^4$ I.E./ml	26	17	6	3

AFP = Alpha-Fetoprotein

initial histology and initial Alpha-fetoprotein level.
Among the 17 patients in whom all residual tumor had been
removed by surgery, 15 patients are alive without evidence
of disease. Of the 13 patients in whom postinductive surgery failed to achieve a complete remission, only 2 are disease free, one patient after additional radiotherapy to the
mediastinum and the second patient after two cycles of ad-

ditional chemotherapy for small pulmonary deposits. All
other patients with residual disease after surgery had local regrowth and died of chemotherapy resistant disease
within 12-14 months. The markers immediately prior to surgery, the results of surgery and the histology of the resected specimens are listed in Table 4. Elevated markers
prior to postinductive surgery are significantly associated
with failure of surgery to achieve complete remission and
to achieve disease-free long term survival (p < .05). The
majority of the patients had fibrotic-cystic or necrotic

TABLE 4

Survival Following Chemotherapy and Surgery

(Median Follow-up 33 mts.)

AFP prior to Surgery	n	NED	LWD	DD
≧ 20 I.E./ml	7	1	1	5
≦ 20 I.E./ml	23	16	5	2

Results of Surgery	n	NED	LWD	DD
PR	13	2	5	6
CR	17	15	1	1

Histology at Surgery	n	NED	LWD	DD
Fibrotic-cystic-necrotic tissue	16	12	2	2
Teratoma	8	4	2	2
Carcinoma	6	1	2	3

tissue in the resected specimen. Of the 17 disease-free
survivors, 12 had no tumor, 4 had mature teratoma and only
1 patient had mature teratoma with malignant foci in the

resected surgical specimen, an indication for subsequent chemotherapy. Three patients out of 6 who had carcinoma in the residual tumor have already died of their disease. In one of these patients a rhabdomyosarcoma was found in the resected tumor mass.

Discussion

Two different groups of patients should be considered for cytoreductive surgery. The first group includes patients who have had a partial remission with primary therapy. The second group includes those who achieved a complete remission after primary chemotherapy, but who relapsed and then achieved a partial remission after salvage chemotherapy (Donohue, 1984). Seventeen of our 30 patients with disseminated nonseminomatous testicular cancer who underwent surgery for residual disease after chemotherapy achieved a complete remission as judged by resection of all gross tumor and negative markers after surgery. The importance of a complete surgical remission is stressed by the poor prognosis of the 13 patients in whom not all gross tumor could be resected. This has also been found by the two most experienced centers (Mandelbaum et al., 1980, Vugrin et al., 1981).

An excessively high level of Alpha-fetoprotein at diagnosis, as seen in 4 of our patients with levels over 10^4 IE/ml, indicates a very poor prognosis (Bagshave et al., 1980) and might indicate a group of tumors resistant to complete eradication by the currently available treatment modalities. Patients with persistently elevated Alpha-fetoprotein levels are poor candidates for postinductive surgery. Only 1 of seven patients achieved a complete remission and 6 patients had residual malignant foci in the resected specimen. Positive markers clearly indicate active tumor and need more aggressive chemotherapy rather than cytoreductive surgery. Surgery can not be considered as an alternative to non-responsive chemotherapy.

As shown in one of our patients with residual rhabdomyosarcoma, the postinductive surgery is designed to completely remove non-germ cell malignancies within germ cell tumors (Ahlgren et al., 1984, Ulbright et al., 1984).

Eight of our 30 patients had mature teratoma in their resected specimen. Gross and histological examination of residual retroperitoneal deposits excised 4-6 months as compared to 4-6 weeks after PVB chemotherapy suggests that residual retroperitoneal mature teratoma existing after chemotherapy can grow and further differentiate (Suurmeijer et al., 1984). This indicates the need for removal of residual disease 1-2 months after completion of chemotherapy. It also prevents the "growing teratoma syndrome" first described by Logothetis et al., 1982.

Patients with residual carcinoma should receive postoperative chemotherapy. Whether patients with residual teratoma would benefit from further chemotherapy remains unanswered.

Aggressive surgery is indicated in patients with advanced bulky disease in whom chemotherapy led to negative markers but not to complete clinical response. An operative mortality of 0 and low morbidity justify this approach which restages the extent of disease, determines the precise pathologic category of the lesions, assesses the need for additional chemotherapy, removes non-germ cell malignancies and prevents the growing teratoma syndrome.

Bibliography

Ahlgren, A.D., Simrell, C.R., Triche, T., Ozols, R., Barsky, S.H. (1984): Sarcoma arising in a residual testicular teratoma after cytoreductive chemotherapy. Cancer 54: 2015-2018.

Carter, S.K. (1983): The management of testicular cancer. Recent Results in Cancer Research, 85: 70-122.

Cavalli, F. (1980): Report of the International Workshop on Staging and Treatment of Testicular Cancer. Europ J Cancer 16, 1367-1372.

Donohue, J.P., Rowland, R.G. (1984): The role of surgery in advanced testicular cancer. Cancer 54: 2716-2721.

Einhorn, L.H., Williams, S.D., Mandelbaum, I., Donohue, J.P. (1981): Surgical resection in disseminated testicular cancer following chemotherapeutic cytoreduction. Cancer 48: 904-908.

Germa, J.R., Begent, R.H.J., Bagshawe, K.D. (1980).: Tumor-Marker levels and prognosis in malignant teratoma of the testis. Br J Cancer 42: 850-855.

Logothetis, C.J., Samuels, M.L., Trindade, A., Johnson, D.E. (1982): The growing teratoma syndrome. Cancer 50: 1629-1635.

Mostofi, F.K., Sobin, L.H. (1977): International histological classification of tumors of testis, No. 16, World
Health Organization, Geneva.

Suurmeijer, A.J.H., Oosterhuis, J.W., Sleijfer, D.Th.,
Schraffordt, K.H., Fleuren, G.J. (1984): Non seminomatous
germ cell tumors of the testis: Morphology of retroperitoneal lymph node metastases after chemotherapy. Europ J
of Cancer and Clin Oncol 20: 727-734.

Stahel, R.A., von Hochstetter, A.R., Largiadèr, F., Schmucki,
O., Honegger, H.P. (1982): Surgical resection of residual
tumor after chemotherapy in nonseminomatous testicular
cancer. Europ J of Cancer and Clin Oncol 18: 1259-1265.

Ulbright, T.M., Loehrer, P.J., Roth, L.M., Einhorn, L.H.,
Williams, St.D., Clark, St.A. (1984): The development of
non-germ malignancies within germ cell tumors. A clinico-
pathologic study of 11 cases. Cancer 54: 1824-1833.

Primary Chemotherapy in Cancer Medicine, pages 359–366
© 1985 Alan R. Liss, Inc.

PERIOPERATIVE CHEMOTHERAPY FOR THE MANAGEMENT OF PRIMARY
LOCAL REGIONAL UROTHELIAL TUMORS

Christopher J. Logothetis, M.D.

Associate Internist/Associate Professor of Medicine
M. D. Anderson Hospital and Tumor Institute
6723 Bertner Avenue, Houston, TX   77030

The chemotherapy of bladder carcinoma has only recently
been recognized as achieving significant responses, which
can be translated into prolonged survival and beneficial
palliative responses to chemotherapy. Initial experiences
with chemotherapy were disappointing. Yagoda, et al. first
demonstrated the ability of cisplatinum to achieve objective
regressions of disease, but he failed to document any
benefit for multiple cisplatinum-based combinations. These
combinations included the additions of Adriamycin and the
addition of Cytoxan sequentially to single-agent cisplatinum.
Conclusion of the initial experience of Yagoda, et al. from
the Memorial Sloan Kettering Hospital was that combination
chemotherapy was not superior to single-agent cisplatinum
therapy. Since then, multiple low-dose chemotherapeutic
regimens have tended to corroborate this data.

The addition of the combination of Methotrexate and
vinblastine to Adriamycin and cisplatinum (MVAC) as proposed
again by the Memorial Sloan Kettering Hospital Group and the
combination of Methotrexate, cisplatinum, and vinblastine as
proposed by the Northern California Oncology Group do
suggests in preliminary analyses that the combination of
Methotrexate, cisplatinum, and vinca alkaloid may add to the
response rate. Such data remains premature, but is encouraging.

In the M. D. Anderson Hospital experience since the
introduction of cisplatinum to the therapy of bladder
carcinoma, a combination of Cytoxan, Adriamycin, and
cisplatinum (CISCA) at relative high dose (Cytoxan 650 mg/m^2,

Adriamycin 50-60 mg/m^2, and cisplatinum 100 mg/m^2) has been employed. Our experience indicates that although complete remissions can be documented, these are only durable in those patients who have nodal metastases only and although high response rates are documented in those patients with distant visceral metastases these tend not to be durable with mean durations of response at approximately one year.

Local regional disease has been managed with the introduction of pelvic arterial infusion at our institution. This combination of pelvic infusion and intravenous therapy results in an apparent increased local control rate. It was again noted that those patients who had local regional disease of advanced urothelial tumors and those patients defined as having unresectable locally advanced disease by evidence of invasion of pelvic visceral or nodal involvement have a high complete remission rate. This complete remission rate was significantly higher than those patients with distant visceral metastases and was far more durable.

Our experience with CISCA chemotherapy for local regional bladder cancer combining intra-arterial and intra-venous chemotherapy currently numbers 38 patients (Table 1).

TABLE 1

Characteristics of 38 Patients with Local or Regional
Disease with i.a. + i.v. CISCA
2/1/82 - 6/29/83

Ages		
Median: 66.75		Range 41 - 82
Sex		
Male: 25		Female: 13
Primary Site		
Bladder : 36		
Ureter: 2		

TABLE 2

Extent of Disease

Disease	Patients		Disease	Patients	
	No.	%		No.	%
*Locally Advanced Disease Only	12	31.6	Local Pelvic Disease + Nodal Mass	26	68.4
Prostatic invasion	3	7.8	Pelvic nodes	15	39.5
Vaginal invasion	1	2.6	Para-aortic nodes	8	21.0
Penile invasion	3	7.8	Mesenteric nodes	1	2.6
Pelvic sidewall fixation	9	23.6	Supraclavicular nodes	2	5.2

* Patients had more than one site of involvement.

Percentage of total number of patients (N = 38).

The clinical presentations of these 38 patients included 12 who had evidence of local pelvic visceral invasion which precluded successful surgical intervention (Table 2). In addition to these 12 patients were 26 patients who had, in addition to local pelvic disease, evidence of gross nodal involvement. These nodes ranged from pelvic nodes, para-aortic nodes, mesenteric nodes, and supraclavicular nodes. The histological distribution of these included 29 who had pure transitional cell carcinomas, 7 who had transition forms of transitional cell carcinomas, and 2 who had pure squamous cell carcinomas. Excluded from these studies were patients with adenocarcinomas who on previous studies were found to be resistant to cisplatinum-based chemotherapy. Transition forms were defined as those patients with transitional cell carcinomas who in addition to the characteristic pathological findings of a transitional cell carcinoma had evidence of squamoid, adenomatous, or spindle transformation. The characteristics of the study population are in Table 1 .

TABLE 3

CISCA Chemotherapy

Intra-arterial and Intravenous

I.V. CISCA

Cytoxan 650 mg/m² B.S.A. Day 1.
Adriamycin 50-60 mg/m² B.S.A. Day 1.
*Cisplatinum 100 mg/m² B.S.A. Day 2.

I.A. CISCA

Percutaneous hypogastric catheter Day 1.
Cytoxan 650 mg/m² B.S.A. Day 1.
Adriamycin 50-60 mg/m² B.S.A. Day 1.
*+Cisplatinum 100 mg/m² B.S.A. via I.A. catheter Day 2.

* Each dose of cisplatinum delivered with forced mannitol
diuresis.

+ Distribution of cisplatinum via each I.A. catheter is
determined by a radionuclide flow study.

The patients were mostly male and the two patients who had
ureteral primary tumors all had arisen in the distal third
of the ureter and presented with local pelvic masses. The
age range was that which was characteristic of urothelial
tumors. Chemotherapy was delivered with combined intravenous and intra-arterial CISCA chemotherapy (Table 3).
Intravenous and intra-arterial CISCA chemotherapy differed,
in addition to the Cytoxan and Adriamycin intravenous cis-
platinum on the second day was delivered intra-arterially
via percutaneously placed intra-arterial catheters. The
dose of cisplatinum was the same in both groups (100 mg/m²).
No attempts at comparing intravenous and intra-arterial
CISCA chemotherapy was done in this study. Those patients
with dominant local regional manifestations of their disease
had their regimen initiated with intra-arterial CISCA
chemotherapy, whereas those patients with dominant nodal
presentations of their disease initiated their regimen with
intravenous CISCA chemotherapy.

The toxicity of this chemotherapeutic regimen was moderate. Culture negative leukopenic fevers occurred in 7.4% of the courses of chemotherapy, and culture positive leukopenic fevers occurred in 16% of the courses of chemotherapy. A total of 115 courses of intravenous CISCA chemotherapy and 48 courses of intra-arterial CISCA chemotherapy were delivered in these 38 patients. Complications of catheter placement occurred in only 2 patients, but in none was severe vascular injury requiring surgery occurred and in neuropathy requiring analgesics occurred in 3 patients and persisted. Renal toxicity occurred in 10 of the cases when defined as a .4 mg% rise in the serum creatinine, but only in 2 of the patients was there a greater than 2 mg% rise in the serum creatinine which persisted. Cardiac toxicity which is defined as a greater than 10% drop in the baseline ejection fraction occurred in only 3 or 7.9% of the patients.

Complete remission occurred in 19 (50%) of those patients treated, whereas 7 (18%) had an objective response. The ability to achieve a complete remission was not determined by prior radiation therapy or prior surgical intervention but was greatly influenced by the histology of the primary (Table 4). Among the patients with pure transitional cell carcinoma, 62% achieved a complete remission, whereas only 14% of those patients with transition forms achieved a complete remission and none of the 2 patients with squamous cell carcinomas achieved an objective response or a complete remission. There is a highly significant difference between the frequency of complete remission and those patients with transition forms and those with primary pure transitional cell carcinomas. The ability to achieve complete remission was independent of the patient's presentation (local regional by virtue of nodal involvement-vs-local regional by virtue of local visceral invasion). Complete remissions were achieved in all categories, both those with pelvic disease, pelvic disease + nodal involvement, and including those patients with locally advanced catastrophic complications as vaginal or penile invasion (Table 5). Patients achieving an objective regression of disease failed to have a survival benefit when compared to those not responding, while patients achieving a complete remission have a mean duration of complete remission of 98 weeks (range 33-172 weeks).

TABLE 4

Histology and Subsequent Response to Chemotherapy

Histologic	No. Patients	Complete Response No. (%)	Objective Response No. (%)	No. Response No. (%)
TCC*	29	18 (62)	6 (21)	5 (17)
				$P<.02$
Transition forms+	7	1 (14)	1 (14)	5 (71)
Squamous cell	2	--	--	2 (100)
Total	38	19 (50)	7 (18)	12 (32)

* Transitional cell carcinoma.
+ Squamoid transformation (5), adenomatous transformation
  (1), spindle variant (1).

Note: Number in parentheses is percentage of total in each
histologic subtype.

TABLE 5

Clinical Presentation of Patients in Complete Remission

Tumor Presentation	No. Patients
Local Disease:	
Pelvic mass	3
Penile invasion	2
Local + Nodal:	
Pelvic mass + pelvic nodes	9
Pelvic mass + para-aortic nodes	2
Pelvic mass + mesenteric nodes	1
Nodal Only*:	
Supraclavicular node (post-cystectomy)	2
Total	19

* Failure of initial surgery.

Upon completion of this study, it became apparent that durable complete remissions could be achieved with CISCA chemotherapy. The inability of other investigators to document a benefit for combination chemotherapy-vs-single-agent chemotherapy could be attributed to two major factors; the treatment of those patients with advanced disease who are less likely to achieve remissions and hence a documented survival enhancement could not be seen, and second, the use of low-dose chemotherapy.

One patient after achieving a complete remission has agreed to a cystectomy and no viable disease was encountered in that patient. The remaining patients have not been managed with consolidation surgery. These encouraging results suggest that primary chemotherapy only without post-chemotherapy radiation therapy or post-chemotherapy surgical exploration may be a correct approach. When recognizing that bladder carcinoma in its local regional presentation is most frequently a systemic disease, the logic for local modalities following chemotherapy for such a clinical presentation can be supported only by a palliative view of this tumor.

These encouraging results with primary chemotherapy only for a select group of patients with local regional disease suggests that patients in the future may be spared the debilitating effects on sexual function and the need for urinary diversion upon the development of more effective chemotherapy.

The role of adjuvant local therapy following initial chemotherapy cannot be assessed. The conclusions of our experience with CISCA chemotherapy for the management of patients with unresectable disease with evidence both of local and distant visceral involvement were; 1) CISCA chemotherapy can achieve complete remissions, 2) complete remissions are dependent on the extent of disease (those patients with local regional disease have a high frequency of complete remissions), whereas those patients with advanced distant disease failed to achieve durable complete remissions, 3) the complete remissions among patients with local regional disease only are durable and do offer the potential for eventual cure, and 4) response rates are histology dependent, that is, that those patients with pure transitional cell carcinoma have a higher frequency of complete remissions than those patients either with transition forms of transitional cell carcinomas or histologic variants such as squamous cell carcinoma and adenocarcinomas of the bladder which appear resistant to cisplatinum-based chemotherapy.

Earlier introduction of chemotherapy may be a further benefit for select patients. It is recognized that those patients who, following a cystectomy, have persistent evidence of lymphatic permeation of tumor, extravesical involvement, or failure to downstage with pre-operative radiation therapy are a group in whom a high relapse rate can be expected. A prospective comparative trial of adjuvant CISCA chemotherapy for five courses delivered for select high-risk patients is being conducted. These patients were to be compared to a group of concurrently treated patients who did not have poor prognostic pathological findings and did not receive adjuvant chemotherapy.

Our preliminary experience is encouraging. In this initial follow-up, patients with poor prognostic pathologic findings at cystectomy who had received adjuvant CISCA chemotherapy have a survival equivalent to those with good prognostic pathological features at cystectomy. No firm statement can be made at present, but the preliminary data suggest a beneficial effect of adjuvant CISCA.

The pessimism in the treatment of bladder carcinoma with chemotherapy appears to be unwarranted. The earlier introduction of chemotherapy in the treatment of bladder carcinoma without compromising the dose of chemotherapy appears to result in a survival benefit. It is yet to be determined whether chemotherapy can be used in place of radiation therapy in a pre-operative setting or whether chemotherapy can replace the role of surgery in those patients with locally invasive disease. It is also not yet established if the effects of chemotherapy merely delay the eventual relapse or result in an increased cure fraction. The ultimate role of chemotherapy in local regional bladder carcinoma and its appropriate integration with radiation and surgery will require further study and a longer follow-up.

SECTION IX
MALIGNANT LYMPHOMA

Primary Chemotherapy in Cancer Medicine, pages 369-374
© 1985 Alan R. Liss, Inc.

COMBINED MODALITY TREATMENT IN STAGE I AND II DIFFUSE
NON-HODGKIN'S LYMPHOMAS

G. Bonadonna M.D., P. Valagussa B.S.,
R. Buzzoni M.D., and E. Bajetta M.D.

Istituto Nazionale Tumori, Milan, Italy

Localized or regionally extended non-Hodgkin's
lymphomas account for 15 to 30% of cases. In approximately
35 to 45% of patients the disease arises in extranodal
sites. Only patients with stage I diffuse histiocytic
lymphoma (DHL) staged through laparotomy and treated with
extensive megavoltage irradiation have a cure of about 90%.
Otherwise, in patients with diffuse pattern of growth irradiation alone is unable to provide a 5-year survival (RFS)
exceeding 60% (stage I 40-60%, stage II 25-35%). For this
reason, chemotherapy is required to kill neoplastic cells
located outside the radiation fields.

Our initial experience with regional irradiation vs irradiation followed by 6 cycles of CVP (cyclophosphamide, vincristine, and prednisone) yielded significantly improved 5-year
RFS and total survival rates in patients treated with the
combined modality approach (Monfardini 1980). Our subsequent
randomized study involved BACOP (bleomycin, Adriamycin,
cyclophosphamide, vincristine and prednisone) versus CVP as
well as chemotherapy preceeding and following radiotherapy.
In fact, in the randomized study testing radiotherapy as
first line treatment 13% of patients showed disease progression, mainly in distant sites, during irradiation or during
the interval between completion of radiotherapy and beginning
of chemotherapy (Monfardini 1980). Furthermore, Adriamycin
and bleomycin containing regimens were shown all over the
world to be superior to CVP in diffuse non-Hodgkin's
lymphomas. Present report further updates our recently
published results (Bonadonna 1984).

PATIENTS AND METHODS

Details concerning patient selection, Rappaport histopathologic classification, staging procedures including laparoscopy and two needle bone marrow biopsies, as well as prophylactic regional radiotherapy, BACOP and CVP combinations were previously published (Bajetta 1981). From July 1976 through November 1983, 159 patients were prospectively randomized. In 23 of 25 patients subjected to laparotomy, surgery was performed because the disease presented as primary neoplasm in the stomach (14 cases), small or large intestine (8 cases), or in the ovary (1 case). The main patient and histopathologic characteristics are presented in Tables 1 and 2. It is important to stress that patients aged over 60 years, systemic symptoms and bulky disease (> 10 cm in largest diameter) were rare findings, while diffuse histiocytic lymphoma accounted for the single most frequent histopathologic subgroup. Only about 10% of the patients were classified as having nodular (follicular) and diffuse pattern of growth. The most frequent primary extranodal site was skin (25% of all extranodal sites), followed by stomach (23%) and intestine (13%).

Prophylactic irradiation to the immediately adjacent and clinically uninvolved lymphoid area(s) was carried out in 138 of 155 (89%) patients. The reasons for avoiding prophylactic irradiation were as follows: primary involvement of skin (11 cases), maxilla (2 cases), bone (2 cases) and upper cervical nodes (2 cases). Three cycles of either BACOP or CVP preceeded and followed the radiation therapy program (Bajetta 1981).

Freedom from progression (FFP), RFS, and total survival were calculated by the use of the product-limit method and computed from the start of treatment. Statistical significance of differences observed was assessed by the use of log-rank test (Peto 1977).

TREATMENT FINDINGS

Comparative complete remission (CR) rates are shown in Tables 3 and 4. The differences between the two treatment groups were minimal and non significant. The 5-year results (Table 5) indicate the superiority of BACOP versus CVP also in the analysis of total survival (74% vs 91%). Furthermore, while the RFS difference between patients with stage I and II remained evident in the CVP group, this difference was

Table 1

MAIN PATIENT CHARACTERISTICS (IN %)

Evaluable patients	CVP group 83	BACOP group 76
Stage I/II	63/37	55/45
Age ≤ 60/ > 60 yr	78/22	84/16
Sex M/F	52/48	63/37
Systemic symptoms	2	2
Bulky disease	8	9
Extranodal	38	38
Waldeyer's ring	19	24

Table 2

COMPARATIVE HISTOLOGY ACCORDING TO RAPPAPORT CLASSIFICATION

	CVP group No.	%	BACOP group No.	%
Histiocytic	35	42	37	49
D Histiocytic	34	41	37	49
Lymphocytic	31	37	26	34
Mixed type	14	17	13	17
Others	3	4	0	
Diffuse	72/80	90	67/76	88
N plus D	8/80	10	9/76	12

N= nodular   D= diffuse

blurred in patients treated with BACOP. In both groups with stage II lymphoma, RFS was related to the number of involved sites (1-3: CVP 58%, BACOP 89%; >3: CVP 25%, BACOP 58%), thus confirming that successes and limits of chemotherapy are influenced by the total tumor volume. No significant RFS differences was observed in patients with DHL (81% vs 88%), nor between patients with nodal or extranodal disease in either treatment group.

Table 3

COMPARATIVE PERCENT COMPLETE REMISSION

	CVP group	BACOP group
Total	94	97
Stage I/II	98/87	100/94
Age $\leqslant$ 60/ >60 yr	92/100	98/92
Sex M/F	93/95	98/96
Bulky disease	100	100
Nodal extent	90	98
Extranodal	100	97
Waldeyer's ring	81	100

Salvage therapy in relapsing patients achieved CR in 76% of evaluable cases failing in the CVP group (most of them were treated with various Adriamycin-containing regimens) and in 56% of those started with BACOP. The median duration of second CR was 20 months (range 7-12) for the CVP group and 8 months for the BACOP group, respectively.

The jatrogenic toxicity can be summarized as follows. Agranulocytosis was not detected in either treatment group. One patient died because of radiation necrosis of the brain stem following a cumulative dose of 4500 rads. Other radiation sequelae were exclusively due to fibrosis (CVP group 4%, BACOP group 9%). Second neoplasms (basal cell carcinoma of the skin and endometrial cancer) were so far detected only in two patients given BACOP plus radiotherapy.

Table 4

COMPARATIVE PERCENT COMPLETE REMISSION
RELATED TO HISTOLOGY

	CVP group	BACOP group
Histiocytic	89	95
D Histiocytic	88	**95**
Lymphocytic	100	100
Mixed type	92	100
Others	100	–
Diffuse	93	97
N plus D	100	100

N= nodular   D= diffuse

Table 5

TOTAL FIVE-YEAR RESULTS. RESULTS ARE IN PERCENT

	CVP group	BACOP group	P
Freedom from progression	57	77	< 0.02
Relapse-free survival	62	79	< 0.03
Stage I	69	81	
Stage II	49	78	
DHL	81	88	
Nodal extent	62	76	
Extranodal extent	61	84	
Total survival	72	88	< 0.06
Survival of complete responders	74	91	< 0.05

CONCLUSIONS

The results of present trial indicate that BACOP plus radiotherapy is superior to CVP plus radiotherapy in the treatment of stage I-II non Hodgkin's lymphomas with diffuse pattern of growth. Therefore, an Adriamycin containing regimen is always indicated in the treatment of all stages of high grade non-Hodgkin's lymphomas, and to avoid early disease manifestations in distant sites combined treatment should be started with chemotherapy. The role of radiotherapy, particularly in stage I diffuse lymphomas, remains important for only 3 of 35 relapses as first manifestation of recurrent disease were documented in irradiated areas (CVP 2, BACOP 1).

On the basis of the reported findings and considering that 5% (CVP) to 12% (BACOP) of patients could not complete the three postirradiation cycles either for refusal or prolonged bone marrow toxicity, our future treatment programs for stage I as well as for stage II with ≤3 involved sites will include 5 to 6 cycles of chemotherapy followed by radiotherapy. The polydrug regimen will be the classical CHOP (cyclophosphamide, Adriamycin, vincristine, and prednisone) which is more simple to administer compared to BACOP. Patients with stage II lymphoma but with > 3 involved cycles will be subjected only to intensive chemotherapy.

REFERENCES

Bajetta E, Buzzoni R, Bonadonna G, et al (1981). Combined radiotherapy-chemotherapy (CVP vs BACOP) in stage I-II diffuse non-Hodgkin's lymphomas. In Salmon S and Jones S (eds): "Adjuvant Therapy of Cancer III", Orlando (Fla), Grune & Stratton, p 107.
Bonadonna G, Bajetta E, Lattuada A, et al (1984). CVP vs BACOP chemotherapy sequentially combined with irradiation in stage I-II diffuse non-Hodgkin's lymphomas. In Jones S and Salmon S (eds): "Adjuvant Therapy of Cancer IV", Orlando (Fla): Grune & Stratton.
Monfardini S, Banfi A, Bonadonna G, et al (1980). Improved five-year survival after combined radiotherapy-chemotherapy for stage I-II non-Hodgkin's lymphomas. Int J Radiat Oncol Biol Phys 6: 125.
Peto R, Pike MC, Armitage P, et al (1977). Design and analysis of randomized clinical trials requiring prolonged observation of each patient. II. Analysis and examples. Br J Cancer 35: 1.

SECTION X
PRIMARY CHEMOTHERAPY

Primary Chemotherapy in Cancer Medicine, pages 377–383
© 1985 Alan R. Liss, Inc.

PRIMARY CHEMOTHERAPY: CONCEPTS AND ISSUES

Franco M. Muggia, M.D.

Rita & Stanley H. Kaplan Cancer Center
NYU Medical Center
New York, NY 10016

Over the past decade therapeutic concepts have gradu-
ally shifted from adjuvant chemotherapy to what I define as
"primary" chemotherapy. One may question the nomenclature
in referring to the application of chemotherapy prior to
surgery or radiation as "primary" chemotherapy. Other terms
such as neoadjuvant chemotherapy or protochemotherapy proposed by Frei (1982) are historically correct but do not
necessarily convey situations when chemotherapy is given
first either as treatment of the primary disease or as the
primary treatment - whatever interpretation one whishes to
take. Whenever possible one may wish to indicate accurately
what role chemotherapy is actually playing, i.e. "induction",
"preoperative", "perioperative" are all terms which may be
used under some circumstances. Finally "upfront" chemotherapy also conveys the critical timing of such treatment.
Nevertheless <u>primary</u> chemotherapy does convey the central
role of such treatment and may be the preferred general
term.

<u>Animal Tumor Models</u>. Adjuvant chemotherapy principles were
derived from animal tumor model studies (Schabel, 1977). In
fact such models contributed in a major way to screening,
to verifying the fractional cell kill hypothesis and dose-
response effect of drugs and to predicting of therapeutic
synergy of drug combinations in addition to laying down the
foundations of adjuvant chemotherapy. The proper sequencing
of therapeutic modalities, on the other hand, is not easily discerned through these models. Therefore one must rely
on human models of disease: that is, on the experience
being recorded through clinical trials. Nevertheless several
assumptions which are invoked in developing principles of

adjuvant chemotherapy come from animal models: 1) the presence of residual micrometastatic disease after surgery, 2)
the relation of relapse rates to delay in treatment (i.e.
age of the tumor), 3) the availability of effective systemic
chemotherapy as a requirement to demonstrate efficacy in adjuvant situations and, 4) the demonstration of greater efficacy with lower tumor burdens.

Interaction Between Modalities. End results of treatment de-
pend not only on the intrinsic efficacy of the drug, but on
the status of the host and on the inherent susceptibility
of the tumor. This interrelationship has been pictured as a
triangle which aptly describes the wide variety of circumstances that affect outcome (Sakurai, 1978). The rationale
for utilizing chemotherapy as the primary modality may be
viewed from this perspective. If the tumor is susceptible
to a drug, the optimal circumstances for tumor eradication
may be present when the host is in the best possible condition. If the host can be rendered in an optimal state
through debulking surgery - as may be possible in most
ovarian carcinomas - then this procedure should probably
precede chemotherapy. A corollary of this relationship is
the great variability of effects from surgery on the host.
To perform an esophageal resection may have quite different
effects on the host than resection of a soft tissue sarcoma.
Moreover, radiation as a local modality has considerably
different effects on the host, and on the tumor than surgery.

Drug factors are also very relevant to the above relationships. Drug distribution depends on blood supply, cell-
cell contacts (e.g. blood-brain barrier) and the physico-
chemical nature of the drug. It is worth reemphasizing as
did Schabel and coworkers (1984) that "an otherwise effective drug will not kill a drug-sensitive tumor cell that it
cannot or does not reach in lethal concentration".

Concepts Supporting "Primary" Chemotherapy
The rational for primary chemotherapy has been emphasized in a number of studies where this strategy appears to
be giving superior results. The major reasons for success
are 1) affecting micrometastases at the earliest possible
time, 2) minimizing the emergence of resistance, 3) maxi-
mizing the optimal conditions of the host and vascularity
of the tumor, 4) enabling one to determine the degree of
responsiveness to systemic therapy and, 5) reducing, obvia-
ting, or delaying the need for local therapies (although
the desirability of this latter achievement has been controversial). The following models of tumor eradication and

growth have been utilized in the development of therapeutic strategies:

1. Spontaneous mutation model advanced by Goldie and Coldman (1979) indicates a decreased probability of cure with increasing cell number. A constant mutation rate per cell generation is believed to be responsible for the random emergence of drug resistant clones. According to this hypothesis it is urgent to begin systemic therapy early during the lifetime of a tumor particularly when the mutation rate constant of a tumor is large.

2. The kinetic model actually consists of two principal alternatives. One expounds the concept of fractional cell kill (Skipper et al, 1964), although allowances have been made for decreased sensitivity at high tumor burdens in relation to a decreased growth fraction. The other kinetic model advanced by Norton and Simon (1977) actually considers that drug-induced cell kill varies during the lifetime of a tumor, with proportionally greater cell kill midway during the exponential phase of tumor growth, and lesser fractional kill during the initial and later phases. This hypothesis actually predicts for more discernible tumor regression at presentation, which is finding supported by some clinical observations.

3. Miscellaneous factors include the role of host status, tumor vascularity, cross-resistance induction, and drug pharmacodynamics and molecular pharmacology of specific compounds. As has been noted the interrelationship between the host, tumor and cytotoxic drugs is a dynamic one and will obviously change with stage of disease. For this reason drug development programs are increasingly mindful of the kind of host where the testing takes place, the type of tumor cell growth (e.g. subcutaneous, ascites, spheroids in ascites) and whether drugs are actually available to the tumors in effective dose levels. A major prediction of the concepts is a close dependence between outcome and stage or tumor burden. Probabilities for cure improve in choriocarcinoma, Burkitt's and other lymphomas, testicular cancer, ovarian cancer, small cell lung cancer and breast cancer when the tumor burden is low (Table 1). In all these conditions chemotherapy has achieved a reproducible level of effectiveness. Where chemotherapy is less effective such as in breast cancer, the evidence has come from adjuvant studies. We have considered here an expanded list of targets including head & neck cancer, and gastrointestinal cancer. This derives both from clearer therapeutic con-

cepts and the expanding availability of more effective
therapies. Specific issues that have arisen will be discussed as illustrative points. Many are clearly discussed in the preceding chapters.

TABLE 1

Examples Concept Predictions

Dependence of outcome on stage/cell number
                            choriocarcinoma
                            Burkitt's & other lymphomas
                            Testicular carcinoma
                            Ovarian cancer
                            Small cell lung cancer
                            Breast carcinoma

General Issues in Primary Chemotherapy.
    Several questions are raised whenever chemotherapy is
adopted prior to locoregional therapy for an apparently
local disease:
1. What are the probabilities for cure from local therapies alone? Surgical treatment is quite effective in
   the early stages of colorectal cancer and moderately
   effective in breast cancer; however in many other
   cancers (i.e. esophagus, lung, osteosarcoma) the risk of
   recurrence even in early stages exceeds 50%. In the
   former conditions possible consequences of the primary
   chemotherapy approach are the masking of the true initial stage, and the exposing of a vast proportion of patients to chemotherapy when the actual risk is low.
   Clearly these problems constitute a major deterrent for
   the use of such an approach.
2. Is there an advantage in terms of tumor control and patients morbidity when the drugs are applied initially
   versus later? Having shown that one may benefit from
   chemotherapy, it becomes relevant to demonstrate that is
   application prior to surgery is more efficacious in
   terms of tumor control and consequently improved survival. However, in most instances trials to prove this
   issue have not been forthcoming. In osteosarcoma results appear to have improved further with the introduction of preoperative treatment. Although such issue
   has not been settled, the feasibility for limb salvage

surgery was enhanced by this strategy. Therefore an advantage of primary chemotherapy may be obtained in terms of lower morbidity if not improved survival. In some circumstances, preoperative chemotherapy brings about some problems: patients with head and neck cancer in particular may refuse operations, and in others the surgeon may perform a less radical operation which, however, one may postulate will bring about a worsening of results. If the result without surgery is equivalent to that obtained by surgical means, then an obvious advantage has been accrued by chemotherapy. Such a principle is being tested in the Veterans Administration trial of chemotherapy and radiation versus surgery in laryngeal cancer.

3. What is the optimal timing of the local therapy following chemotherapy? A special category of this issue is simultaneous radiation and chemotherapy. This last strategy is attractive in conditions where chemotherapy does not appear effective enough and with certain drugs that may be synergistic with radiation. In esophageal cancer chemotherapy appears to effectively downstage the tumor; however, pathologic complete remissions are rare. A role for simultaneous radiation and chemotherapy may also be worth exploring in lung cancer and head and neck cancer. Beyond this special situation, the crucial question addressed by many pioneers in this area is when to introduce the local intervention. In breast cancer one cycle of preoperative chemotherapy is being studied by the Vancouver group but was not enough in the Hellenic trial and obviously insufficient to achieve CR in the NCI trial. In lung cancer, the Dana Farber trial has modified their initial approach to include several additions cycles of chemotherapy prior to thoracotomy. In head and neck cancer, one trial sponsored by the National Cancer Institute did not indicate an advantage for one cycle of chemotherapy prior to surgery and radiation versus the local modalities alone. However, more cycles may be needed as demonstrated in the trials at Wayne State and analyzed as time required to complete remission. When radiation is also te be added, the problem of timing becomes even more complex. It is of interest that in head and neck cancer, response to chemotherapy predicts for response to radiation as well.

The timing of ancillary local therapies, is also an issue: for example when should prophylactic brain irradiation be given in lung cancer? or when should intraperitoneal therapy begin if used as consolidation in intra-abdominal malignancies?

Special Issues:

Several points have been established or raised by primary chemotherapy experience. These are included among the following areas of disease:

1. Osteosarcoma: limb preservation has become feasible, and chemotherapy appears to be adding to overall survival. Part of this success might be attributed to the preoperative treatment, but this point has not been established.

2. Ewing's sarcoma: the ability to delay local therapy by beginning with chemotherapy may allow the latter to proceed with greater intensity. The suggestion of an increase in survival needs to be confirmed.

3. Breast cancer: in locally advanced disease the ability to delay local therapy may prove beneficial in allowing greater intensity of chemotherapy; also local therapy may eventually perhaps be obviated. In earlier stages the advantage of beginning with chemotherapy is being addressed through clinical trials.

4. Lung cancer: increased responsiveness to chemotherapy is being reported in patients with localized disease prior to any treatment. This may render disease resectable; however, whether cures result from such an approach must be confirmed. If radiation is the only local approach, the sequence of chemotherapy followed by radiation may be better tolerated than vice versa.

5. Head and neck, and esophageal cancers: downstaging of disease has been demonstrated but impact on survival is uncertain. However, preliminary results raise hopes that chemotherapy may contribute to better long terms results, otherwise deemed unlikely by the usual adjuvant therapies.

6. Gynecologic cancer: the concept of surgical debulking even in situations where resection is not easily achieved has been accepted in ovarian cancer; however, this may be questioned to an increasing degree as chemotherapy efficacy improves. Trials in cervical cancer are ongoing but impact of chemotherapy is uncertain.

7. Gastrointestinal cancer: in tumors other than esophagus, the trials are hampered by the limitations of chemotherapeutic efficacy vis-a-vis its toxicity. In gastric cancer, however, some hope that preoperative chemotherapy may contribute to enhanced resectability has been raised.

8. Testicular cancer: in these patients chemotherapy is very effective and truly constitutes the primary modali-

ty for non-seminomatous tumors (after orchiectomy). This situation may also increasingly pertain to bulky seminomas in lieu of radiation. The roles for surgery - usually as salvage - are increasingly well described in the experience at MD Anderson and the Swiss group.

9. Bladder cancer: impressive results are being reported from chemotherapy as the primary treatment in selected patients with invasive, unresectable bladder cancer. Future studies in this disease are eargerly awaited.

Conclusions

Chemotherapy prior to local therapy is being widely a-dopted in the treatment of a wide variety of solid tumors. Definitive studies indicating an advantage for such strategy are mostly not available. However, important observations are being made concerning factors contributing to chemosensitivity and resistance, the relationship of surgery to development of metastases, and other important concepts of tumor biology. Such observations will contribute both to improving results by the careful integration of available anticancer therapies and to the future of drug development.

References

Frei E, III. Clinical cancer research: Embattled species. Cancer. 50:1797-1799, 1982.

Schabel FM, Jr. Surgical adjuvant chemotherapy of metastatic murine tumors. Cancer. 40:558-568, 1977.

Schabel FM, Jr, Griswold DB, Corbett TH, and Laster WR, Jr. Increasing the therapeutic response rates to anticancer drugs by applying the basic principles of pharmacology. Cancer (Supplement). 54:1160-1167, 1984.

Goldie JH, and Coldman AJ. A mathematic model for relating the drug sensitivity of tumors to their spontaneous mutation rate. Cancer Treat Rep. 63:1727-172, 1979.

Skipper ME, Schabel FM, Jr., and Wilcox WS. Experimental evaluation of potential anticancer agents. XII. On the criteria and kinetics associated with "curability" of experimental leukemia. Cancer Chemotherapy Reports. 35:3-111, 1964.

Norton L, Simon R. Tumor size, sensitivity to therapy and design of treatment schedules. Cancer Treat. Rep. 61:1307-1317, 1977.

Sakurai Y. Development of cancer chemotherapy in Japan. In: Advances in Cancer Chemotherapy. SK Carter, et al (Editors. Japan Scientific Society Press, Tokyo, pp. 3-10, 1978.

Primary Chemotherapy in Cancer Medicine, page 385
© Alan R. Liss, Inc.

CLOSING REMARKS

Jacques A. Wils

Department of Internal Medicine,
Laurentius Hospital, 6043 CV Roermond,
The Netherlands

This symposium which has focussed on combined-modality
treatment of various malignant diseases using chemotherapy
as a first line, has now come to an end. A great deal of
fascinating data has been presented. For some diseases,
this approach can already be regarded as standard treatment,
while for others only the coming years will show if first
line chemotherapy is of major benefit.
You have heard that there will be a similar symposium within
6 weeks in Vancouver, organized by Dr. Goldie and Dr. Ragaz.
The ideas for this and the Vancouver meeting emerged independently and we were not aware of each other's activities
in organizing these meetings until we met at the ASCO 1984
in Toronto. It would be interesting to organize the next
meeting on this topic together, perhaps within a few years
somewhere in the mid-Atlantic. I prefer the Bahama's especially at this time of the year. This would cut down ex-
penses and reduce the number of the ever increasing oncology
meetings.
I would now like to thank all the contributors, chairmen and
the scientific committee for having made this meeting what
it has been, and I would like especially to thank Farmitalia
Carlo Erba, Bo Häggström, Jan Smeets and Rene Fuchs and his
staff for their considerable efforts and support. Without
them this symposium would not have been possible and I will
call upon them again for the next symposium in two or three
years.

Index